NUTRITION BILL OF RIGHTS

framed by

The American Dietetic Association
1976–America's Bicentennial Year

the Right to Good Nutrition

Every American has the right to optimum nutritional health

the Right to Food Choices

Every American has the right to access to a variety of safe foods that will promote good nutrition and improve resistance to disease.

the Right to Nutrition Information

Every American has the right to nutrition education—to make informed choices from available foods; to have protection against food and nutrition misinformation.

THE AMERICAN
DIETETIC ASSOCIATION

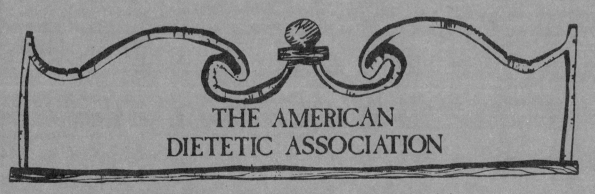

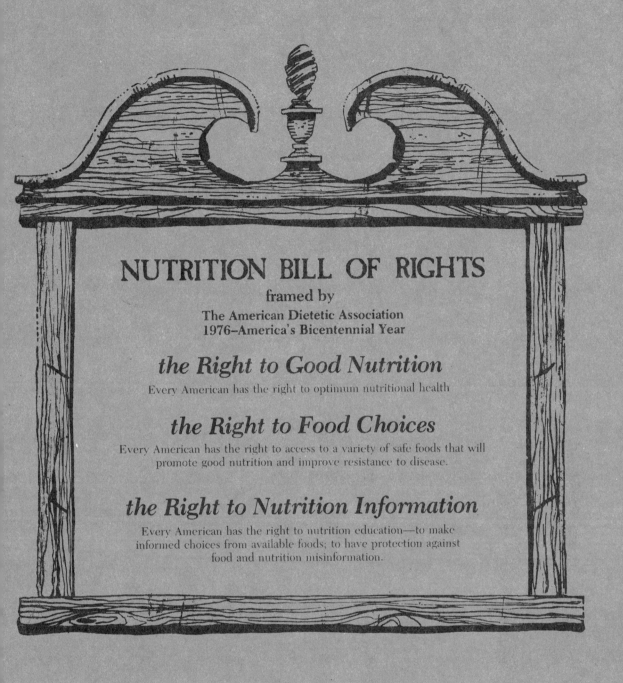

Shackelton's

NUTRITION ESSENTIALS AND DIET THERAPY

Fifth Edition

Charlotte M. Poleman, B.S., R.D.
Dietetic Consultant and Nutrition Counselor
Ithaca, New York
Formerly Head, Dietary Department
Lakeside Nursing Home
Ithaca, New York

Christine Locastro Capra, M.A., R.D.
Clinical Dietitian
The Faxton Hospital and Children's Hospital and Rehabilitation Center
Utica, New York

1984
W. B. SAUNDERS COMPANY
Philadelphia □ London □ Toronto □ Mexico City □ Rio de Janeiro □ Sydney □ Tokyo

W. B. Saunders Company: West Washington Square
Philadelphia, PA 19105

1 St. Anne's Road
Eastbourne, East Sussex BN21 3UN, England

1 Goldthorne Avenue
Toronto, Ontario M8Z 5T9, Canada

Apartado 26370—Cedro 512
Mexico 4, D.F., Mexico

Rua Coronel Cabrita, 8
Sao Cristovao Caixa Postal 21176
Rio de Janeiro, Brazil

9 Waltham Street
Artarmon, N.S.W. 2064, Australia

Ichibancho, Central Bldg., 22-1 Ichibancho
Chiyoda-Ku, Tokyo 102, Japan

Library of Congress Cataloging in Publication Data

Shackelton, Alberta Dent.
Shackelton's Nutrition: essentials and diet therapy.

First-4th eds. published as: Practical nurse nutrition education.
Includes index.
1. Diet therapy. 2. Nutrition. I. Poleman, Charlotte M. II. Capra, Christine L. III. Shackelton, Alberta Dent. Practical nurse nutrition education. IV. Title. V. Title: Nutrition essentials and diet therapy. [DNLM: 1. Nutrition—Nursing texts. 2. Diet therapy—Nursing texts. QU 145 S524p]
RM216.S447 1984 613.2 83-14468
ISBN 0-7216-7280-9

Shackelton's Nutrition: Essentials and Diet Therapy ISBN 0-7216-7280-9

Last digit is the print number: 9 8 7 6 5 4 3 2 1

This book is dedicated to the memory of

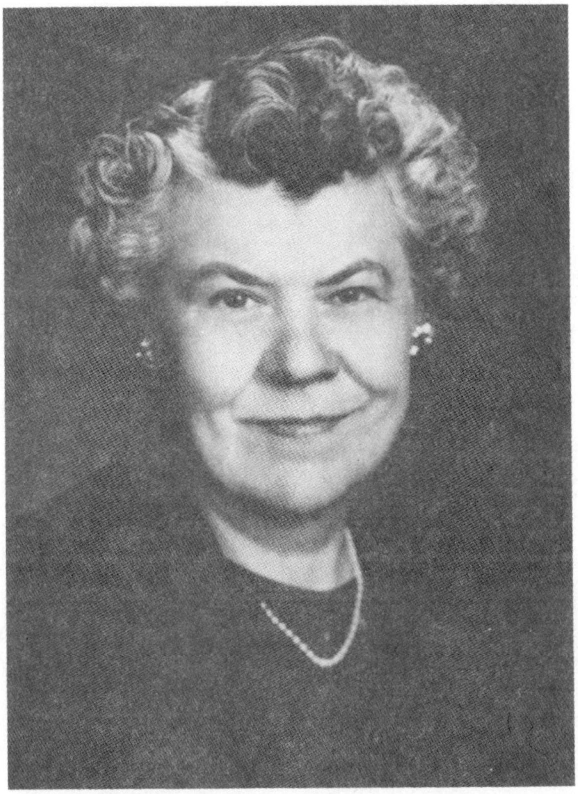

ALBERTA DENT SHACKELTON

Born November 28, 1896
Died March 2, 1978

PREFACE

The fifth edition of *Practical Nurse Nutrition Education* is now *Shackelton's Nutrition: Essentials and Diet Therapy.* The title change reflects the current authors' dedication to the memory of Alberta Shackelton, the original author. The new title also indicates the wider audience for whom the book is intended.

This edition continues to provide up-to-date, concise, and easy-to-follow basic principles of nutrition and their application in all areas of nutritional care. It is intended for practical, associate-degree, and baccalaureate-degree nursing students. It is well suited for students of dietetic technology and other health care fields. The information presented can be used by the professional or the layman to improve nutritional practices in the clinical or home setting. This book has been written from the viewpoints of both hospital and nursing home dietitians to show the flexibility of nutritional care planning. The authors hope that this text will promote a better understanding of the importance of meeting individual nutritional needs.

The question-answer format has been retained. The material is still presented in three sections: Normal Nutrition, Therapeutic Nutrition, and Food Preparation and Service. Units and parts have been replaced by chapters. The addition of the chapter outline provides the reader with a quick summary of the major topics that will be discussed. Valuable suggestions from the previous edition have been incorporated into this edition. Larger print makes the book easier to read. A Teacher's Guide provides the instructor with sample test questions and suggested audio-visual aids. The "Terms to Understand" are fully defined in the text or in the glossary at the back of the book. There are more pictures, graphs, tables, and charts than in previous editions.

Chapter Four, Nutrition in the Life Cycle, has been expanded to include nutritional guidelines for athletes. Sound, basic nutrition information is presented to help combat many common myths in this area. Section Two, Therapeutic Nutrition, now includes a discussion of the nutritional problems and needs during cancer treatment. Many practical suggestions are outlined. Methods of nutritional assessment and support have received special emphasis, since these areas have seen the greatest advances in recent years and have become nutrition specialties. Nutritional interventions for coping with various types of physical stress such as the trauma of surgery, burns, and fractures are also discussed. This material may be of greatest interest to the more advanced student.

Section Three, Food Preparation and Service, now includes a discussion of therapeutic menu planning and food sanitation. The Appendix has a more expanded list of sources of nutrition information and nutrition materials available free of charge or at minimal cost.

The authors wish to acknowledge the persons who have in some way contributed to the outcome of this edition. First, we wish to thank Mr. Horace Shackelton, whose kindness and interest in the book have been a continuing source of inspiration throughout its development. The enthusiasm, ideas, and support of the following people are also greatly appreciated: Deborah Hailston-Jaworski, Jean Cobb, Diane Blodgett, Sally Hoffmeister, Gwen Ball, and Judy Watkins.

We would also like to thank our families, including our husbands, Tom and Marty, for their encouragement and continued support throughout the process of this revision.

Special acknowledgement goes to Katherine Pitcoff, Nursing Editor at W. B. Saunders, who has been a constant source of ideas, enthusiasm, patience, and understanding. Her efforts and skills are greatly appreciated.

Permission to use photographs and published materials is gratefully acknowledged.

CHARLOTTE M. POLEMAN
CHRISTINE L. CAPRA

CONTENTS

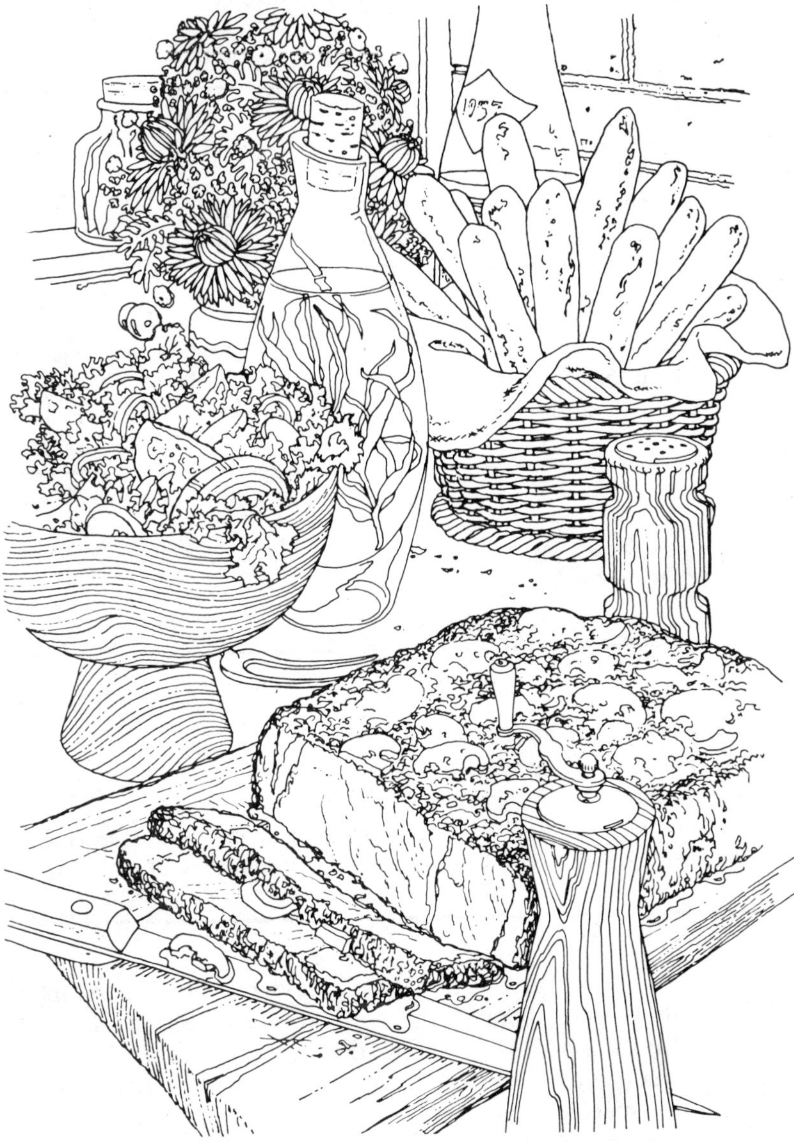

Section One
NORMAL NUTRITION

OBJECTIVES

To understand
- ☐ The basic principles of normal nutrition.
- ☐ The relationship of good nutrition to optimal health.
- ☐ The amounts and kinds of foods needed in the daily diet.
- ☐ Programs in public health and community nutrition.

To apply
- ☐ Basic nutrition principles to the nutritional and psychological needs of the individual throughout the life cycle.
- ☐ Knowledge of nutritional needs to meal planning for individuals and family.

Introduction

OBJECTIVES

To understand
- ☐ How nutrition developed as a science.
- ☐ The basic terms in the study of nutrition.
- ☐ Who are the nutrition "experts."
- ☐ The importance of teamwork in delivering optimum nutritional care.
- ☐ The attitudes and understanding necessary for the study of nutrition.

HOW HAS NUTRITION DEVELOPED AS A SCIENCE?

From early times people have been interested in the food they consume, its passage through the body and its effects. It has been said by some writers that the history of the world might be written in terms of food, starting with the use of wild native foods and the beginning of food cultivation, followed by specific health values ascribed to foods by early philosophical and biblical writers.

In the 1600s, with the development of chemistry and other fields of science, some of the questions about food began to be answered. The contributions of Antoine Lavoisier in the late 1700s sparked the beginning of nutrition study. Lavoisier is credited with recognizing the role of respiration in food metabolism. He is called the "father of nutrition science." Other important contributions were made by Lusk, Atwater, McCollum, Benedict, Rose, Rubner, and countless others.

At the beginning of this century, interest in nutrition was primarily concerned with how much energy (calories) humans need and how carbohydrates, proteins, and fats compare in energy value. Proteins became the target of specialized studies. Minerals were discovered subsequently. Almost simultaneously with their discovery came that of vitamins. To follow later were amino acids, fatty acids, trace mineral elements, enzymes, hormones, and so on.

As can be seen in the accompanying figure, available information has been put to use to improve the quality of life. The public has come to realize that not just food but the kinds of food one consumes can make a difference.

The science of nutrition has come of age.

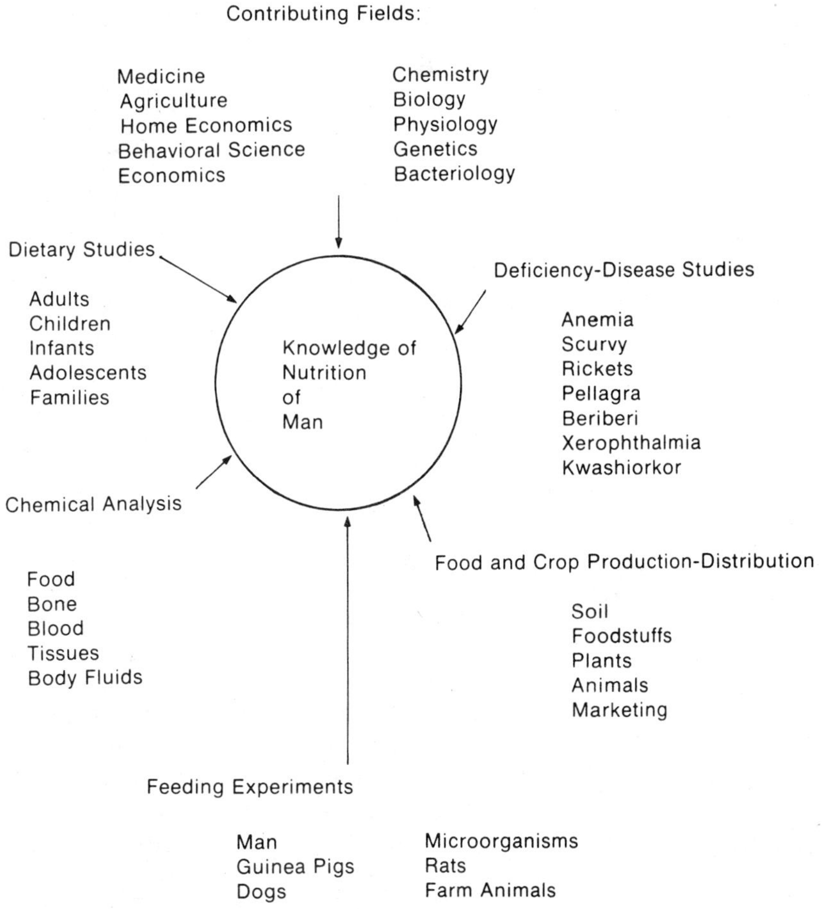

Methods and areas of investigations that lead to the development of the science of nutrition. (From M. V. Krause and L. K. Mahan, *Food, Nutrition, and Diet Therapy*, 6th ed. W. B. Saunders Company, Philadelphia, 1979; after M. E. Lowenberg, *Food and Man*, John Wiley & Sons, New York).

WHAT ARE THE BASIC TERMS TO UNDERSTAND IN NUTRITION STUDY?

1. *Food* is any substance taken into the body that will help to meet the body's needs for energy, maintenance, and growth.
2. *Nutrition* is the sum of the processes by which the body utilizes food for energy, maintenance, and growth.
3. *Malnutrition* is a state in which a prolonged lack of one or more nutrients retards physical development or causes the appearance of specific clinical conditions (anemia, goiter, rickets, etc.).
4. *Optimum Nutrition* means that a person is receiving and utilizing the essential nutrients to maintain health and well-being at the highest possible level. It provides for a reserve.
5. *Nutritional Status* is the condition of the body as it relates to the consumption and utilization of food.
   a. "Good nutritional status" refers to the intake of a balanced diet containing all the essential nutrients to meet the body's requirements for energy, maintenance, and growth (see nutritional assessment, p. 177).
   b. "Poor nutritional status" refers to an inadequate intake (or utilization) of nutrients to meet the body's requirements for energy, maintenance,

and growth. A person who is suffering from malnutrition is in poor nutritional status (see nutritional assessment, p. 177).

6. *Nutrient* is a chemical substance present in food that is needed by the body. Included in the more than 50 nutrients needed by the body are proteins, carbohydrates, fats, minerals, vitamins, and water.
7. *Nutritional Care* is the application of nutrition knowledge to the feeding of people.

WHO ARE THE NUTRITION EXPERTS?

Increasingly, the public is demanding to know more about the foods they eat and how they affect health and well-being. This growing interest in the field of nutrition has attracted a large number of individuals. Nutrition counseling should be sought only from those with appropriate credentials.

The *registered dietitian* (R.D.) is recognized as a nutrition expert. All registered dietitians must successfully complete at least four years of specialized study at an accredited college or university as well as clinical training before or after the baccalaureate degree. Many registered dietitians hold a master's or doctorate degree.

"Registered dietitians are experts in understanding, interpreting and determining a person's nutritional needs in both health and disease. They understand the relationship between the elements of food and the body's needs. They are educated to assess conditions which are less well-known to the public but are nonetheless important. These areas include knowledge of eating patterns; environmental factors, such as how food is procured, and social, ethnic, economic and cultural factors that affect food selection."[1]

As knowledge in the field of nutrition grows, so does the responsibility of the dietitian. Dietitians exhibit their expertise in various settings — communities, clinics, academic or research institutions, and food industries, to name a few.

The *dietetic technician* has a two-year degree in a food-related area from an accredited college and performs his or her duties under the supervision of a registered dietitian.

When seeking advice in the field of nutrition ask someone who truly qualifies as a nutrition expert—**the registered dietitian.**

TEAMWORK: THE OPTIMAL DELIVERY OF NUTRITIONAL CARE

The dietitian assesses patient needs and implements a nutritional care plan to meet those needs. Although the dietitian is responsible for the nutritional care of the patient, the support of other members of the health care team—physician, nurse, pharmacist, and social worker—is necessary. It is only through a team effort that the patient will receive optimal nutritional care.

Physician. The physician orders the type of nutritional care the patient is to receive. Information is gathered from the patient's medical history, physical examination, and laboratory values. If there is reason to suspect that the patient is not in good nutritional status, further nutritional assessment is done by the dietitian. It is important that the physician reinforce the importance of whatever type of nutritional care the patient is to receive (regular diet, 4-gram sodium, tube feeding, etc.). The physician must be open to the suggestions and findings of other health professionals in order for the patient to receive the best possible medical and nutritional care.

Nurse. Because of their close and continuous association with patients, nurses provide valuable input regarding the patient's nutritional progress.

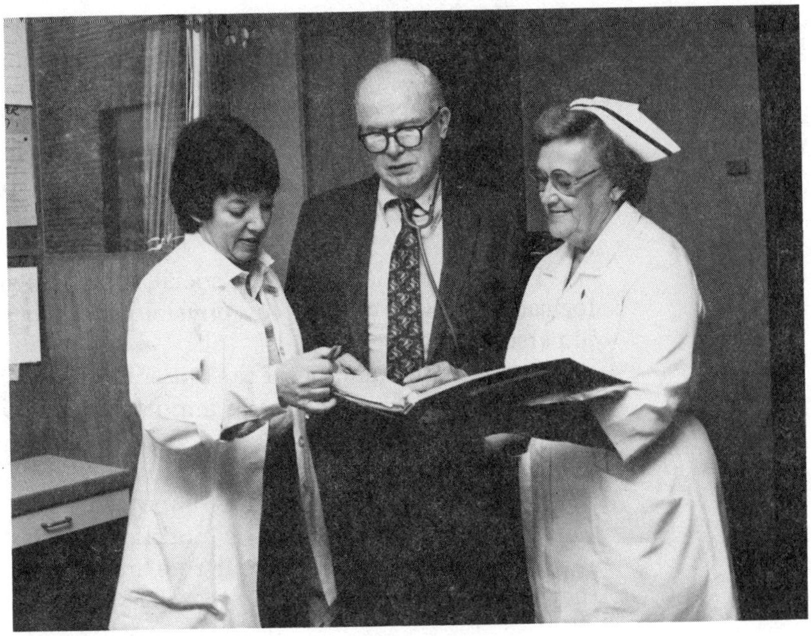

A dietitian, doctor, and nurse discuss a patient's progress using the medical chart. (Courtesy of The Faxton Hospital, Utica, New York.)

They can emphasize to the patient the need for the nutritional care that is to be delivered. Nurses provide assistance at mealtime and are aware of the patient's acceptance or rejection of the nutritional care plan. They consult with the dietitian about nutritional problems so that the dietitian's expertise can be used to solve these problems. Because of limited staff, the dietitian is not always available to visit every patient. Many times, through early recognition and referral of nutrition problems by the nurse, the overall quality and scope of nutritional services offered by the dietitian is enhanced.[3]

Social Worker. The social worker provides information regarding the patient's family and financial situation. If, upon discharge, the patient is unable to prepare meals or, because of limited income, to purchase the necessary food, the social worker can arrange for assistance. The dietitian should be notified of such situations so that discharge diet instructions can be appropriately made.

Pharmacist. The pharmacist is responsible for preparing the nutritional solutions the physician orders. These solutions are administered through veins or enteral routes (see Nutritional support, p. 215). The dietitian makes sure that these solutions are providing adequate nutrients for the patient and consults with the physician and pharmacist about changes in solutions when necessary.

Because of specialized knowledge about drugs and their actions, the pharmacist is able to serve as a resource concerning drug and nutrient interactions.

WHAT ATTITUDES AND UNDERSTANDING WILL BE HELPFUL AS YOU STUDY NUTRITION?

1. An appreciation of the role of nutrition for optimal health, efficiency, longevity, and enjoyment of life for everyone, including yourself and family.
2. An appreciation of the importance of the right kinds and amounts of foods daily for good nutrition for yourself, your family, and your patients.
3. An appreciation of the role of nutrition in the total care of the patient: to maintain good nutrition through an illness, to improve the patient's state of nutrition when necessary, or as a single or one of several therapeutic measures.
4. An appreciation of the social, racial, religious, economic, and psychological factors, as well as the physiological factors, in feeding both well and ill persons.
5. An understanding of the patient's well-established patterns of eating.
6. An appreciation of the importance of *your* having the right attitude toward food and nutrition habits for success in feeding patients and their willingness to accept diet modifications.
7. An appreciation of the importance of the normal basic diet as a foundation for any therapeutic modification.
8. An appreciation of your role and responsibility in educating patients, their families, and community members in good nutrition habits.

WHAT KNOWLEDGE AND SKILLS WILL BE OF VALUE IN MEETING PATIENTS' NEEDS?

Knowledge of:

1. Characteristics of good and poor nutritional status.
2. Nutrients for good nutrition and their functions in the body.
3. Nutritive values of foods in the various food groups.
4. Nutritional needs of individuals in different age groups and under varying activities.
5. Daily food guides for good nutrition.
6. Ways the normal diet is modified for therapeutic purposes.
7. Principles of meal planning for nutritional adequacy and palatability.
8. Food economics and selection.
9. Principles of food preparation for economy, retention of nutrients, and palatability.
10. Food fads and fallacies.
11. Agencies concerned with problems of nutrition and health.
12. Diseases that require diet modification and what is involved in the therapy.
13. Basic relationships between food and drugs.

Skills:

1. Ability to recognize outward signs of good and poor nutrition.
2. Ability to apply basic principles of nutrition to the wise selection of your own daily foods and to those of your family.
3. Ability to plan adequate and palatable meals for yourself and family.
4. Ability to prepare simple, nutritious meals, as necessary.
5. Ability to serve food attractively and correctly to yourself, your family, and patients.
6. Ability to make simple modifications in the normal diet to conform to doctor's therapeutic diet orders; or to adapt a family meal for the family member requiring nutritional therapy.
7. Ability to answer questions of patients regarding food and nutrition and help them understand reasons for their nutritional therapy and the need for their cooperation.

8. Ability to report to physician and dietitian about a patient's dietary problems and needs.

9. Ability to give a patient assistance at mealtime.

10. Ability to advise on nutritional care at home.

11. Ability to evaluate the adequacy of the food served on the tray and consumed by the patient.

WHAT IS YOUR NUTRITIONAL I.Q. AS YOU BEGIN NUTRITION STUDY?

Some of the following statements are true; some are false. Read each question and then check your answer in the appropriate column before you consult the list of correct answers at the bottom of page 9.

	True	False
1. Toasted bread has the same number of calories as untoasted bread.	____	____
2. Rice, spaghetti, and macaroni have the same food value as potatoes.	____	____
3. Brown eggs have the same nutritive value as white eggs.	____	____
4. Gelatin is a "good" source of protein.	____	____
5. Fish and celery are brain foods.	____	____
6. Everyone should eat a good source of protein such as milk, eggs, meat, fish, or poultry at every meal.	____	____
7. More food is needed when studying for examinations.	____	____
8. A daily diet for reducing should have adequate amounts of protein, minerals, and vitamins but furnish less than the daily requirements for kcalories.	____	____
9. Proteins and starches should not be eaten in the same meal.	____	____
10. Margarine and butter contain the same number of calories.	____	____
11. Vegetable juices have magic health-giving properties.	____	____
12. Frozen orange juice has the same food value as fresh orange juice.	____	____
13. All fruits and vegetables should be eaten raw.	____	____
14. Sour cream contains the same number of calories as sweet cream.	____	____
15. Milk and cheese are constipating foods.	____	____
16. One never outgrows the need for milk in the diet.	____	____
17. "Wonder foods" such as yogurt and blackstrap molasses help keep one young and fit.	____	____
18. Water is fattening.	____	____
19. There is no danger in eating fish or seafood and milk, or milk and cherries, or milk and tomatoes in the same meal.	____	____
20. A well person who eats the right kinds and amounts of foods every day does not need to take vitamin pills.	____	____
21. Skipping meals is a good way to lose weight safely.	____	____
22. One must not drink water when trying to lose weight.	____	____
23. No food can be considered "fattening" or "slenderizing."	____	____

24. Natural sweets like honey have fewer calories and less carbohydrate than sugar. ____ ____

25. Craving for a certain food does not mean that the body needs it. ____ ____

26. Pasteurized milk has the same food value and is safer than unpasteurized milk. ____ ____

27. Drinking water at meal time may aid digestion if it is not used to wash down food. ____ ____

28. There is no danger in using aluminum cooking utensils in food preparation. ____ ____

29. Vegetables eaten whole or simply cut up for preparation are more nutritious than if put through a vegetable juicer. ____ ____

30. People need calcium (milk) in their diets even after they are full-grown adults and their bones are formed. ____ ____

31. A teenager needs more milk every day than a preschooler. ____ ____

32. A combination of honey and vinegar has special healthful properties. ____ ____

33. Only a doctor can determine whether a person needs to take vitamin pills or concentrates. ____ ____

34. "Fad diets" for reducing are not only ineffective for permanent weight reduction but they may be dangerous as well. ____ ____

35. A daily diet containing the right amounts of milk, some meat or fish or poultry or eggs, fruits, vegetables, and enriched or whole-grain breads and cereals will provide all the nutrients needed for good nutrition. ____ ____

36. Most diseases are due to faulty diet. ____ ____

37. At least one serving of a "good" protein should be eaten at every meal. ____ ____

38. "Starve a fever and feed a cold." ____ ____

39. Foods grown in poor soil or where chemical fertilizers are used have lower nutritional value than those grown in good soil. ____ ____

40. True weight loss cannot be accomplished by reducing the amount of water in the diet. ____ ____

41. "Enriched" foods are valuable in the diet because they contain added nutrients in kinds and amounts. ____ ____

42. Brittle fingernails are improved by taking some gelatin in fruit juice several times daily. ____ ____

43. Poor diets eaten by teenagers are deficient in several important nutrients. ____ ____

44. Fruit juices cause an "acid reaction" in the body. ____ ____

45. Some foods rich in vitamin C should be eaten daily as the body cannot store this vitamin. ____ ____

46. Grape juice, beef juice, tomato juice, and beets are high in iron. ____ ____

47. Orange juice loses vitamin C if exposed to air in an opened container. ____ ____

48. Prunes, bran, and so on are "sure cures" for constipation. ____ ____

49. Starches are "fattening." ____ ____

50. One should eat a wide variety of foods daily to meet nutrient requirements as specified by the RDA. ____ ____

51. Dietary supplements alone can prevent, treat, or cure disease. ____ ____

52. Diabetes is caused by eating too much sugar. ____ ____

53. Tea has almost as much caffeine as coffee. ____ ____

54. Vitamin E prevents heart disease, cancer, impotency, and circulatory problems. ____ ____

55. Women need more iron than children. ____ ____

56. Beet and turnip greens contain large amounts of vitamin A. ____ ____

Number correct answers ____
Number incorrect answers ____

How good do you think your Nutrition Score is?

Correct answers:

1. T	9. F	17. F	25. T	33. T	41. T	49. F
2. F	10. T	18. F	26. T	34. T	42. F	50. T
3. T	11. F	19. T	27. T	35. T	43. T	51. F
4. F	12. T	20. T	28. T	36. F	44. F	52. F
5. F	13. F	21. F	29. T	37. T	45. T	53. T
6. T	14. T	22. F	30. T	38. F	46. F	54. F
7. F	15. F	23. T	31. T	39. F	47. T	55. T
8. T	16. T	24. F	32. F	40. T	48. F	56. T

MY "FOOD AND NUTRITION EXPERIENCE" DIARY

To help make you "food and nutrition-minded" as you study nutrition, (1) jot down below any out-of-class food and nutrition comments, questions, or experiences you encounter in discussions with individuals and later as you give nutritional care to patients (checking menus, setting up and/or observing and serving trays, feeding patients, etc.) and (2) assemble in a notebook (preferably), folder, or file box any available food and nutrition booklets, clippings, or other printed materials.

Date	*Food and Nutrition Experience*	*Comments*

REFERENCES

1. *Dietitians: The Professionals in Nutritional Care*, Brochure no. 1077. American Dietetic Association, Chicago, 1977.
2. A. Henneman et al., "Teaching Nutritional Assessment to Nursing Students," *Journal of the American Dietetic Association*, Vol. 78, No. 5, 1981, p. 498.

Food, Nutrition, and Health

1

CHAPTER OUTLINE

RELATION OF NUTRITION TO HEALTH
- Factors Affecting Health
- Functions of Food
- Nutrition Studies and Surveys
- World Food Problems and Agencies

GUIDES FOR GOOD NUTRITION
- Description and Purpose of Dietary Guidelines
- How to Use Food Guides
- Resources for Determining the Nutritive Value of Food

PUBLIC HEALTH AND COMMUNITY NUTRITION
- Relation of Food and Nutrition to Public Health
- Nutrition Education Concepts and Application of Knowledge
- Nutritional Labeling
- Additives
- Consumer Food Protection Agencies and Organizations

OBJECTIVES

☐ To understand the meaning of health and good nutritional status.
☐ To learn how to apply various food guides.
☐ To become acquainted with the agencies and programs that promote good nutrition and health.

TERMS TO UNDERSTAND

Dietary guidelines
Food and Nutrition Board (FNB)
Food fad
Health
Holistic health
Nutrition quack
Nutritional status
National Academy of Sciences (NAS)
National Research Council (NRC)
Public health
Recommended Dietary Allowances (RDA)
The Basic Four Food Groups

Relation of Nutrition to Health

HOW IS HEALTH DEFINED?

Health, as defined by the World Health Organization of the United Nations, is "a state of complete physical, mental, and social well-being, and not merely the absence of disease or infirmity."[1] While it is possible to have good nutrition without good health, the best or optimal health is impossible without good nutrition.

Great progress has occurred over the past 75 years in the improvement of the general level of health. The increase in longevity is one example, the average life span being considerably greater now than in the early 1900s. The control of preventable disease, particularly in the case of children, and also better nutrition for all are considered reasons for this increase in longevity. "Curative" medicine has been largely replaced by "preventive" medicine or, as termed by some, "productive health."

Public health is the field of medicine that is concerned with safeguarding and improving the health of the community as a whole.

Holistic health is a system of preventive medicine that takes into account the whole individual, promotes personal responsibility for well-being, and acknowledges the total influences—social, psychological, and environmental—that affect health, including nutrition, exercise, and mental relaxation.

WHAT FACTORS AFFECT ONE'S STATE OF HEALTH?

Many factors affect one's state of health, such as proper functioning of all body organs, posture, good health and hygiene habits, a good mental attitude, and the correction of remediable defects. Figure 1–1 indicates that the same factors that promote good nutrition also promote good health. It is generally agreed that one of the most important environmental factors affecting the health of an individual, a community, or a nation is good nutrition.

Optimal (best or most favorable) health is founded on good nutrition. Eating the right kinds and amounts of food and following good dietary habits throughout the entire life cycle means healthier bodies and minds, greater vitality and energy, greater resistance to disease, efficiency, happiness, and longevity. The role played by food in promoting and maintaining good health is therefore, a major one. In other words, "food becomes our nutrition." Its role in fulfilling nonmetabolic needs of social, socioeconomic, and emotional types needs to be recognized as well.

Personal aspects of good nutrition are far-reaching for the individual, since the assurance of one's own good health favors accomplishment and happiness. Good nutrition is likewise a community asset, paying valuable dividends. Continuing awareness of its importance has resulted in some improvements in dietary habits for many and lessened manifest nutritional deficiencies. However, there is still room for dietary improvement, as a fairly large percentage of the population of every community exhibits partial dietary deficiencies. The international aspects of good nutrition are evidenced in the many world nutrition betterment programs under way.

Insufficient food (calories) and deficiencies of protein, minerals, and vitamins in the diet all affect physical fitness and work capacity. It has even been demonstrated that mental ability, associated with personality changes, as well as physical ability may be affected by a very poor diet.

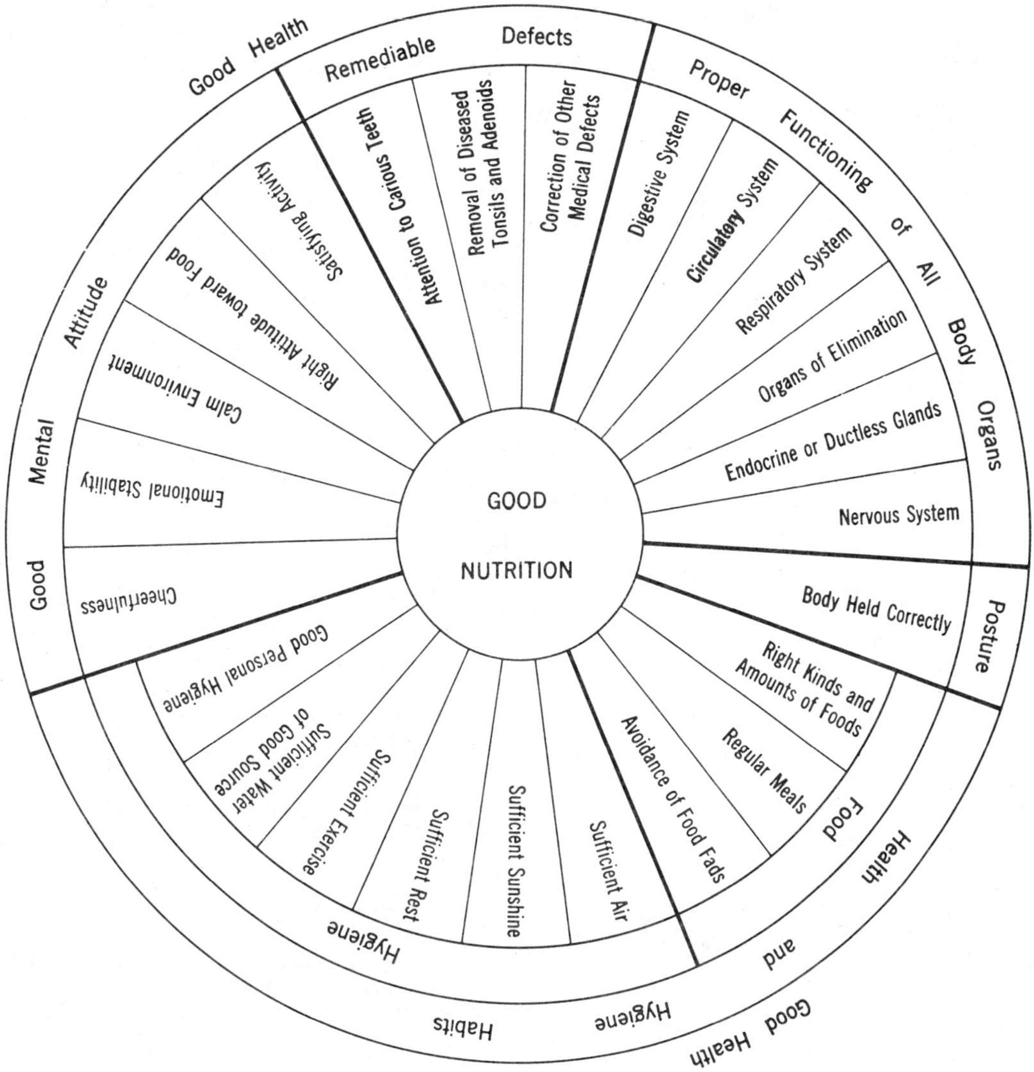

Figure 1–1. Factors in health and nutrition. (From M. T. Dowd, and A. Dent, *Elements of Foods and Nutrition*, 2nd ed. John Wiley & Sons, New York.)

WHAT ARE THE FUNCTIONS OF FOOD IN NUTRITION?

As defined earlier, food is any material, solid or liquid, which after ingestion, digestion, and absorption from the intestinal tract is used to build and maintain body tissues, regulate body processes, and supply energy (calories). Any given food is a mixture of certain elements such as the minerals (calcium, phosphorus, sodium, iron, etc.), certain compounds (carbohydrates, fats, proteins, some vitamins), and water, any of which is called a nutrient.

A nutrient is, therefore, any substance that performs one or more functions in the body. Nutrients include carbohydrates, fats, proteins, minerals, vitamins, and water. Some nutrients function in more than one way. Any single food might contain only one nutrient (carbohydrate in sugar) or several nutrients (protein, fat, calcium, vitamin A in milk). A variety of foods in the diet in the correct amounts will provide all the necessary nutrients (about 50 when the various amino acids, minerals, and vitamins are counted) in the correct amounts.

TABLE 1-1. Functions of Food in Nutrition

Function in Nutrition	Nutrients	Foods
1. Build and repair body tissue	Proteins	Meat, fish, poultry, eggs, milk, cheese, dried peas and beans, cereals, breads
	Minerals—Calcium	Milk, cheese, ice cream, collards, kale, mustard greens, turnip greens
	Iron	Lean meat, liver, eggs, green leafy vegetables, whole-grain and enriched cereals, dried peas and beans, dried fruits
2. Regulate body processes	Water	
	Minerals	See above.
	Vitamins—Vitamin A	Whole milk, butter, eggs, liver, dark-green and yellow vegetables, fortified margarine, deep-yellow or orange fruits
	Vitamin D	Vitamin D–fortified milk, fish liver oils, sardines, salmon, tuna, small amounts in eggs
	Thiamine	Meat (pork=high), fish, poultry, whole-grain and enriched bread and cereals
	Riboflavin	Milk, cheese, ice cream, meats, fish, poultry, eggs, liver, kidney
	Niacin	Lean meat, poultry, peanuts, beans, peas, whole-grain and enriched cereal products
	Ascorbic acid	Citrus fruits, strawberries, cantaloupe, tomatoes, green peppers, broccoli, raw greens, cabbage, new potatoes
	Proteins	See above.
3. Furnish energy	Carbohydrates	Sugars, sweets, molasses, flour, flour products, potatoes, starchy vegetables, and fruits
	Fats	Butter, margarine, shortenings, salad dressing, oils, meat fats, bacon, nuts, cream
	Also proteins to some extent; expensive source	See above.

Table 1-1 shows the functions of food, the nutrients performing these functions, and the common food sources of the nutrients.

WHAT ARE THE CHARACTERISTICS OF GOOD NUTRITIONAL STATUS (NORMAL NUTRITION) AND HOW ARE THEY APPRAISED?

Easily Observable Characteristics

Correct weight for height and age
Bones straight and without enlargements
Broad chest
Well-shaped head
Straight back with no protruding shoulder blades

Less Easily Observable Characteristics

Sense of well-being
Absence of fatigue and tiredness
Good appetite
Restful sleep
Normal functioning of all processes: circulation, respiration, digestion, metabolism, elimination

Flat abdomen
Firm muscles
Smooth, clear, slightly moist skin of good color
Smooth glossy hair
Bright and alert eyes and expression
Well-formed jaws
Good posture
Unobstructed breathing
Teeth well placed in jaws and free from caries
Cheerful disposition

Nutritional status is appraised by:

1. Determination of overweight and underweight, often by measurement of skin-fold
2. Clinical examination with special attention to the condition of skin, eyes, mouth, tongue, gums, teeth, and muscles
3. Blood pressure and pulse rate
4. Biochemical tests on the blood for various constituents associated with health, such as hemoglobin, serum vitamin A, vitamin C, plasma protein, serum albumin, and hematocrit
5. Tests of urine samples for urinary riboflavin, thiamine, creatinine, and glucose
6. Correlation of the above with a dietary history

WHAT STUDIES OVER THE YEARS SHOW THAT FOOD REALLY MAKES A DIFFERENCE IN HEALTH?

1. Recent studies indicate that previously malnourished children (particularly those malnourished in late infancy and early childhood) who receive sensory stimulation, along with adequate nutrition, show some evidence of "catch-up" in intellectual development.[2]
2. Other studies are cited in which vitamin and mineral supplementation during pregnancy apparently reduced the incidence of toxemia and prevented edema and rises in blood pressure. Also, a review of worldwide epidemiological data reveals that populations with relatively low daily calcium intakes (240 to 368 mg) have a greater incidence of eclampsia (1.59 to 12.0 per cent) than do populations with relatively high daily calcium intakes (884 to 1100 mg calcium daily, and an eclampsia incidence of 0.4 to 0.9 per cent).[3]
3. A controlled study, as well as observation during and following World War II, demonstrated clearly that poorly fed people are affected mentally as well as physically.[4]
4. Studies of industrial workers in various sectors of the United States economy reveal that many people consume inadequate diets, with resulting poor nutritional status.[4]
5. Increases in maternal weight gain were shown to accompany significant and desirable increases in infant birth weight.[5]

AMERICAN DIETARY HABITS AND NUTRITIONAL STATUS

The average American diet, as measured by the food available for consumption, is varied and sufficient to feed our population well. But how well do Americans really eat and how good is their nutritional status? With our abundant food supply, are we the best-fed nation in the world?

Nutrition surveys indicate how dietary habits affect nutritional status. The poor results of many surveys since 1940 have stimulated nutrition education programs and have given impetus to the enrichment of bread and flour and the fortification of foods. Surveys have also indicated the need for school breakfast and lunch programs and have provided data for new educational materials and for the Food Stamp Program.

In 1965, a nationwide dietary survey showed that only half of United States households had diets that met the Recommended Dietary Allowances (RDA) for seven nutrients. As a result, nutrition programs for people of all ages and income levels were intensified, and the consumption of milk, enriched grain products, and other foods rich in required nutrients was encouraged.

Improvement was shown in a later nationwide survey in 1977, which revealed that the food used by households had a higher nutrient density than the food used in 1965. The consumption of dark-green vegetables which, if not overcooked, have a high content of vitamins A and C, increased, as did the use of fruits, especially citrus fruits. The use of bread and cereals declined, as did fat consumption. Calcium consumption still remained low. The survey also showed that women of lower socioeconomic status are less likely to breast-feed their children than women of higher socioeconomic status,[7] which affects infant nutrition.

Ten State Nutrition Survey (TSNS)

In 1968–70 the U. S. Department of Health, Education and Welfare conducted a survey in low-income areas of ten states to assess the nutritional status of the nation. Twelve nutrients were studied, and it was found that there was an unexpectedly high prevalence of conditions associated with malnutrition. Social, cultural, and geographic differences apparently affected nutritional status as well.

Health and Nutrition Examination Survey (HANES)

The first Health and Nutrition Examination Survey (HANES), held between 1971 and 1975, studied 30,000 people between the ages of 1 and 74; the second HANES was conducted between February 1976 and March 1980. All income levels were studied, but nutritional problems were found to be more prevalent and acute among the poor. Iron-deficiency anemia was discovered in all age groups, especially among the young. Obesity, poor growth, and dental caries were also evident.

National Food Consumption Survey

The United States Department of Agriculture (USDA) conducts a national food consumption survey approximately every 10 years. The latest of these surveys was carried out in 1977–78 and indicated that elderly women had significantly low intakes of calcium and vitamin B_6. Other data from this survey revealed that the diet of those with low incomes had improved since the previous USDA survey. The improvement was attributed to food assistance programs. Generally, the intakes of pyridoxine (vitamin B_6), magnesium, iron, and zinc were shown to be below the RDA levels. There was evidence of an excessive intake of calories, fat, cholesterol, sugars, salt, and alcohol.

Preschool Nutrition Survey

The Preschool Nutrition Survey was conducted in 1968–70 and showed that many children had low intakes of ascorbic acid or were anemic or both. Significantly, as the socioeconomic status of the family increased, the nutritional status of the children improved.

America is the "land of plenty," but the goals of the right kind and sufficient amount of food and optimum nutrition for every American have not been completely realized. In order to achieve these goals, U.S. households need to become more aware of the foods that make up a good diet, be motivated to choose these foods, and be financially able to buy them.

WHAT U.S. AGENCIES HELP TO IMPROVE NUTRITION?

Several food assistance programs of the Food and Nutrition Service of the USDA have been effective in improving the nutritional status of people who are too poor, too young or old, or too handicapped to provide fully for themselves. These programs are operated through federal, state, and local governments and are activated locally, by public officials, private organizations, and volunteer citizens. Food for Families provides (1) donated foods, (2) food stamps to low-income families at home, and (3) supplemental foods for health or selected highly nutritious foods to needy pregnant women, new mothers, and infants and young children. Child Nutrition Programs include (1) school breakfast, (2) school lunch in elementary and secondary public and nonprofit schools, and (3) preschool summer food service and meals to preschool children in day-care centers and similar organized away-from-home activities.[7,8]

The Consumer and Food Economics Research Service and the Food and Nutrition Service of the USDA are interested in the nutrition of the American family. Three other federal agencies, the Children's Bureau, Food and Drug Administration, and Public Health Service, conduct nutrition research or provide services or both. A list of other federal, state, and local governmental agencies, nongovernmental organizations, educational and industrial institutions, and private agencies interested in the nutritional welfare of the American family can be found on p. 37.

WHAT ARE WORLD PROBLEMS IN NUTRITION AND WHAT ARE THE INTERESTED AGENCIES?

In less well-developed countries, a large number of people are estimated to be undernourished, malnourished, and hungry. The problem is greatest among women and children. People are hungry not only because there is not enough food but also because they are too poor to purchase the food that is available. The general consensus is that the situation is worse in Africa than in other countries.

The four basic ways of dealing with the international hunger problem are through:

1. Donation of food by various groups
2. International efforts that target the food to vulnerable groups of people such as women and children
3. Promotion of agricultural production, food technology, and better and more complete use of the country's own food resources
4. Economic assistance

The United States has developed various programs and campaigns that assist developing countries in combating malnutrition. The U.S. Foreign Aid and Food for Peace programs and activities of the Agency for International Development (AID) are coordinated with United Nations agencies or "multilateral institutions." The governments of many nations contribute to the organizations that distribute food or money for the purpose of improving nutritional standards. Some of these agencies are:

FAO, the United Nations Food and Agriculture Organization, which studies various aspects of world food problems, especially raising nutrition standards by improving the growth, distribution, and storage of food.

WHO, the World Health Organization, which concerns itself with worldwide health problems, especially those that relate to nutrition.

UNESCO, the United Nations Educational, Scientific and Cultural Organization, which is interested in improving the standard of living of people all over the world through science education and by eliminating illiteracy.

UNICEF, the United Nations International Children's Emergency Fund, which has directed the distribution of milk to children all over the world through emergency relief, school feeding, and maternal and child health care centers.

Private voluntary organizations also help to combat international malnutrition. *OXFAM–UK,* which was founded in England as the Oxford Famine Society, donates money and services for agricultural development. *CARE* is an organization that receives food from the Food for Peace Program for relief activities.

The *World Bank* lends money to developing countries. Its agricultural and nutritional divisions sponsor international projects.

Study Questions and Activities

1. List some characteristics of good nutritional status under the following headings: appearance, physical well-being, mental health.
2. What are the functions of food in nutrition? Which nutrients perform each function?
3. Be able to cite several instances which show that a change in diet improves nutrition.
4. What progress has been made toward the improvement of American dietary habits and nutritional status as a result of nutrition surveys?
5. What are the two main reasons that hunger is prevalent in less well-developed countries?

Guides for Good Nutrition

WHAT ARE DIETARY GUIDELINES AND WHAT IS THEIR PURPOSE?

Since World War II, dietary guidelines based on the Recommended Dietary Allowances have been important in formulating national and international food and nutrition policies. Before 1960, the primary goal of guidelines was to ensure growth and development and to improve resistance to disease through adequate nutrition. Currently the emphasis is on reducing the incidence of chronic and degenerative diseases. In addition to the Food and Nutrition Board of the National Academy of Sciences, the American Medical Association (AMA), the U.S. Department of Agriculture (USDA), the U.S. Department of Health and Human Services (DHHS) and the governments of Canada, Australia, and Norway have influenced public health by establishing dietary guidelines that emphasize the need to consume a varied diet with adequate calories and nutrients in order to maintain health and body weight. All the dietary guidelines agree that people at risk on the basis of family history, elevated blood pressure, diabetes, and blood lipid profiles should follow individualized professional dietary advice as a part of convalescent care. All of the agencies that offer guidelines also recommend reducing the fat content of the diet from 40 per cent to 35 per cent of energy intake. In general, moderation is the key word for the guidelines.

The USDA's *Guide to a Better Diet* (previously called *A Daily Guide*) was developed over 25 years ago. It is a simple, organized method that may be used in applying the dietary guidelines (See p. 24 and Fig. 1–2 for further details). Whereas the dietary guidelines were developed to discourage excesses in the diet, the Four Food Groups system of the *Guide to a Better Diet* illustrates how to meet minimum daily requirements.[10] Guides similar to the Basic Four Food Groups are used in many countries, varying only slightly, depending upon food habits and food availability.[11]

DIETARY GUIDELINES FOR AMERICANS

The following guidelines were developed in 1980 by the USDA/DHHS. These guidelines are used for generally healthy Americans and stress good eating habits based on moderation and variety.[8,9]

1. *Eat a variety of foods*
2. *Maintain ideal weight*
3. *Avoid foods high in fat, especially saturated fat and cholesterol**
4. *Eat foods with adequate starch and fiber*
5. *Avoid too much sugar*
6. *Avoid too much sodium*
7. *If you drink alcohol, do so in moderation*

EAT A VARIETY OF FOODS

Most foods contain more than one nutrient, but no single food provides all the necessary nutrients in the correct amounts for good health. Milk, for instance, contains very little iron or vitamin C. The greater the variety of foods in the diet, the less likely either a deficiency or an excess of any single nutrient will develop. Variety also reduces the likelihood of exposure to excessive amounts of contaminants in any single food item.

One way to assure variety, and with it a well-balanced diet, is to select foods each day from each of the following major groups:

Fruits	Milk, cheese, and yogurt
Vegetables	Meats, poultry, fish, and eggs
Whole-grain and enriched breads, cereals, and grain products	Legumes (dry peas and beans)

To assure an adequate diet for an infant, unless there are special problems, breast-feeding is recommended. Other foods are delayed until the infant is 3 to 6 months old, and neither salt nor sugar need be added to the food.

MAINTAIN IDEAL WEIGHT

If weight loss is recommended, it should be done at a rate of 1 to 2 pounds a week until the goal is reached. The process of losing weight successfully depends on good eating habits, which include eating slowly, preparing smaller portions, and avoiding "seconds." It is important to increase physical activity; eat less fat and fatty foods; and less sugar and sweets; and avoid too much alcohol.

*The USDA/DHHS guidelines are the only guidelines that recommend reducing cholesterol intake.

AVOID FOODS HIGH IN FAT, ESPECIALLY SATURATED FAT AND CHOLESTEROL

To avoid consumption of too much fat, especially saturated fat and cholesterol, lean meat, fish, poultry, and legumes are recommended as protein sources. Eggs and organ meats such as liver should be eaten in moderation.

EAT FOODS WITH ADEQUATE STARCH AND FIBER

More complex carbohydrates (starches) are recommended, and this can be achieved by substituting starches for fats and sugar and by selecting foods that are good sources of fiber and starch, such as whole-grain breads and cereals, fruits and vegetables, beans, peas, and nuts.

AVOID TOO MUCH SUGAR

To avoid excessive consumption of sugar, it is recommended that less refined sugars and foods containing sugars be used. Fresh fruits or fruits canned without sugar or in light syrup rather than in heavy syrup should be selected. Food labels will indicate sugar content. In the development of dental caries, how often and the form in which sugar is eaten are just as important as how much is eaten.

AVOID TOO MUCH SODIUM

To avoid too much sodium, only a small amount of salt should be used in cooking and only a little salt, if any, added at the table. Consumption of salted potato chips, pretzels, nuts, and popcorn; condiments such as soy sauce, steak sauce, and garlic salt; cheese; pickled foods; and cured meats should be limited. It is important to read food labels carefully to determine the amounts of sodium in processed foods and snack items. One can learn to enjoy the flavor of foods without salt.

IF YOU DRINK ALCOHOL, DO SO IN MODERATION

Alcoholic beverages tend to be high in calories and low in nutrients. Vitamin and mineral deficiencies occur commonly in heavy drinkers, in part because of poor intake but also because alcohol alters the absorption and use of some essential nutrients.

DIETARY GUIDELINES TO REDUCE CANCER RISK

In 1982 the National Academy of Sciences (NAS) suggested what people should and should not eat to reduce the risk of cancer. The committee studied the results of hundreds of cancer studies, and Dr. Clifford Grobstein concluded that there is increasingly impressive evidence that food does affect the chances of developing cancer.[12] The guidelines and recommendations are as follows:

1. Eat less fatty meat and high-fat dairy products, which have been linked to cancer of the breast and colon.
2. Cut back on salt-cured and smoked foods such as ham, bacon, bologna,

and frankfurters, which have been implicated in cancer of the esophagus and stomach.

3. Drink only moderate amounts of beer, wine, or hard liquor. Excessive drinking, especially in combination with smoking, is said to increase the risk of cancer of the upper gastrointestinal and respiratory tract.

4. Eat fruits and vegetables and whole-grain cereal products daily. Consuming a diet rich in vitamin C (tomatoes, peppers, citrus fruits) may lower the risk of cancer of the esophagus and stomach. Vegetables such as carrots, spinach, and broccoli are rich in carotene, a precursor of vitamin A, and may be protective against cancer of the lung, breast, bladder, and skin. The panel advised against trying to prevent cancer by taking high-dose vitamin supplements.[12]

DIETARY GOALS FOR THE UNITED STATES—WHAT ARE THEY?

In January 1977, the Senate Select Committee on Nutrition and Human Needs issued "Dietary Goals for the United States." The six goals were meant to be applied to the country as a whole and are as follows:

1. Increase carbohydrate consumption to account for 55 to 60 per cent of energy (caloric) intake.
2. Reduce saturated fat consumption to account for about 10 per cent of total energy intake and balance with polyunsaturated and monounsaturated fats, which should each account for about 10 per cent of energy intake.
3. Reduce cholesterol consumption to about 300 mg a day.
4. Reduce sugar consumption by almost 40 per cent, to account for only about 15 per cent of total energy intake.
5. Reduce salt consumption by about 50 to 85 per cent, to approximately 3 gm a day.

To achieve these goals, the Committee suggested the following changes in food selection and preparation:

1. Increase consumption of fruits, vegetables, and whole grains.
2. Decrease consumption of meat, and increase consumption of poultry and fish.
3. Decrease consumption of foods high in fat, and partially substitute polyunsaturated fat for saturated fat.
4. Substitute nonfat milk for whole milk.
5. Decrease consumption of butterfat, eggs, and other high-cholesterol sources.
6. Decrease consumption of sugar and foods high in sugar content.
7. Decrease consumption of salt and foods high in salt content.

The Committee states that "although genetic and other individual differences mean that these guidelines may not be applicable to all, there is substantial evidence indicating that they will be generally beneficial."[12a]

WHO SETS STANDARDS FOR NUTRIENT REQUIREMENTS?

The National Academy of Sciences (NAS) was established in 1863 to provide advice to the federal government. This private society is composed of over 1,100 distinguished scholars in the fields of science and technology. The National Research Council (NRC) was organized in 1916 at the request of President Woodrow Wilson as a branch of the National Academy of Sciences to assist in the solution of problems created by World War I. In 1940, as a result of anticipated involvement of the United States in World

War II, the Food and Nutrition Board (FNB) of the NAS was appointed to advise the government on food and nutrition matters. This group scientifically developed a guide for planning and procuring food supplies for the national defense. The FNB first published this guide, called *Recommended Dietary Allowances*, in 1943 to "provide standards serving as a goal for good nutrition." The report has been revised at approximately five-year intervals as additional data have become available.[13]

WHAT ARE RECOMMENDED DIETARY ALLOWANCES?

Recommended Dietary Allowances (RDA) are the levels of intake of essential nutrients considered, in the judgment of the Committee on Dietary Allowances of the FNB on the basis of available scientific knowledge, to be adequate to meet the known nutritional needs of practically all healthy persons.[13] They are used as a guide to determine the nutritional adequacy of the diet.

The RDA are recommendations for the average daily amounts of nutrients that population groups should consume over a period of time. They should not be confused with requirements for a specific individual, because these vary considerably and are ordinarily unknown. Problems such as premature birth, inherited metabolic disorders, infections, chronic diseases, and the use of medications require special dietary and therapeutic measures. The RDA (with the exception of total energy intake) are estimated to exceed the requirements of most healthy individuals.

The ninth edition of *Recommended Dietary Allowances* was published in 1980, and a summary chart appears on the inside of the front cover of this text. Nutritional requirements differ with age, sex, body size, and physiological state, and therefore the RDA are presented for various age and weight groups and for males and females. Modifications required under special circumstances have not been listed. The following changes were made in the 1980 revision:

1. The allowance for vitamin C (60 mg for adults) has been raised. This increase permits the maintenance of a satisfactory body pool of ascorbic acid for several weeks and 85 per cent absorption efficiency. This allowance may increase the nutritional status for iron in some groups.
2. Vitamin E requirement is dependent on the amount of polyunsaturated fatty acids (PUFA) ingested. A diet low in PUFA will have a lower requirement for vitamin E. The values in the table should be considered as average intakes in balanced diets in the United States, but the adequacy of these intakes will vary if the PUFA content deviates significantly from that which is customary. The allowance has been lowered on the basis that there is no clinical or biochemical evidence that vitamin E status is inadequate in normal ingestion of balanced diets.
3. Iodine allowance has been increased somewhat.
4. Folacin allowance for infants is lowered slightly.
5. The allowance for energy is treated differently from the allowances for specific nutrients. Energy needs vary from person to person, depending on physical activity and the characteristics of the individual. Therefore, the average energy needs for each age and sex group should be used only as guidelines.

A new feature in the ninth edition of *Recommended Dietary Allowances* is the inclusion of recommendations for a number of nutrients in addition to the 18 essential nutrients covered in previous editions. These additional nutrients are known to be essential, but the requirements have been less accurately quantified. Present knowledge is sufficient, however, to provide a range within which lies the requirement. It is considered that intakes below the lower end of the range are likely to lead to deficiency and that intakes above the upper limit may give rise to toxic effects, especially so for trace elements.

How Are the Recommended Dietary Allowances Used?

The RDA are used by federal, state, and local health and welfare agencies in licensing and certification standards for group care facilities such as day-care centers, nursing homes, and residential homes. The RDA are, in fact, the basis for virtually all feeding programs.[11] They are used to interpret food consumption records, to evaluate the adequacy of food supplies in meeting nutritional needs, to plan and procure food supplies for groups, to establish guides for public food assistance programs, to evaluate new food products developed by industry, to establish guidelines for nutritional labeling of foods, and to develop nutrition education programs.

How Are the Recommended Dietary Allowances Determined?

In establishing the RDA, the Committee thoroughly reviews and evaluates all available data, published and unpublished. The Committee then arrives at a consensus and sets the RDA (except for energy) at a value above the average requirement.

The allowance refers to the amount of nutrient that must be consumed in order to insure that the requirements of most people are met. The amount by which the allowance is set above the average requirement varies from nutrient to nutrient.[13] For some nutrients there is limited information about the variability of individual requirements, and judgments must be made.

How are Recommended Allowances Translated into Foods for the Day?

The technical information supplied by *Recommended Dietary Allowances*, sometimes referred to as "The Nutrition Yardstick," must be interpreted in terms of a selection of foods to be eaten daily if it is to be valuable from a practical standpoint. The RDA should be met by consuming a wide variety of acceptable, palatable, and economically attainable foods, and not through supplementation or use of fortified foods. Various basic diet patterns may be devised to serve as guides in food selection.

The U.S. Department of Agriculture's "Guide to a Better Diet" (see Fig. 1–2) shows one way to choose daily foods wisely. Most foods contain more than one nutrient but no single food provides all the necessary nutrients in the correct amounts for good health. With the help of this guide, it is possible to obtain all the nutrients needed daily from a variety of common foods.

Table 1–2 provides an evaluation of the foundation of an adequate diet for an adult.

WHAT ARE THE DANGERS OF CONSUMPTION OF EXCESS NUTRIENTS?

A substantial proportion of the population consumes an excess over the RDA for several nutrients without evidence of adverse effects. However, not all nutrients are well tolerated if as much as two to three times the RDA is consumed. For example, a high intake of vitamins A and D and certain trace elements can be toxic. Also, an energy intake in excess of the requirement is highly undesirable, since it will lead to obesity.

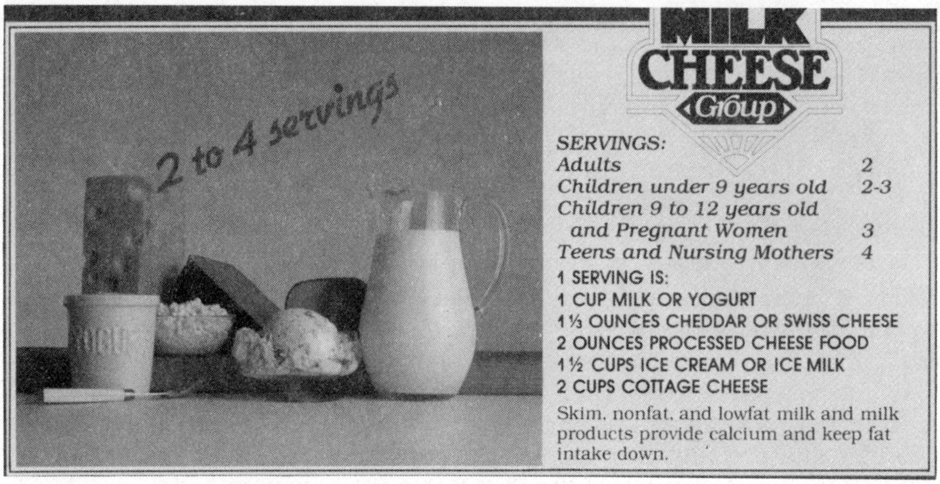
2 to 4 servings
CHEESE
Group
SERVINGS:
Adults 2
Children under 9 years old 2-3
Children 9 to 12 years old and Pregnant Women 3
Teens and Nursing Mothers 4
1 SERVING IS:
1 CUP MILK OR YOGURT
1 1/3 OUNCES CHEDDAR OR SWISS CHEESE
2 OUNCES PROCESSED CHEESE FOOD
1 1/2 CUPS ICE CREAM OR ICE MILK
2 CUPS COTTAGE CHEESE
Skim, nonfat, and lowfat milk and milk products provide calcium and keep fat intake down.

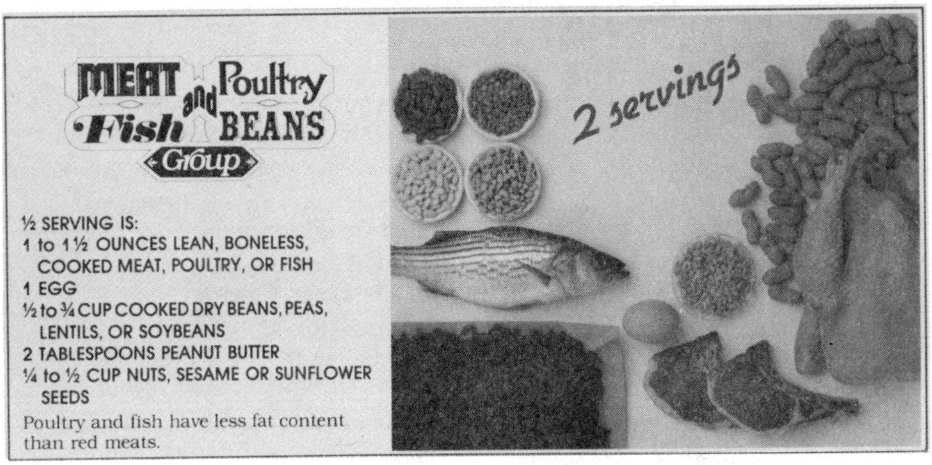
MEAT and Poultry
Fish BEANS
Group
2 servings
1/2 SERVING IS:
1 to 1 1/2 OUNCES LEAN, BONELESS, COOKED MEAT, POULTRY, OR FISH
1 EGG
1/2 to 3/4 CUP COOKED DRY BEANS, PEAS, LENTILS, OR SOYBEANS
2 TABLESPOONS PEANUT BUTTER
1/4 to 1/2 CUP NUTS, SESAME OR SUNFLOWER SEEDS
Poultry and fish have less fat content than red meats.

Figure 1–2. The Four Food Groups of the "Guide to a Better Diet." (From the U.S. Department of Agriculture, Washington, D.C.)

Even though there are many who ardently encourage the public to ingest large quantities of vitamins and minerals, the Committee on Dietary Allowances of the FNB is not aware of convincing evidence that the consumption of an excess of any one nutrient or combination of nutrients will have any unique nutritional benefit.[13]

HOW IS THE GUIDE TO A BETTER DIET USED?

The *Guide to a Better Diet* (Fig. 1–2) was formulated by nutrition scientists who combined the nutrient needs of people and the nutritive values of foods into a diet plan. Foods in the guide are grouped into four food groups according to their main contributions to the diet (Table 1–3).

The Basic Four Food Groups system is used as a way of translating the RDA into a meaningful system that can be used in planning diets. It is easy to choose a variety of favorite foods from the guide and stay within the

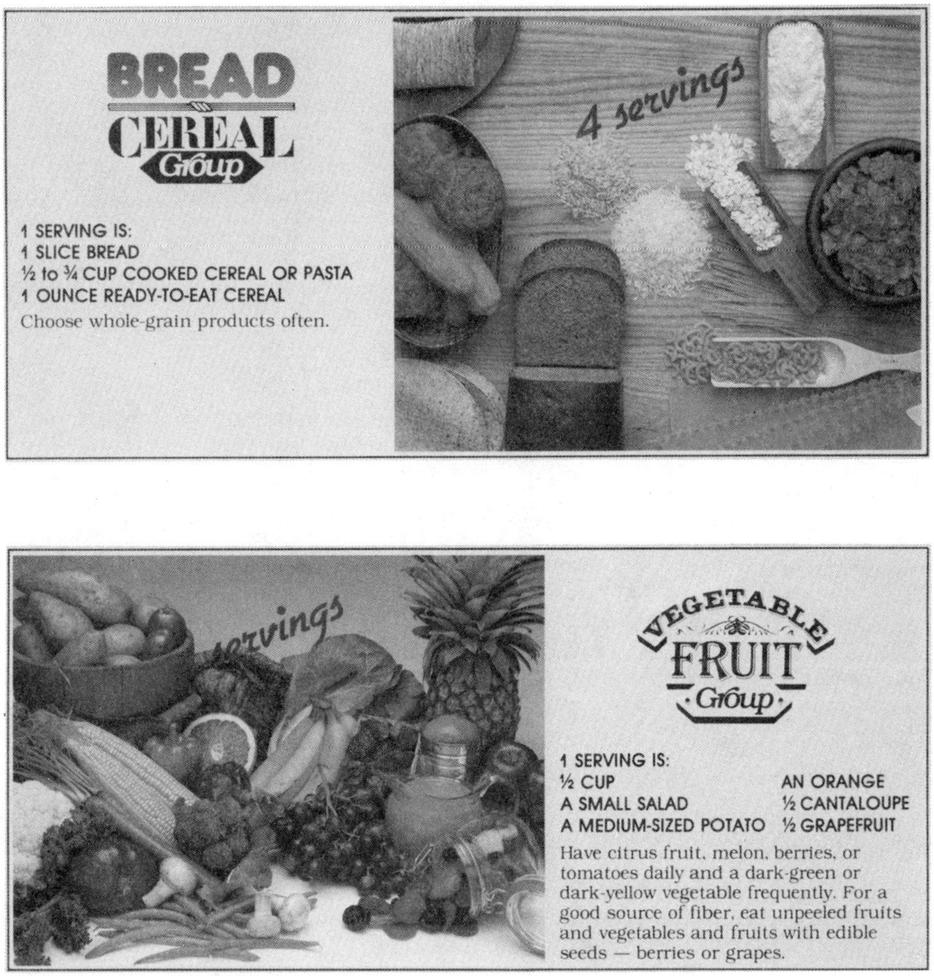
BREAD
CEREAL
Group
4 servings
1 SERVING IS:
1 SLICE BREAD
½ to ¾ CUP COOKED CEREAL OR PASTA
1 OUNCE READY-TO-EAT CEREAL
Choose whole-grain products often.
servings
VEGETABLE
FRUIT
Group
1 SERVING IS:
½ CUP
A SMALL SALAD
A MEDIUM-SIZED POTATO
AN ORANGE
½ CANTALOUPE
½ GRAPEFRUIT
Have citrus fruit, melon, berries, or tomatoes daily and a dark-green or dark-yellow vegetable frequently. For a good source of fiber, eat unpeeled fruits and vegetables and fruits with edible seeds — berries or grapes.

Figure 1–2. *Continued*

family budget, and at the same time be assured of getting all the nutrients in the right amounts.[14] The choices should be made according to the individual's eating style and needs. The suggested number of servings from the four food groups will comprise a total of about 1200 calories. However, foods can be added to the foundation diet if more calories are needed. For instance, everyone needs the same nutrients throughout the life cycle, but there are times when the body needs larger amounts, as during growth and convalescence. In general, boys, men, large people, and those who are very active have greater requirements for energy (calories) and nutrients than girls, women, small people, and inactive people, respectively.

It is wise to have some meat, poultry, fish, eggs, or milk at each meal. There is a fifth group composed of fats, sweets, and alcohol. It provides calories but few nutrients and should be used with caution. The fats in the diet should include some vegetable oil.[15]

TABLE 1–2. Evaluation of the Foundation of an Adequate Diet for an Adult*

Food	Average Serving: *Household Measure*	Average Serving: *Weight (gm)*	Kilocalories	Protein (gm)	Fat (gm)	Carbohydrate (gm)	Minerals: *Calcium (mg)*	Minerals: *Iron (mg)*	Vitamins: *A (I.U.)*	Vitamins: *Ascorbic Acid (mg)*	Vitamins: *Thiamine (mg)*	Vitamins: *Riboflavin (mg)*	Vitamins: *Niacin (mg)*
Milk (whole or equivalent)	1 pt	488	300	16	16	22	582	.2	620	4	.18	.8	.4
Meat group													
Eggs	1	50	80	6	6	1	28	1.0	260	0	.04	.15	tr.
Meat, poultry, fish[1]	3 oz (cooked)	85	322	19	26	0	9	2.0	23	—	.09	.19	4.6
Vegetable–fruit group													
Vegetables:													
Deep green or yellow[2]	1 salad or cooked	50 raw or 70 cooked	23	.9	tr.	5	20	.5	2596	9	.03	.06	.3
Other cooked[3]	½ cup	85	52	2.5	tr.	13	19	1.1	300	4.8	.04	.26	.4
Potato, peeled and boiled	1 medium	122	90	3	tr.	20	8	.7	tr.	22	.12	.05	1.6
Fruits:													
Citrus[4]	1 serving	125	50	.3	tr.	13.5	23	.4	284	50	.07	.03	.31
Other (fresh and canned)[5]	1 serving	135	99	.4	tr.	25	8	.6	235	6	.03	.04	.36

Bread–cereal group													
Cereal (whole-grain and enriched)[6]	½ cup cooked	25 (dry)	80	2.2	1	16	6	.65	1180	4.5	.20	.18	1.5
Bread (whole-grain and enriched)	3 slices 1 whole wheat 2 white	78	170	7	3	40	90	2.0	tr.	tr.	.29	.15	2.4
Totals[7]			1266	57.3	52	180.5	793	9.61	5498[8]	100.3	1.09[9]	1.9	11.9[10]
Recommended Daily Dietary Allowances†													
Man (age 23–50; wt, 154 lb; ht, 69 in)			2700	56.0			800	10.0	5000	60	1.4	1.6	18
Woman (Age 23–50; wt, 128 lb; ht, 65 in)			2000	44			800	18.0	4000	60	1.0	1.2	13

*Data from *Nutritive Value of Foods*, Home and Garden Bulletin No. 72, U.S. Department of Agriculture, 1979.
[1]Evaluation based on figures for cooked (lean and fat) beef, lamb, and veal.
[2]Evaluation based on lettuce, cooked carrots, green beans, winter squash, and broccoli.
[3]Evaluation based on average for cooked peas and beets.
[4]Evaluation based on Florida oranges and white and pink grapefruit; whole and juice.
[5]Evaluation based on canned peaches, applesauce, raw pears, apples, and bananas.
[6]Evaluation based on oatmeal and corn flakes.
[7]With the addition of more of the same foods, or other foods, to meet calorie requirement, the totals will be increased.
[8]With the use of liver this figure will be markedly increased.
[9]With the use of pork, legumes, and liver this figure will be markedly increased.
[10]The average diet in the United States, which contains a generous amount of protein, provides enough tryptophan to increase the niacin value by about a third.
[11]These figures are expressed as niacin equivalents, which include dietary sources of the preformed vitamin and the precursor, tryptophan.
†Recommended Dietary Allowances, National Research Council, Washington, D.C., 1974.

TABLE 1–3. A Description of the Four Food Groups

Milk Group

Some milk every day for everyone:
- 2 to 3 cups for children under 9
- 3 or more cups for children 9 to 12
- 4 or more cups for teenagers
- 2 or more cups for adults
- 3 or more cups for pregnant women
- 4 or more cups for nursing women

Use: Milk, fluid whole, evaporated, or skim; dry; or buttermilk

Cheese and ice cream may replace part of milk on basis of calcium content as follows:

1-inch cube cheddar-type cheese = ½ cup milk

½ cup cottage cheese = ⅓ cup milk

2 tablespoons cream cheese = 1 tablespoon milk

½ cup ice cream = ¼ cup milk

1 cup yogurt = 1 cup milk

Meat Group

2 or more servings every day

Use beef, veal, lamb, variety meats such as liver, heart, kidneys
Poultry and eggs; fish and shellfish
Alternates—dry beans, dry peas, lentils, nuts, peanuts, peanut butter

Count as one serving: 2 to 3 ounces of lean cooked meat, poultry, or fish—all without bone; 2 eggs; 1 cup cooked dry beans, dry peas, or lentils; 2 tablespoons peanut butter.

Vegetable–Fruit Group

4 or more servings every day including:

(1) 1 *serving* of a *good* source of vitamin C
OR
2 *servings* of a fair source of vitamin C

(2) 1 *serving at least every other day*, of a *good* source of vitamin A, such as dark-green or deep-yellow vegetables

(3) The remaining 1 to 3 servings may be any vegetable or fruit including those that are valuable for vitamin C and vitamin A

Count as one serving: ½ cup vegetable or fruit or a portion as ordinarily served, such as 1 medium apple, banana, orange, or potato, or half a medium cantaloupe or grapefruit, or juice of 1 lemon.

Bread–Cereal Group

4 servings or more daily. Or, if no cereals are chosen, have an extra serving of bread or baked goods which will make at least 5 servings from this group daily.

Use: all breads and cereals that are whole-grain, enriched, or restored (check label to be sure); breads, cooked cereals, ready-to-eat cereals, cornmeal, crackers, flour, grits, macaroni, spaghetti, rice, noodles, rolled oats, quick breads, and other baked goods if made with whole-grain or enriched flour. Parboiled rice and wheat may also be included in this group. Count as one serving: 1 slice of bread, 1 oz ready-to-eat cereal, ½ to ¾ cup cooked cereal, cornmeal, grits, macaroni, noodles, rice or spaghetti.

HOW DO THE FOUR FOOD GROUPS SUPPLY NEEDED NUTRIENTS?

The Food Value Wheel (Fig. 1–3) is a handy visual reminder of *nine* of the nutrients for which allowances have been recommended, and the food group which is the major source of each nutrient. The outside rim shows the four food groups. The inner rim of the wheel lists the name of nine key nutrients for which complete analytical data regarding food supply and human needs are available. (See RDA 1980 for additional nutrients.) These recommendations are standards of plenty. They represent the amount of a nutrient required by the body plus extra amounts to provide for times of increased need and the wide differences between individual needs. At present, it is probable that diets furnishing adequate amounts of the nutrients on the Food Value Wheel will also supply sufficient quantities of all other nutrients needed by normally healthy individuals.

The selection, preparation for cooking, and principles underlying correct food preparation will be discussed more fully in Section Three.

In studying nutrition, many resources, including food composition tables, are used. Knowledge of food values is important no matter what approach is used in learning about food selection for good health, whether it be food

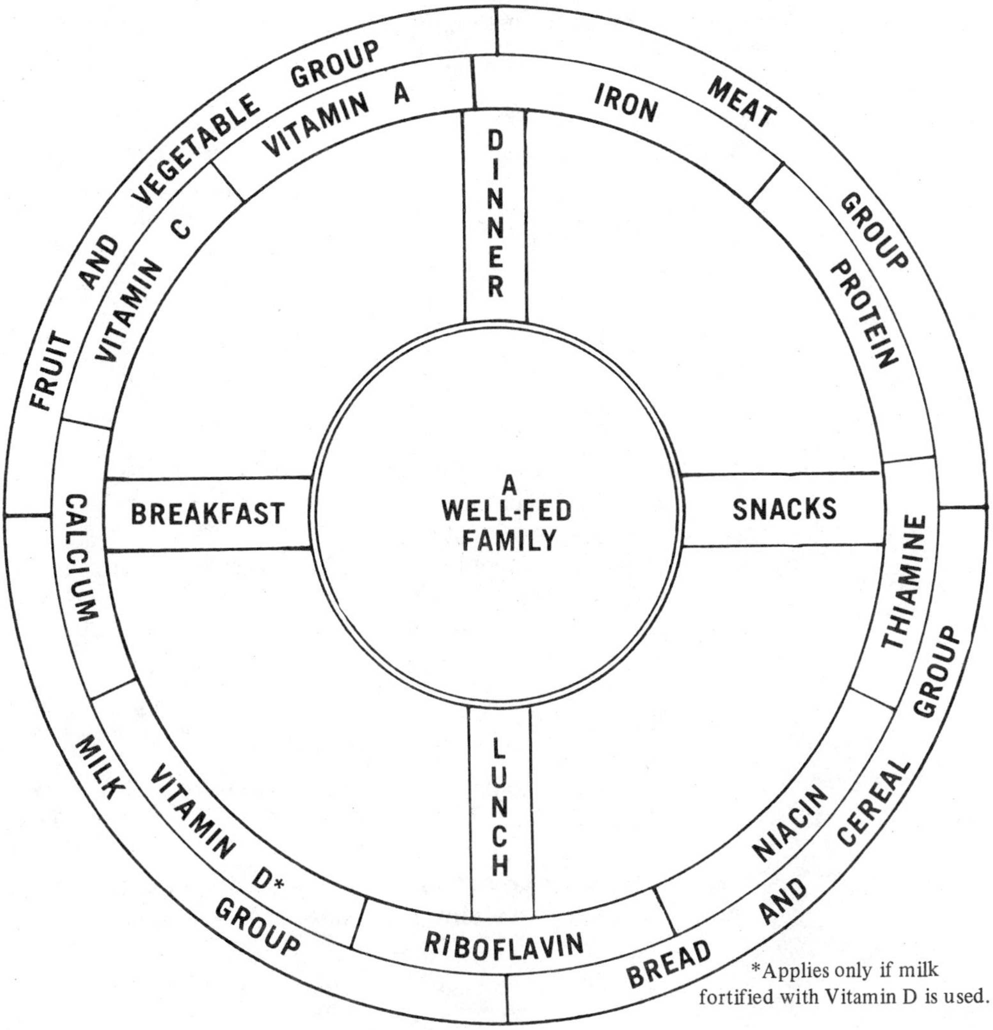

Figure 1–3. A Food Value Wheel. (From Home Economics Extension Leaflet 25. New York State College of Home Economics, Ithaca, New York.)

guides or nutrients in foods, as in nutrition labeling. Food value tables vary in meaning, but the shorter versions are satisfactory for most purposes. See Appendix 6 for the nutritive value of some foods and a list of additional resources for food values.

Study Questions and Activities

1. What is meant by Recommended Dietary Allowances?

2. Underline in *red pencil* the figures in the table of Recommended Dietary Allowances on the inside of the front cover, which indicate the requirements for calories and each of the nutrients listed for a person of your age (in other words, *your* daily requirements for calories and all nutrients)

and jot them down below. You will be referring to these figures throughout the course.

My RDA:

Kcalories	________	Thiamine	________ mg
Protein	________ gm	Vitamin B_6	________ mg
Vitamin A	________ IU	Vitamin B_{12}	________ μg
Vitamin D	________ IU	Calcium	________ mg
Vitamin E	________ IU	Phosphorus	________ mg
Ascorbic Acid	________ mg	Iodine	________ μg
Folacin	________ gm	Iron	________ mg
Niacin	________ mg	Magnesium	________ mg
Riboflavin	________ mg	Zinc	________ mg

3. Why is breakfast such an important meal of the day? What constitutes a good breakfast? What are some of the dangers of skipping breakfast or eating an inadequate breakfast?

4. Complete the accompanying food selection score card.

Can you see further improvements which it might be desirable for you to make in your daily food selection?

5. This menu was eaten by a teenager:

Breakfast:	Lunch:	Dinner:
Banana	Hot dog on roll	Broiled hamburger
Corn flakes	Relish	Baked potato and margarine
Cream and sugar	Chocolate cake	Harvard beets
Toast, butter, and jelly	Coke	Cherry pie

Judge the meals according to the Four Food Group Diet Plan.

List the foods and amounts lacking for a teenager.

Food Selection Score Card

Score your diet for each day and determine your average score for the week. If your final score is between 85 and 100, your food selection standard has been good. A score of from 75 to 85 indicates a fair standard. A score below 75 indicates a low standard.

Maximum Score for Each Food Group	Credits	Columns for Daily Check
20	Milk Group: Milk (including foods prepared with milk as cheese and ice cream) Adults: 1 glass, 10; 1½ glasses, 15; 2 glasses, 20 Children: 1 glass, 5; 1½ glasses, 10; 2 glasses, 15; 4 glasses, 20*	
25	Meat Group: Eggs, Meat, Cheese, Fish, Poultry, Dry Peas, Dry Beans, and Nuts 1 serving of any one of above, 10 1 serving of any two above, 20 If liver (beef, lamb, pork, or calf's) or kidney is used, extra credit, 5	

Food Selection Score Card (*Continued*)

Maximum Score for Each Food Group	Credits	Colums for Daily Check
35	Vegetable–Fruit Group: Vegetables: 1 serving, 5; 2 servings, 10; 3 servings, 15 Potatoes may be included as one of the above servings If dark green or deep-yellow vegetable is included, extra credit, 5 Fruits: 1 serving, 5; 2 servings, 10 If citrus fruit, raw vegetable, or canned tomatoes are included, extra credit, 5†	
15	Bread–Cereal Group: Bread—dark whole grain, enriched or restored Cereals—dark whole grain, enriched or restored 2 servings of either, 10; 4 servings of either, 15	
5	Water (total liquid including milk, coffee, tea, or other beverage): Adults: 6 glasses, 2½; 8 glasses, 5 Children: 4 glasses, 2; 6 glasses, 5	
100	Final Score	

*Count ½ cup milk in soups, puddings, cream pies.
†Count ½ serving vegetables in soups or fruit in salad.
Deductions from final score: Each meal omitted, 10; Meals at irregular hours, 5; "Snacking" between meals, 5; Excessive soft drinks, 10.

Public Health and Community Nutrition

HOW IS FOOD RELATED TO PUBLIC HEALTH?

The health of a community depends on a safe food and water supply. There are many agencies that promote good sanitation practices with respect to food handling in order to prevent disease and control epidemics. These agencies are concerned with all aspects of food quality, including food preservation and food additives, and are also concerned with the prevention of both natural and bacterial food poisoning, water-borne diseases, and the dangerous effects of pesticides.

The United States Public Health Service, which is the principal health agency of the federal government, concerns itself with all factors affecting the health of people, including nutrition. Other federal and various state and local agencies—official, voluntary, professional, and industry-sponsored—are also concerned with factors affecting health and nutrition.

For the public to become better informed about nutrition, the following basic concepts need to be taught:

1. Nutrition is the way the body uses food.
   - We eat food to live, to grow, to keep healthy and well, and to get energy for work and play.

2. Food is made up of different nutrients needed for growth and health. Nutrients include proteins, carbohydrates, minerals, and vitamins.
   - All nutrients needed by the body are available through food.
   - Many kinds and combinations of food can lead to a well-balanced diet.
   - No food, by itself, has all the nutrients needed for full growth and health.
   - Each nutrient has specific uses in the body.
   - Most nutrients do their best work in the body with other nutrients.
3. All persons, throughout life, have need for the same nutrients but in varying amounts.
   - The amounts of nutrients needed are influenced by age, sex, activity, and state of health.
4. The way food is handled influences the amount of nutrients in food, its safety, quality, appearance, taste, acceptability, and cost.
   - Handling means everything that happens to food while it is being grown, processed, stored, and prepared for eating.[16]

HOW IS NUTRITIONAL KNOWLEDGE USED TO IMPROVE HEALTH?

Nutritional Studies

Unfortunately, people are not always motivated to adopt nutritionally sound food practices when selecting foods. A homemaker may accept the idea that sound food practices will provide healthful benefits but may find, after trying to implement knowledge of nutrition, that the practices are too time-consuming or too expensive, or that the family is not happy with new foods. Thus nutritional knowledge may appear inconsistent with food practices. Knowledge of nutrition may be an insufficient basis for convincing others that sound health and dietary practices are important.[17]

On the other hand, a study by the USDA showed that Americans are sensitive to health and nutrition concerns when they buy food. Almost two-thirds of those surveyed said they had adjusted household diets in the past three years for health or nutrition reasons, including weight reduction or maintenance reduction of sugar and fat intake. Fiber, apparently, was not a prominent factor in the selection of foods.[18]

Nutrition Labeling

Nutrition labeling was developed by the Food and Drug Administration (FDA) and the food industry for the purpose of providing the public with nutrition information. Nutrition labeling is required if a nutrient has been added to a food or if a nutrition claim is made about the food, but otherwise it is voluntary. Figure 1–4 shows some examples of nutrition labeling.

The United States RDA* were developed by the FDA for use in nutrition labeling. These replace the minimum daily requirements (MDR) and are set high enough to meet the needs of most healthy people in the United States. The highest values for nutrients in the RDA table established by the Food and Nutrition Board of the National Academy of Sciences are used in each of four groupings: (1) adults and children over 4 years of age, (2) infants up to 1 year of age, (3) children under 4 years of age, and (4) pregnant women or lactating women.

*Not to be confused with the FNB–RDA discussed earlier in the chapter.

PASTEURIZED
HOMOGENIZED
VITAMIN D
MILK

NUTRITION INFORMATION
Per Serving

SERVING SIZE	ONE CUP
SERVINGS PER CONTAINER	8
CALORIES	150
PROTEIN	8 GRAMS
CARBOHYDRATE	11 GRAMS
FAT	8 GRAMS

Percentage of U.S. Recommended Daily Allowances (U.S. RDA)

PROTEIN	20	VITAMIN D	25
VITAMIN A	4	VITAMIN B_6	4
VITAMIN C	4	VITAMIN B_{12}	15
THIAMINE	6	PHOSPHORUS	20
RIBOFLAVIN	25	MAGNESIUM	8
NIACIN	*	ZINC	4
CALCIUM	30	PANTOTHENIC ACID	6
IRON	*		

*Contains less than 2% of the U.S. RDA of these nutrients

MILK, VITAMIN D_3 ADDED

ENRICHED WHITE BREAD
Nutrition Information, per serving
Serving Size = 2 slices (Approx. 2 oz.)
Servings per Container = 8

	2 Slices per serving	6 Slices per day
CALORIES	140	420
PROTEIN, grams	4	12
CARBOHYDRATE, grams	27	81
FAT, grams	2	6
PERCENTAGE OF U.S. RECOMMENDED DAILY ALLOWANCES (U.S. RDA)		
PROTEIN	6	15
VITAMIN A	0	0
VITAMIN C	0	0
THIAMINE	15	45
RIBOFLAVIN	10	30
NIACIN	10	30
CALCIUM	6	20
IRON	8	25

Ingredients: Flour, water, sugar, vegetable shortening, yeast, salt, yeast nutrients, niacinamide, iron, thiamine chloride, and riboflavin, calcium propionate (a preservative)

Net Wt. 16 oz. (1 lb.)

Figure 1–4. Examples of nutrition labeling from a milk carton and a bread wrapper.

The consumer who eats a wide variety of foods and who takes advantage of nutrition labeling will be assured of getting a well-balanced, healthful diet. The following information must appear in a standard design and in the same order on all labels:[19]

1. Nutrition information for one-serving amounts
2. The size of a serving
3. Protein, carbohydrate, and fat in grams
4. Protein as to percentage of the U.S. RDA
5. Seven vitamins and minerals and their percentage of the U.S. RDA
6. *Optional:* Twelve other vitamins and minerals
7. *Optional:* The percentage of calories from fat and amounts of fatty acids, cholesterol, and sodium

Nutrition labeling is a valuable tool in learning to apply nutrition information in a practical way. For example, nutrition labels are used to:

1. Identify foods that are major sources for important nutrients.
2. Compare and contrast the nutrient composition of a variety of foods.
3. Choose foods that provide the best nutritional value for cost.
4. Choose foods that provide the best nutrient:calorie ratio.
5. Estimate the nutritional adequacy of a day's food intake.
6. Make appropriate additions or substitutions to improve a nutritionally inadequate diet.
7. Select foods for therapeutic restrictions as prescribed by the physician, such as foods for low-sodium and calorie-controlled diets.[20]

FOOD ADDITIVES

According to law, an additive is "any substance the intended use of which results or may reasonably be expected to result directly or indirectly in its becoming a component or otherwise affecting the characteristics of any food."[21] For example, nitrites are added to prevent botulism in cured products; ascorbates and other ingredients, to maintain quality. Only minute quantities of these additives are used and usually in lower amounts than might exist naturally in many food products.

The 1958 Food Additives Amendment was designed to protect the consumer. Because of this legislation, additives used in processed food must be proved safe by industry before they can be incorporated into any food product. The USDA requires that additives meet the following requirements:

1. They are approved by the FDA and are limited to specific amounts.
2. They meet a specific, justifiable need in the product.
3. They do not promote deception as to product freshness, quality, or weight.
4. They are truthfully and properly listed on the product label.

FUNCTIONS OF ADDITIVES[22]

Additives are used in food to:

1. Improve nutritional value of certain foods (e.g., the addition of thiamin, riboflavin, niacin, and iron to flour and cereal).
2. Maintain appearance, palatability, and wholesomeness in certain foods by preventing food spoilage caused by molds, bacteria, and yeast, for example.
3. Enhance flavor of certain foods. For example, cloves, ginger, and cinnamon are additives in spice cake and gingerbread.

4. Give a characteristic color to certain foods.
5. Maintain a desired consistency in foods.
6. Control acidity or alkalinity in certain foods (e.g., baking powder, a leavening agent, in cakes).
7. Serve as maturing and bleaching agents.
8. Help retain moisture.

HOW DOES FOOD LEGISLATION PROTECT THE CONSUMER?[23]

The United States Government is extensively involved in food and nutrition policy at the federal, state, and local levels and plays a major role in protecting the consumer's right to buy safe, wholesome food. An example of an important decision made by the Congress is the 1958 Delaney Amendment of the Food, Drug and Cosmetic Act, which prohibits the intentional addition to food of any substance shown to cause cancer in man or animals. Table 1–4 gives examples of major federal laws affecting food and nutrition policy.

The executive and judiciary branches are also involved in protecting the consumer. An Executive Order in 1979 requires all agencies to have a plan for obtaining consumer input on proposed regulations. Congress approves budgets for activities of regulatory agencies and gives authority to several agencies within the executive branch to make food and nutrition policies. The courts become involved with food and nutrition issues if certain laws, regulations, and penalties are questioned.

The public has become increasingly aware of food and nutrition issues over the past decade. Many people, for example, show considerable concern over the role that cholesterol, saccharin, and nitrites have in the relationship of diet to health. New problems have been identified as the food system has become more complex and as nutrition, food science, and technology have

TABLE 1–4. Examples of Major Federal Laws Affecting U.S. Food and Nutrition Policy

Federal Food, Drug and Cosmetic Act (1938) authorizes the Food and Drug Administration to oversee processing and labeling of foods in terms of safety, quality, and standards.

Agricultural Marketing Act (1946) authorizes the Department of Agriculture to inspect, grade, and certify all agricultural products.

Delaney Amendment (1958) prohibits addition to food of any substance shown to cause cancer in man or animals.

Fair Packaging and Labeling Act (1965) authorizes Food and Drug Administration to regulate certain aspects of food labeling.

Egg Products Inspection Act (1970) requires inspection of egg products and surveillance of egg shells.

Federal Meat Inspection Act (1970) requires inspection of all meats and meat products for wholesomeness.

Poultry Products Inspection Act (1971) requires inspection of all poultry and poultry products for wholesomeness.

Food and Agricultural Act (1977) sets policies related to price and income supports for farmers, grain reserves, food assistance programs, research, and extension.

Saccharin Study and Labeling Act (1977) prohibited the Food and Drug Administration's proposed ban on saccharin and required the National Academy of Sciences to study food safety issues.

advanced. New laws and agencies have been developed to attempt to resolve these problems as they have come to light.

City, state, and federal governments together provide food protection services. At the state and local levels, commercial trade of foods between states is controlled by certain federal agencies. Food production and sales within a state are regulated by the state's Department of Agriculture and Markets. And any mandatory inspection of food, wherever it is prepared, manufactured, processed, or sold is for the consumer's benefit.

Table 1–5 lists food and nutrition–related responsibilities of federal agencies.

HOW IS NUTRITION RELATED TO PUBLIC HEALTH PROGRAMS?

Preventive health programs and disease control have always been the responsibility of health departments — national, state, and local. With the growth of the science of food technology and the science of nutrition and the more effective use of our better knowledge in preventive medicine, nutrition and nutrition education have become the added responsibility of health departments and other agencies interested in the health of people.

Although deficiency diseases are either eliminated or better controlled in our country by improved agricultural procedures, improved economic conditions, enrichment programs, and increased attention to nutrition needs, nutrition education continues a never-ending process both to maintain what

TABLE 1–5. Food and Nutrition–Related Responsibilities of Federal Agencies

Bureau of Alcohol, Tobacco and Firearms (BATF) — regulation of alcoholic beverages.

Consumer Product Safety Commission (CPSC) — safety of food handling equipment.

Department of Agriculture (USDA)

- *Economics Research Service* (ERS) — analyses and reporting of food situation and outlook.
- *Food and Nutrition Service* (FNS) — administration of Food Stamp, School Lunch, Women, Infants and Children, and Donated Food Programs.
- *Food Safety and Inspection Service* (FSIS) — inspection and labeling of meat, poultry, and eggs; grading of all foods; nitrite in cured meats and poultry.
- *Human Nutrition Information Service* (HNIS) — food consumption standard tables for nutritive value of food, and educational materials.
- *Science and Education Administration* (SEA) — Extension Service, Agricultural Research Service, Cooperative State Research Service, National Agricultural Library.

Department of Health and Human Services (HHS)

- *Centers for Disease Control* (CDC) — analyses and reporting of incidence of food-borne diseases.
- *Food and Drug Administration* (FDA) — food labeling, safety of food and food additives, inspection of food processing plants, control of food contaminants, food standards.
- *National Institutes of Health* (NIH) — research related to diet and health.

Environmental Protection Agency (EPA) — standards for drinking water and water pollution, use of pesticides on food crops.

Federal Trade Commission (FTC) — food advertising, competition in food industry.

National Marine Fisheries Service (NMFS) — inspection, standards, and quality of seafood.

Occupational Safety and Health Administration (OSHA) — employee safety in food processing plants.

is good and to improve where needed, to promote a longer, healthier life by the application of the principles of good nutrition.

The health and well-being of infants and their mothers were probably the first angles of nutrition to be included in public health and nutrition programs. Prenatal and well-baby clinics were established to help improve the health of these two groups and to provide continuing education for them.

Nutrition services have expanded over the years to give attention to health and nutrition needs of various age groups in the United States and other types of groups in the total population — schoolchildren, teenagers, senior citizens, industrial workers, and special population groups throughout the country. Also, increased attention is given to persons living in situations where group feeding is involved — orphanages, nursery and other schools, day-care centers, homes for the handicapped, nursing homes, homes for the aged, summer camps, public institutions, and the like.

Some state and local agencies and nongovernmental organizations which include nutrition services in their programs are listed in Table 1–6; and

TABLE 1–6. State and Local Agencies and Nongovernmental Organizations That Provide Nutrition Services

Governmental

State and Local Levels

Departments of Agriculture
State extension services
State experiment stations
State universities — Departments of Food and Nutrition
Departments of Welfare
Departments of Health
Department of Education

Nongovernmental

National Level

American Medical Association Council on Foods
National Academy of Sciences, National Research Council, Food and Nutrition Board
American Red Cross
Professional Organizations
- American Medical Association
- American Dietetic Association
- American Home Economics Association
- American Dental Association
- American Public Health Association
- American Heart Association
- American Nurses' Association
- American Institute of Nutrition

Funds and Foundations
- Milbank Memorial Fund
- Nutrition Foundation
- Ford and Rockefeller Foundations

Metropolitan Life Insurance Company
Society of Nutrition Education
Industry-sponsored
- American Dry Milk Institute
- National Dairy Council
- Cereal Institute
- National Livestock and Meat Board

State and Local Levels

Educational agencies
Social agencies
Civic groups
United Community Services
Industry sponsored
American Red Cross
Infant Welfare Organizations
Church groups

federal agencies, in Table 1–5. (International organizations are discussed on pages 17–18.) The nutritional services of these agencies are actively carried out in the form of community programs. The aim of these programs is to improve the nutrition of those of all age groups, ethnic backgrounds, and economic levels through research, technology, and food distribution. Legislation has made funds available for professionals to carry out varied activities of state nutrition programs, day-care centers, the WIC (Women, Infants, and Children) program, Dial-a-Dietitian, and heart disease control programs. The national nutrition policy of providing the population with a balanced diet at a reasonable cost is the foundation of the programs striving to meet the nation's food needs.

Specific Programs and What They Do

Day-care centers help meet nutritional needs of children of working mothers by supplying breakfast, lunch, and snacks.

WIC program is administered by the Food and Nutrition Service of the U.S. Department of Agriculture and serves infants and children from birth to 5 years of age and women who are pregnant or nursing. Nutrition counseling and supplemental foods are provided without charge if financial and residency requirements are met and if the women and children are considered to be nutritional risks. The program's goal is to reduce the incidence of infant deaths, birth defects, mental retardation, and slow learning.

Heart disease control programs are important in providing diet counseling to individuals who are at a high risk for coronary or cardiovascular disease. Ways to control hypertension are also suggested.

Dial-a-Dietitian program provides dietitians to answer questions about diet and food and nutrition by telephone in many cities in the United States.

Project Head Start is a federally funded program that combines nutrition, social services, parent involvement, and health services with an educational program for the benefit of preschool children and their families. Nutritious daily meals and snacks are included.

Expanded Food and Nutrition Education for the Poor (EFNEP) is administered by the Cooperative Extension Service of the U.S. Department of Agriculture and provides training to nutrition aides so that they may assist families in planning nutritious low-cost meals.

Homemaker services are available for the home-bound person.

Meals on Wheels is a federally funded program that provides meals delivered to older persons who are unable to cook for themselves.

There also is legislation that Congress and the state legislatures have enacted in order to authorize and finance nutrition programs. Examples are: (1) Medicare, (2) Maternal and Child Health Welfare, (3) Commodity Distribution Program, (4) Child Nutrition Act of 1966, (5) Title VII of the Older Americans Act, which established Nutrition Programs for the Elderly, Food Stamps, Portable Meals program, and Home, Health and Neighborhood Aids, and (6) Community Group Feeding Plans.

WHAT IS THE IMPORTANCE OF THE SCHOOL LUNCH PROGRAM IN COMMUNITY NUTRITION EDUCATION?

The school lunch furnishes a large share of the child's daily nutrition needs if eaten regularly and completely. It is supplemented by the home diet. In addition to being an important factor in improving nutrition of children and their performance in school, it provides an educational experience for forming good habits and can have far-reaching effects on nutrition in the family and community.

In 1946, the United States Congress passed the National School Lunch

Act, which provided, on a permanent basis, federal aid to state and community lunch programs in the form of financial assistance by cash reimbursement (matched in amount with funds from state sources) and also foods suitable for the school lunch program purchased and distributed by the U.S. Department of Agriculture. A local sponsor or sponsoring agency is required for a school operating under this act and lunches must meet certain nutritional standards. Operation on a nonprofit basis and availability of lunches to all children regardless of ability to pay and without discrimination are also requisites. The total amount of money and food a school may receive depends on the type of lunch served (with the highest rate of reimbursement going for the complete lunch), the amount spent for food, the need for aid, and the number of lunches served to the children. Over the years the school lunch has become an essential part of the whole educational program.

The National School Lunch Act was designed to (1) provide nutritious, reasonably priced lunches to schoolchildren and children in residential child care institutions; (2) contribute a better understanding of good nutrition; and (3) foster good food habits. Nationwide, approximately 3 million breakfasts and 26½ million lunches are served daily to students.

There is much public interest in nutrition, and schools are expected to provide nutrition education, to provide nutritious meals and to operate lunchrooms that truly are nutrition laboratories. Furthermore, the school has a responsibility for safeguarding the health of today's children. School food service has thus become a basic part of the nutrition and education program of the schools. The growing school breakfast program has expanded this role. Both programs reflect advances in knowledge of food, nutrition, and food service management.[24]

HAVE FEDERAL FOOD PROGRAMS BEEN EFFECTIVE?

The American Dietetic Association has stated that "an adequately nourished body is essential to physical and emotional health and contributes to readiness for learning. All children need adequate food and educational opportunities to learn good food habits." This philosophy has been the framework for school nutrition programs. The government has increasingly supported child nutrition programs since 1970, but public and government priorities have changed. Controlling the size of government and the growth of federal spending is a widespread concern. The Field Foundation Report "Hunger in America; The Federal Response," published in 1979, concluded that federal programs over the last decade have helped in solving the problems of hunger and malnutrition. However, the future success of the programs depends both on the extent of government assistance and on how effectively and efficiently public funds are used.[25]

WHY IS FOOD AND NUTRITION MISINFORMATION A PROBLEM IN COMMUNITY EDUCATION AND HOW CAN IT BE COMBATED?

Food fads and nutritional quackery have multiplied as the science of nutrition has grown. It is probably not too far from the truth to say that every scientific finding in nutrition has been converted into misinformation by the food faddist or nutritional quack for his own ends. A trained person can easily differentiate between the accurate and the unsound. Unfortunately, the lay person is not always able to do this. In addition, the dramatic (but misleading) manner in which fads and fallacies (sometimes with a grain of truth in them) are propounded, with zip and emotional appeal, shrouds the falseness. As many as 200 fallacies regarding food and nutrition were listed in one report, from very simple, harmless ones to those of dangerous proportions.

Anything that is out of line with current scientific evidence is considered misinformation. Some fallacies are furthered by the nutritional or food quack who pretends to be a specialist in the field of food, nutrition, or medicine or by the food faddist who follows and advocates with great enthusiasm certain food customs and habits. No single food is essential to health, but some 60 nutrients now recognized by nutrition scientists are essential. These nutrients may be obtained by eating a varied diet. The food faddist would have one believe otherwise. He either makes exaggerated claims for the value of certain foods or advocates the omission of other foods from the diet because of the harmful properties he believes they possess. Another type of food faddist emphasizes "natural" or "organic" foods and wishes them to be consumed in place of others. Special devices of one kind or another, either with or without an accompanying food fad, are another stock-in-trade of the faddist.

The food quack of today has been likened to the patent medicine man of yesterday, except that he uses a lot of scientific jargon (important sounding to the untrained ear) to sell the product, be it a "special food," "special food preparation," "special diet," "special regime," or a book, magazine, or reducing gadget. It is wise to be suspicious of any writer, lecturer, or TV speaker who makes claims contrary to accepted information, claims wholesome food to be harmful or undesirable in some way, uses a scare technique in regard to health, claims to be a scientist or authority, claims association with an unheard-of organization, makes extravagant or unscrupulous claims or attacks on the Food and Drug Administration or a medical, public health, or nutrition authority. One should also be suspicious of any material that comes from an anonymous source.

Nutrition authorities agree that more widespread and more effective dissemination of sound scientific information on nutrition is necessary to combat food and nutrition misinformation. The Food and Drug Administration of the U.S. Department of Health and Human Services has long been concerned about the promotion of food supplements as cure-alls for conditions which require medical attention. Misleading promotion of food supplements violates federal law. It is carried on in the following ways:

1. So-called "health food lecturers" who claim, directly or indirectly by inference, that the products they are promoting are of value in preventing and curing disease, when in fact they are ineffective for such purposes.
2. Door-to-door sales agents posing as nutrition experts.
3. Pseudo-scientific books and journals frequently recommending some particular food or combination and often written by persons with little nutrition background or training. These may include advertisements for various products in which the publisher has a commercial interest.

False ideas about food are the stock in trade of the food faddist and the following four ideas are used by practically all operators in the field:

1. Myth that all diseases are due to faulty diet.
2. Myth that soil depletion causes malnutrition.
3. Myth that overprocessing of foods is causing malnutrition.
4. Myth of subclinical deficiencies.

Nutrition authorities agree that the best way to buy vitamins and minerals is in the packages provided by nature — vegetables, fruits, milk, eggs, meat, fish, and whole-grain and enriched breads and cereals. The normal American diet now includes such a variety of foods that most persons can hardly fail to have an ample supply of the essential food constituents. The public should distrust any suggestion of self-medication with vitamins and minerals to cure diseases of the nerves, bones, blood, liver, kidneys, heart, or digestive system. See page 23 for a discussion of excess nutrient intake.

Study Questions and Activities

1. List all the reasons you can think of why persons take up food fads.
2. What are the signs of a food faddist?
3. Why is self-medication dangerous?
4. Become familiar with the food fad or fad diet assigned you by the instructor so you may report about it to the class. Be sure you can refute the fad or fad diet.
5. What laws in your state safeguard food and health?

Visit the health department in your city. Learn about any nutrition activities that are conducted by the department.

Are there other organizations in your city that carry on nutrition programs?

What are they and what do their nutrition programs cover?

REFERENCES

1. *World Health Organization—What It Is, What It Does, How It Works.* World Health Organization, Geneva, 1956.
2. "Infant and Child Nutrition: Concerns Regarding the Developmentally Disabled," *Journal of the American Dietetic Association,* Vol. 78, No. 5, May 1981.
3. *Nutrition News,* Vol. 45, No. 2, April 1982.
4. M. V. Krause and L. K. Mahan, *Food, Nutrition and Diet Therapy,* 7th ed. Philadelphia, W. B. Saunders Company, 1984.
5. A. Gormican, J. Valentine, and E. Satter, "Relationships of Maternal Weight Gain, Prepregnancy Weight, and Infant Birthweight." *Journal of the American Dietetic Association,* Vol. 77, No. 6, Dec. 1980.
6. *Nutrition News,* Vol. 43, No. 1, April-May 1980.
7. *Tools to Fight Malnutrition.* Food and Nutrition Service, U.S. Department of Agriculture, Washington, D.C., 1970.
8. A. E. Harper and E. J. McCollum, *Food and Nutrition News.* Vol. 52, No. 4, Mar.-April 1981.
9. *Nutrition and Your Health, Dietary Guidelines for Americans,* U.S. Department of Agriculture and U.S. Department of Health and Human Services, Washington, D.C., 1980.
10. *Nutrition and the MD,* Vol. 7, No. 12, Dec. 1981.
11. *Nutrition News,* Vol. 42, No. 3, Sept.-Oct. 1979.
12. *U.S. News and World Report,* "What's Safe to Eat—And What Isn't," June 28, 1982, p. 6.

12a. U.S. Senate Select Committee on Nutrition and Human Needs, "Dietary Goals for the United States." Government Printing Office, Washington, D.C., rev. 1977.

13. *Recommended Dietary Allowances,* 9th ed. Food and Nutrition Board, National Research Council, Washington, D.C., 1980.
14. *Family Fare—A Guide to Good Nutrition,* HG. No. 1. U.S. Department of Agriculture, Washington, D.C., rev. 1978, p. 2.
15. *Food for Fitness—A Daily Food Guide,* Leaflet No. 424, U.S. Department of Agriculture, Washington, D.C., 1973.
16. M. M. Hill, "Nutrition Education," *Nutrition Program News,* Sept.-Dec. 1976.
17. E. A. Yetley and C. Roderick, "Nutritional Knowledge and Health Goals of Young Spouses," *Journal of the American Dietetic Association,* Vol. 77, No. 7, July 1980, pp. 31–41.
18. *Nutrition Notes 83,* United Fresh Fruit and Vegetable Association, Winter 1981.
19. *Nutrition Labels and U.S. RDA,* DHEW Publication No. (FDA) 76-2042. U.S. Department of Agriculture, Washington, D.C., 1976.
20. *Nutrition Source Book,* National Dairy Council, 1980.

21. D. M. Kinsman, "A Fresh Look at Processed Meats," *Food and Nutrition News*, Vol. 53, No. 5, May-June 1982. National Livestock and Meat Board.
22. *Food Additives—Everyday Facts*, Manufacturing Chemist Association.
23. C. A. Bisogni and P. F. Thonney, "The Government Gets into the Act," Unit IV-3 in *Nutrition; A Holistic Approach*, in A. Gillespie and B. Mayfield, eds. Inservice Training by Mail, Division of Nutritional Services, Cornell University, Ithaca, New York.
24. G. Applebaum, "School Lunch—Changes and Challenges," *Nutrition News*, Vol. 45, No. 1, Feb. 1982, p. 1. National Dairy Council.
25. A. G. Vaden, *The Professional Nutritionist*, Winter 1981, p. 10.

Nutrients

2

CHAPTER OUTLINE

CARBOHYDRATES
- Sources
- Role in Dental Health
- Functions
- Dietary Fiber

FATS
- Types
- Functions
- Requirements
- Sources

PROTEINS
- Types
- Functions
- Requirements
- Sources

ENERGY REQUIREMENT
- Daily Energy Needs
- Calorie Content of Foods
- Calories for Activities

MINERALS AND WATER
- Functions
- Requirements
- Sources
- Deficiencies

VITAMINS
- Functions
- Requirements
- Sources
- Deficiencies/Toxicity

UTILIZATION OF NUTRIENTS
- Digestion
- Absorption
- Metabolism
- Drug-Diet Interactions

OBJECTIVES

To understand:

☐ Nutrients and their characteristics, functions, recommended dietary allowances, and food sources.

☐ How the body utilizes nutrients.

To apply:

☐ Knowledge of nutrients in evaluating one's own diet for adequacy.

☐ Knowledge of nutrients in maintenance of optimal health and prevention of disease.

TERMS TO UNDERSTAND

Absorption	Digestion	Kwashiorkor
Alkaline-ash	Electrolytes	Legumes
Amino acid	Energy	Marasmus
Anabolism	Enrichment	Metabolism
Anemia	Enzyme	Osmosis
Antibodies	Essential amino acid	Osteomalacia
Avitaminosis	Essential fatty acid	Osteoporosis
Basal metabolism	Fiber	Peristalsis
Beriberi	Goiter	pH
Carbohydrate	Glycogen	Polyunsaturated fat
Catabolism	Hemoglobin	Precursor
Cellulose	Hormone	Protein
Cholesterol	Hydrogenated fat	Saturated fat
Complete protein	Hypervitaminosis	Toxicity
Dehydration	Incomplete protein	Unsaturated fat
Dietary fiber	Kilocalorie	

Carbohydrates

WHAT ARE CARBOHYDRATES?

Carbohydrates, mostly plant products in origin, include sugars, starches, and cellulose and are composed of the elements carbon, hydrogen, and oxygen. Carbohydrates are formed by all green plants by a complex process known as photosynthesis. In this process sugar is first formed from carbon dioxide and water in a series of reactions, one or more of which are dependent upon the aid of sunlight and the green plant pigment known as chlorophyll. Some of the sugar remains in the plant sap; the rest of the sugar units can be converted into starch and other carbohydrates, even of very complex form. The dry matter of most plants is largely carbohydrate and provides energy directly when eaten as food by man and animals.

HOW DO CARBOHYDRATES FEATURE IN DIETS?

Cereals and cereal products, fruits, vegetables, sugars, and syrups are the chief sources of carbohydrates in the average diet. For a very large part of the world, grains of one sort or another and root vegetables constitute a major food source, ranging from an approximate 50 per cent in the American diet to a much higher proportion — as much as 80 per cent — in other countries. Wheat in the form of breads, cereals, and pastas (macaroni, noodles, spaghetti) feature prominently in the Western world; corn, in the diet of Indians in America as well as in the diet of blacks in the South; wheat and rye, in Europe; wheat and rice, in the Near East; and rice, in the diet of Orientals.

Carbohydrates are the most readily available and easily digested of the energy foods and, in the case of breads, cereals, and potatoes, are inexpensive. For this reason, they feature largely in diets at lower economic levels.

They are also generally popular and palatable. Cereals can be grown almost everywhere and can be transported and stored easily. Refined sugar and starches, such as cornstarch, are the only pure carbohydrate foods.

Dietary fiber (the sum of indigestible carbohydrate and carbohydrate-like components of food) consumption has decreased in developed countries since the turn of the century. Some claim that the incidence of various diseases such as diverticulosis, cardiovascular disease, colonic cancer, and diabetes is inversely related to dietary fiber consumption.[1]

WHAT IS THE ROLE OF CARBOHYDRATE IN DENTAL HEALTH?

There is a relationship between the form and frequency of carbohydrate intake and dental caries. Sugar-containing foods that stick to the teeth are more harmful than liquid sweets such as soft drinks. There is continuous acid production in the mouth when sweetened food is eaten frequently over a period of time. Therefore, it is less harmful to consume sugar as part of a meal than as a between-meal snack. The presence of other foods stimulates saliva flow, which helps neutralize food particles and wash them away. Raw fibrous foods which require more chewing also stimulate saliva flow and are often recommended as between-meal substitutes for sweets. If sugar is present in these foods, it is usually at a fairly low concentration.[2]

WHAT ARE DIFFERENT TYPES AND SOURCES OF CARBOHYDRATES?

Carbohydrates are either small single units (molecules) or larger units, consisting of two or several units, or still larger and more complex ones, consisting of many small units linked together. Those which have special significance in nutrition are the simple sugars—glucose, fructose, and galactose; the double sugars—sucrose, lactose, and maltose; and the more complex forms—starch, glycogen, and cellulose.

Simple Sugars (Monosaccharides)

Glucose (grape sugar, corn sugar, dextrose) is found in fruits, certain roots, corn, and honey. It is less sweet than table sugar and is a very inexpensive form of sugar. It is the form of sugar in the blood, as it is the end product of all carbohydrate digestion. It is also the form in which carbohydrates are absorbed, because it is the only fuel the central nervous system can use. Glucose is given for immediate energy (by mouth or intravenously), as it is ready for utilization by the body. It is stored as glycogen in the liver.

Fructose (fruit sugar) is found in honey and in many fruits and vegetables. It is combined with glucose in table sugar and gives honey its characteristic flavor.

Galactose is produced from lactose in milk, but does not occur free in nature.

Sorbitol, a sugar alcohol, is also a simple sugar but without nutritive value. It is sometimes used as a "non-nutritive" sweetener in "dietetic" foods.

Double Sugars (Disaccharides; Changed to Simple Sugars in Digestion)

Sucrose (cane sugar, beet sugar, table sugar) is found in sugar cane, sugar beets, molasses, maple sugar, and maple syrup, and in many fruits and vegetables.

Lactose (milk sugar) is produced only by mammals. It is less soluble and less sweet than cane sugar, and is digested more slowly.

Maltose (malt sugar) is found in malt and malt products. It is made from the starch available in sprouting grain and is not found free in nature. It is formed when starch is changed to sugar during digestion and appears with dextrin (a polysaccharide) in infant formulas.

Complex Compounds (Polysaccharides; Many Simple Sugar Units Combined)

Starch is the form of the reserve store of carbohydrates in plants (grains, seeds, roots, potatoes, green bananas, and other plants) and is changed into glucose during digestion (through intermediate steps of dextrin and maltose).

Glycogen ("animal starch") is the body's reserve form of carbohydrate, stored in the liver, and is quickly changed to and from glucose as necessary.

Cellulose (fiber) is found in the pulp and skins of fruits and vegetables, the structural parts of plants, and the coverings of seeds and outer covering of nuts. It is indigestible, so it provides bulk and stimulation for the intestinal tract. Agar-agar and pectin (hemicelluloses related to cellulose) absorb water and add bulk to the intestines. Pectins in fruits and seeds are used in making jelly, and agar-agar is used as a thickening agent.

Dextrin is formed from starch breakdown by heat or by enzymes during digestion. For example, starch is converted to dextrin in the toasting of bread.

HOW DO CARBOHYDRATES FUNCTION IN NUTRITION?

The *primary function* of carbohydrates is to meet the body's specific needs for energy. After these needs are met, carbohydrates are comparable to fats in protein-sparing action. Carbohydrates are readily converted to energy. One gram of carbohydrate yields 4 kilocalories (kcalories), and carbohydrates provide 46 per cent of the calories in the average American diet.

Other functions of carbohydrates are

1. To *spare* the burning of protein for energy (protein has more important functions)
2. To *aid* in the more efficient and complete oxidation (burning) of fats for energy
3. As *sugar*, to produce energy quickly
4. As *starch*, to provide an economical and abundant source of energy after change to glucose
5. As *lactose*, carbohydrate has a certain laxative action (remains in the intestines longer and encourages desirable bacterial growth) and aids in the absorption of calcium
6. As *cellulose* (insoluble and indigestible), it aids in the normal functioning of the intestines.

WHAT ARE COMMON FOOD SOURCES OF CARBOHYDRATES?

PLANT SOURCES

Cereal grains. Rice, wheat, corn, oats, rye, barley, buckwheat, and millet also contain, in addition to starch, some protein, minerals, and vitamins. Whole-grain and enriched sources contain iron and B-complex vitamins.

Vegetables. Green leafy vegetables are the lowest in carbohydrates. Roots, tubers, and seeds contain more carbohydrate; starchy vegetables—corn, dried peas and beans, and potatoes—contain the most. Sugar in fresh green peas changes to starch after harvesting. Vegetables also contain cellulose.

Fruits. Fruits contain a large proportion of water. Their carbohydrate content is mostly sugar and, except in dried fruits, it is low. Starch in immature bananas changes to sugar in ripening. Fruits do contain some cellulose. Nuts contain 10 to 20 per cent carbohydrate (and are also high in protein and fat).

Sweets. Ordinary table sugar, molasses, maple syrup and sugar, corn syrup, honey, and sorghum syrup are poor sources because they are concentrated with "empty" calories.

ANIMAL SOURCES

There are none of importance except possibly lactose in milk. Traces of glycogen are found in meat, poultry, fish, and eggs, and small amounts are available in liver and scallops.

WHAT IS THE DAILY CARBOHYDRATE REQUIREMENT?

If carbohydrate intake is limited, the body is capable of converting amino acids and the glycerol of fats into glucose. Therefore, there is no specific dietary requirement for carbohydrate. However, it is desirable to include a reasonable proportion of the caloric intake in the form of carbohydrate. The ingestion of 50 to 100 gm of digestible carbohydrate per day can prevent ketosis, excessive breakdown of tissue protein, loss of cations, especially sodium, and involuntary dehydration.[1]

WHAT HAPPENS TO CARBOHYDRATES IN THE BODY?

Carbohydrates are easily digested and the degree of absorption is high. Digestion of starch starts in the mouth and is completed in the small intestine. Double sugars are digested in the small intestine (Fig. 2–1).

Simple sugars like glucose and fructose are ready for absorption in the digestive tract. Double sugars like sucrose must be changed to simple sugars for absorption. Complex carbohydrates like starch require two steps in digestion for their change to simple sugar (glucose) for absorption in the intestinal

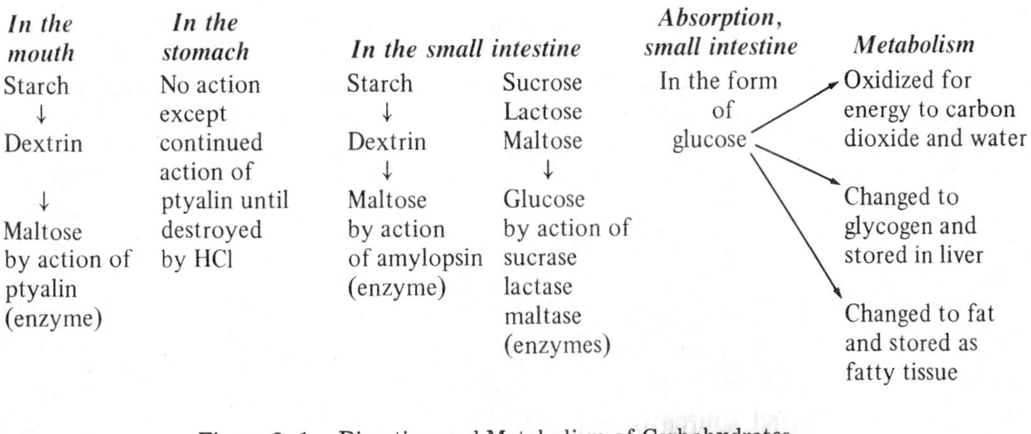

Figure 2–1. Digestion and Metabolism of Carbohydrates.

tract. Cooking starch facilitates digestion, as it breaks down the cell walls, making easier the action of digestive enzymes. Cellulose (fiber) is indigestible and passes through the intestinal tract unchanged.

Glucose, formed from all carbohydrate in food eaten, is absorbed into the blood stream through the walls of the small intestine and metabolized as shown in Figure 2-1.

WHAT IS MEANT BY "ENRICHMENT"?

Whole-grain products contribute not only considerable amounts of carbohydrate to the diet but also some protein and appreciable amounts of some minerals and vitamins. When milled to produce the popular white product with better keeping quality (with removal of bran layers and germ), most of the B vitamins—thiamine, riboflavin, and niacin—and iron are lost. The addition of these nutrients in synthetic form to cereals and their products, or *enrichment*, to replace those removed in the milling process is now approved. It is estimated that about 80 to 90 per cent of the flour and bread on the market are enriched.

WHAT IS DIETARY FIBER?

Dietary fiber is all of the indigestible carbohydrate and carbohydrate-like components of food including cellulose, lignin, hemicelluloses, pentosans, gums, and pectins. How much of each of these substances is present determines the character of the fiber of each plant. Whole-wheat bread, apples, and cabbage each contribute fiber to the diet, but the benefit of each varies because their fiber composition is different. Therefore, it is important to eat a variety of whole grains, fruits, and vegetables. Laboratory methods to measure the dietary fiber in foods are still being established. Nutritionists are working to develop a system that can be applied to all foods. Different methods of measurement will give different results.[2] Dietary fiber differs from crude fiber, which reflects only a portion of the cellulose and lignin in foods. Although the body has no enzymes to digest dietary fiber, intestinal muscular contractions reduce cellulose to smaller proportions, and digestive juices and bacterial action soften tough fibers.

WHAT ARE SOME HEALTH BENEFITS OF DIETARY FIBER IN THE DIET?

Even though fiber is not a nutrient, it is an important part of the diet. Fiber provides bulk by absorbing water and therefore aids in eliminating wastes from the body, thus preventing constipation. The fiber in cabbage is easily broken down by bacteria in the large intestine and fermentation occurs. This process promotes the growth of useful bacteria that can alter potentially harmful substances.

There are theories that fiber has a role in preventing diverticular disease, gallstones, and cancer of the colon, and it has also been said to reduce cholesterol levels.[2]

WHAT ARE THE REQUIREMENTS FOR DIETARY FIBER?

The Food and Nutrition Board of the National Academy of Sciences has not recommended a specific level of dietary fiber. For the general population, however, moderate increases in dietary fiber consumption are desirable. There must be a healthy balance. Large amounts of bran, the most concentrated source of food fiber, are known to cause diarrhea and other health problems. In fact, nutritional deficiencies may result from too much fiber because certain minerals such as iron and zinc can bind with fiber and become unavailable to the body.[3] See Table 2–1 for the dietary fiber content of selected foods.

Study Questions and Activities

1. What are the different kinds of carbohydrates?
2. In what ways, other than providing energy, are carbohydrates important in the diet?
3. Why is an excess of sugars and sweets in the diet undesirable?
4. What is the meaning of dietary fiber?
5. What changes would you make in the following meals to increase the fiber or cellulose content?

(1)	(2)	(3)
Applesauce	Tomato juice	Mixed fruit juice
Corn flakes	Meat loaf	Creamed chicken on steamed rice
Cream and sugar	Mashed potatoes	Hubbard squash
Enriched toast	Buttered carrots	Muffin and butter
Butter and jelly	Roll and butter	Baked caramel custard
Milk or coffee	Lemon meringue pudding	Coffee
	Tea	

TABLE 2–1. Dietary Fiber in Selected Foods*

Food Group	Serving Size	Gm Dietary Fiber per Serving
Breads and cereals†		
Enriched white bread	1 slice	0.38
Whole-wheat bread	1 slice	1.70
Bran cereal, shredded form	1/3 cup	6.13
Corn flakes	1 cup	1.05
Puffed wheat	1 cup	1.07
Rolled oats, uncooked	1/3 cup	1.67
Shredded wheat	2/3 cup	4.13
Vegetables‡		
Broccoli, cooked	1/2 cup	3.17
Cabbage, cooked	1/2 cup	2.06
Carrots, raw	1 medium	2.43
Lettuce, raw	2 leaves	0.23
Peas, canned	1/2 cup	6.00
Fruits‡		
Apples, unpeeled	1 medium	2.22
Apples, peeled	1 medium	2.13
Banana	1 medium	2.08
Peach	1 medium	2.28
Strawberries	1/2 cup	1.58

*From *Food for Health: The Carbohydrate Connection—The Knack of Snacking.* Cornell Cooperative Extension, Division of Nutritional Sciences, Cornell University, Ithaca, New York, 1979.

†Adapted from values of Peter Van Soest, Department of Animal Sciences, New York State College of Agriculture and Life Sciences, Cornell University, Ithaca, New York.

‡Adapted from values of D. A. Southgate, Medical Research Council, Cambridge, England.

Fats

WHAT ARE FATS?

Fats constitute a second group of nutrients that provide energy in the diet. They and certain fat-like substances are classified as lipids. Fats are compounds of fatty acids—three molecules of fatty acids and one molecule of glycerol (triclycerides)—which, like carbohydrates, contain carbon, hydrogen, and oxygen but in different proportions. When oxidized, they give about 2¼ times more energy than carbohydrates. Most of the fats in foods occur as triglycerides.

The kinds and types of fatty acids present in a fat determine whether it is liquid or solid at room temperature, its flavor, and other properties. Common fats found in foods include stearin (stearic acid) in beef suet and other animal fats, palmitin (palmitic acid) in both animal and vegetable fats, olein (oleic acid) in almost all fats and oils, and butyrin (butyric acid) in butter.

Fat-like substances having important roles in the body include phospholipids (fat plus the mineral phosphorus) and sterols (ergosterol in plants; and cholesterol, either free or combined with fatty acids as cholesterol esters, in animal tissues).

HOW DO FATS FEATURE IN DIETS?

Approximately one-third to one-half of the total caloric intake in the American diet comes from fat, a figure that is high compared with that of other countries. Only about 10 to 20 per cent of the caloric intake comes from fat in diets in European and Asian countries. The consumption of fats, both in kind and amount, has increased in our country during the past 50 years. More oils and margarines, but less butter, are now used; the greater consumption of meat, poultry, fish, and milk has increased fat intake from these sources as well.

WHAT ARE THE DIFFERENT KINDS OF FAT?

Any fats that remain fluid at ordinary room temperature are called oils; those that remain solid are called fats. For convenience, food fats are classed as "visible" fats (those purchased and used as fats) and "invisible" fats (those that are parts of natural foods) (Table 2–2).

TABLE 2–2. "Visible" and "Invisible" Fats

"Visible" Fats		"Invisible" Fats	
Bacon	Salt pork	Meat	Eggs
Lard	Salad dressings	Fish	Baked goods
Oils	Other shortenings	Poultry	Cream
Margarine	such as cooking fats	Whole milk	Cheese
Butter		Ice cream	Nuts

Hydrogenated fats are made by treating liquid fats—vegetable oils such as cotton, corn, soybean, etc.—with hydrogen to produce a plastic fat for cooking purposes or a table fat for a butter substitute. Cooking fats and margarines found on the market, each under a different trade name, are examples of this type of fat. Margarines may be further treated for use as table fats by churning with cultured milk to improve flavor and fortifying with the vitamin A equivalent of butter.

WHAT DO "SATURATED" AND "UNSATURATED" FATS MEAN?

Fatty acids, a variety of which are present in different food fats, are classified as "saturated" and "unsaturated" depending on the absence or presence of double bonds between the carbon atoms in the molecule. No hydrogen can be added to saturated fatty acids, as they have no double bonds. The predominance of saturated fatty acids makes a fat solid. Hydrogen atoms can, however, be added to unsaturated oleic acid with its one double bond (*mono*unsaturated) or to linoleic acid and linolenic acid with 2 and 3 double bonds, respectively (*poly*unsaturated). This makes possible the conversion of oils into plastic fats (margarines) by hydrogenation as mentioned previously.

Food fats contain a mixture of both kinds of fatty acids. If saturated acids predominate, the fat is solid and called a saturated fat; if unsaturated acids predominate, the fat is called a polyunsaturated fat. Researchers are now interested in the possible consequences of consumption of polyunsaturated fatty acids (PUFA) above that amount required for preventing deficiency symptoms.

The relative amounts of fatty acids in foods and diets is referred to as a P/S ratio (P = polyunsaturated/S = saturated fatty acids). A ratio of polyunsaturated fat to saturated fat (P/S) less than 2:1 is generally considered undesirable.

Some of the margarines available are made by combining vegetable oils containing unsaturated fatty acids with just enough hydrogenated fat to get the right plastic state. These margarines have more of the free unsaturated fatty acids. The labels on such margarines will list the liquid oil first, may be marked "high in polyunsaturates," and may also state the amount and type of fatty acids present. Tub margarines are sometimes preferred to stick margarines because they are generally thought to have a more favorable P/S ratio.

Saturated fats are found in animal products such as whole milk, cream, butter, cheeses made from whole milk, egg yolk, meat, and lard, and margarine, hydrogenated shortening, chocolate, and rich desserts.

Polyunsaturated fats are found in vegetable oils (including safflower, corn, cottonseed, soybean, and sesame oils), fish, salad dressings, mayonnaise, and certain margarines.

WHAT ARE ESSENTIAL FATTY ACIDS?

Essential fatty acids are necessary for the nutritional well-being of all animals. The principal ones for the human are linoleic and arachidonic acids. They have multiple purposes, including (1) the maintenance of the functioning and integrity of cellular and subcellular membranes, (2) cholesterol metabolism regulation, and (3) acting as precursors of a group of hormone-like compounds (prostaglandins). Vegetable oils are the primary source of linoleic acid in the diet. The recommended intake of essential fatty acids for a population having a high fat intake, as is currently found in the United States is 8 to 10 per cent of dietary calories.[1] Essential fatty acids are not synthesized in the body and must be supplied by food.

WHAT SHOULD ONE KNOW ABOUT CHOLESTEROL?

Cholesterol, one of the "fat-like" sterols, is found in various concentrations in all animal tissue and the blood and has important functions in the body, food intake or synthesis within the body being responsible for its presence. A fatty deposit containing cholesterol (which interferes with the flow of blood) is characteristic of a cardiovascular disease known as atherosclerosis, the exact cause of which is unknown.

Cholesterol has an essential role in the structure of sex and adrenal hormones and is converted to vitamin D_3 by the action of ultraviolet light on the skin. It is stored in the liver and also occurs in the form of a lipoprotein in the blood in the amount of less than 10 per cent of total body cholesterol.[4]

HOW DO FATS FUNCTION IN NUTRITION?

The *primary function* of fat is to serve as a concentrated source of heat and energy (1 gram of fat yields 9 kcalories, more than twice that of carbohydrate). About one-third to one-half of the kcalories in the current American diet comes from fat. The body cells, except for the cells of the nervous system and erythrocytes, can use fatty acids directly as a source of energy. In addition, fats function to:

1. *Furnish* essential fatty acids
2. *Spare* burning of protein for energy
3. *Add* flavor and palatability to the diet
4. *Give satiety* value to the diet (fats slow the digestive process and retard the development of hunger)

Animal fats and fortified margarines not only contain some of the fat-soluble vitamins (A, D, E, and K), but also aid in their absorption. They also play a role in the absorption of fatty acids. Excess fat, stored in the body as adipose tissue, insulates and protects organs and nerves. Fats also lubricate the intestinal tract, and the phospholipids have an important role in metabolism.

WHAT ARE REQUIREMENTS FOR FATS?

There are no specific requirements for fat other than meeting the body's need for the essential fatty acids, usually found in a diet containing 15 to 25 gm of appropriate food fats.[1]

WHAT ARE COMMON FOOD SOURCES OF FAT?

Animal sources		*Plant sources*	
Whole milk	Bacon	Vegetable oils—corn, cotton, peanut, etc.	
Butter	Cheese	Margarines	Salad dressings
Lard	Cream	Chocolate	Nuts, Olives
Meat fats	Egg yolk	Peanut butter	Avocadoes

It is important to note that mineral oil, frequently used in salad dressings, is not a food fat, as it cannot be digested and utilized by the body. Its use as a substitute for salad oils should be avoided as it interferes with the absorption of fat-soluble vitamins in the intestine. When used as a laxative, if at all, it should never be taken near mealtime.

In the mouth	*In the stomach*	*In the small intestine*	*Absorption, small intestine*	*Metabolism*
No action	Emulsified fats ↓ Fatty acids and glycerol by action of gastric lipase	Fats, after emulsification by bile ↓ Fatty acids and glycerol by action of pancreatic and intestinal lipase	In the form of fatty acids and glycerol which are recombined into a new fat during absorption	New fat ↓ oxidized for energy to carbon dioxide and water or stored as fatty tissue Some fat combines with phosphorus to form phospholipids

Figure 2–2. Digestion and Metabolism of Fats.

WHAT HAPPENS TO FATS IN THE BODY?

Fats, being insoluble in water, require special treatment in the gastrointestinal tract so that their end products can be absorbed through the intestinal wall. No digestion of fat takes place in the mouth. Only finely emulsified fats such as are found in butter, cream, and egg yolk can be digested in the stomach. For the most part, fats are digested in the small intestine by enzymes from the pancreatic juice after the fats have been emulsified by bile and bile salts. Fats are changed to glycerol and fatty acids during digestion (Fig. 2–2).

Fatty foods are digested without difficulty but they require a longer time for digestion than do carbohydrates. Softer fats are more completely digested and absorbed than harder fats. Fried foods are not necessarily indigestible but are more slowly digested.

The presence of carbohydrates in the diet is necessary for the complete oxidation of fats in the tissues; otherwise, acetone bodies accumulate, resulting in ketosis.

Study Questions and Activities

1. What important functions, in addition to energy, are performed by fats?
2. How do fats and carbohydrates compare in energy value?
3. Name several plant sources of fats; several animal sources.
4. What is the calorie value of a food that contains 12 gm of fat and 25 gm of carbohydrate?
5. If you require 2000 calories and 25 per cent or one-quarter of the calories should come from fat, how many *grams* of fat will be in your diet?

Proteins

WHAT ARE PROTEINS?

Proteins are complex food substances (nutrients) made up of amino acids composed of carbon, hydrogen, and oxygen, the same elements found in carbohydrates and, *in addition, nitrogen.* The presence of nitrogen makes them different from carbohydrates and fats: proteins are capable of building body tissues in addition to furnishing heat or energy. Sulfur, phosphorus, and iron may also be present.

Twenty-two amino acids—called "building stones" or units—are known to be physiologically important and are found in different amounts and combinations in food proteins. Eight of these amino acids are called "essential" and must be supplied adequately in the daily food of the adult. At least one additional one, and possibly a second, are needed for growth in children. These "essential" or "indispensable" amino acids cannot be synthesized by the body in adequate amounts.

Plants are able to build their own protein from the nitrogen in certain substances in the soil, carbon dioxide from the air and with water, the energy needed for this process being supplied by the sun. Animals and humans must get their protein preformed from plants and other animals. These preformed proteins are then digested and the end products used to build special types of body proteins as necessary.

HOW DO PROTEINS FEATURE IN DIETS?

In the United States there are adequate sources of good quality protein and, on the whole, the average person probably eats a sufficient amount. The total amount of protein as a source of energy in the American diet has remained at 11 to 12 per cent in this century. Some studies show, however, that the amount of protein may be inadequate in the diet of some persons, for economic or other reasons. In many parts of the world, protein may be adequate but of poor quality; in still other parts, there is a definite shortage of protein foods and this constitutes a health hazard. Also, many countries lack sufficient information about their protein food supply and how to use it. Superstition and poor sanitary conditions may also account for inadequate consumption of protein. In some instances, limited available sources may be too expensive for low-income groups.

Short stature is a characteristic of peoples in areas where protein is derived largely from plant sources; in other parts, meat featured in diets means taller stature and stronger, healthier physiques. A protein nutrition problem due to a very restricted intake in many of the newly emerged and emerging nations is the deficiency seen in children—kwashiorkor—resulting in retarded growth and development, lowered resistance to disease, loss of appetite, changes in skin and hair, and severe edema. Treatment of this condition with reconstituted nonfat dry milk brings improvement as does a product—INCAPARINA—developed in some areas from a combination of inexpensive local grain and vegetable protein sources by the Institute of Nutrition of Central America and Panama (INCAP).

Various divisions of the United Nations are interested in developing locally produced vegetables as sources of protein in underdeveloped areas, with financial support arranged by various national and international organizations. The right combination of vegetable protein sources can provide a protein of better quality than that present in any single vegetable.

WHAT ARE THE DIFFERENT KINDS OF PROTEINS?

The nutritional quality of a protein depends on the assortment of amino acids in the protein. On this basis, a protein is referred to as being a "complete" or an "incomplete" one.

A "complete" protein will contain the amino acids necessary both for growth and for maintenance and repair of body tissues and is said to have a high "biologic" value. Generally speaking, animal sources of protein—meat, fish, poultry, eggs, milk and its products—contain complete proteins.

An "incomplete" protein will maintain life (repair worn-out tissue) but it will not support growth because it lacks the amino acids required for building (growth). Vegetable and other plant sources contain incomplete proteins of poor "biologic" value. Incomplete proteins can be supplemented by complete proteins from animal sources as in cereal and milk, toast and eggs, and macaroni and cheese. The protein quality of bread can be improved by making it with milk instead of water.

If people knew exactly how to combine cereals, vegetables, and other plant sources in the right mixtures and amounts, they could provide themselves with the right assortment of amino acids to meet their protein needs. This is not practical or desirable for most people, of course, and so the daily diet should contain both animal sources of protein (about one-third of the total requirement) and some plant sources. It is desirable to have some animal protein in every meal, the total daily amount being divided about equally among the three meals of the day.

HOW DO PROTEINS FUNCTION IN NUTRITION?

Protein is a part of all protoplasm in every living cell in muscles, organs, and glands and is found in all body fluids except bile and urine. Protein in the diet provides nitrogen to be utilized in the synthesis of body proteins and other nitrogen-containing substances and is involved in a variety of important metabolic functions:

1. It is essential for life, supplying material to repair or replace worn-out tissues.
2. It is essential for growth, supplying material for tissue building.
3. It supplies some energy (4 calories per gram) but it is an expensive source.
4. It supplies certain essential substances necessary for the construction and proper functioning of important body compounds (enzymes, hormones, hemoglobin, antibodies, other blood proteins, glandular secretions).
5. Certain amino acids play very special and vital roles in nutrition.

To carry out tissue-building functions efficiently and adequately, it is essential that all the necessary amino acids for the building at hand be present simultaneously. This is another reason why it is important to have the day's supply of protein about equally divided among the three meals. Sufficient amounts of carbohydrates and fats to provide for energy needs will prevent some of the protein needed for building and repair from being diverted for energy.

WHAT ARE RECOMMENDED DIETARY ALLOWANCES FOR PROTEIN?

The protein allowance for maintenance nitrogen equilibrium is based on a requirement of 0.45 gram per kilogram of body weight per day.[1] This requirement is increased 30 per cent to take account of the loss of efficiency of the standard reference protein (whole egg). This results in an allowance of 0.6 gm/kg body weight/day of high-quality protein. However, 0.8 gm/kg body weight/day is allowed for the mixed protein diet of the United States. Thus, the allowance for a 70 kg man is 56 gm of protein per day; that for a 55 kg woman, 44 gm.

For infants, the allowances are based on the amount of protein provided by the quantity of milk required to ensure a satisfactory rate of growth. This is estimated to be 2.24 gm/kg/day during the first month of life and falls gradually to about 1.5 gm/kg/day by the sixth month.

The protein requirement during growth is higher than that in adulthood, since nitrogen must be provided for the formation of new tissue. The allowances for children and young people are calculated from information on growth rates and body composition. The allowances decrease gradually from 2.0 gm/kg/day at 6 months to 1 year to .8 gm/kg/day at age 18.

During pregnancy an additional 30 gm of protein is recommended. This is based on nitrogen retention of 16 mg/kg body weight/day and on 50 per cent utilization of dietary protein. The dietary protein allowance for the lactating woman is 20 gm/day more than that for the nonpregnant and nonlactating woman.

Protein requirement is increased in any condition in which the body protein is broken down, as in hemorrhage, burns, poor protein nutrition previous to surgery, wounds, and long convalescence. Deficiency of protein over a long period of time results in weight loss, reduced resistance to disease, skin and blood changes, slow wound healing, and a condition known as nutritional edema.

Diets rich in protein, especially animal protein, are generally beneficial, since they contain adequate amounts of important trace nutrients such as zinc, iron, and some vitamins.[1]

Exercise in itself does not increase the need for protein if the diet contains sufficient carbohydrate and fat to meet increased energy needs. As energy foods are added to the diet to meet energy requirements, some increase in protein foods will occur naturally.

WHAT ARE COMMON FOOD SOURCES OF PROTEIN?

There are two types of sources for proteins, animal and plant. Animal sources are complete and therefore more expensive than plant sources, which are incomplete.

Animal sources. These include milk, cheese, eggs, meat, fish, and poultry. These complete protein sources supply the nutritionally essential amino acids and should provide about one-third of the daily dietary protein. Complete proteins are also called "high-quality" proteins. It should be noted that gelatin, although an animal source, lacks several essential amino acids and is therefore incomplete.

Plant sources. These include vegetables (generally poor sources except for legumes—dry peas, beans, lentils, and peanuts), cereals, breads, and nuts. These incomplete protein sources lack one or more of the nutritionally essential amino acids and are inadequate for building purposes. They need to be supplemented in the diet with complete proteins, although they may supplement each other, combining as "complementary" proteins. Soybeans, although of plant origin, contain high-quantity and high-quality protein.

Table 2–3 shows the protein content of some basic four foods, and Table 2–4 shows the RDA for protein.

WHAT HAPPENS TO PROTEINS IN THE BODY?

The proteins in the daily diet must be broken down into their component parts, the amino acids, by digestion before the body can absorb them into the blood from the small intestine and use them. Digestion of protein is started in the stomach by enzymes in the gastric juice and is continued (and completed) in the small intestine by enzymes from the pancreatic and intestinal juices (Fig. 2–3).

TABLE 2–3. Protein Content of Some Basic Four Foods

Food Group	Serving Size	Protein (gm)	% RDA* 44 gm	% RDA* 56 gm
Milk and Dairy				
Milk	1 cup	9	20	16
Cottage cheese	1/4 cup	8	18	17
Cheese	1 oz	7	15	12
Yogurt	1 cup	10	22	17
Meat and Alternates				
Veal	3-1/2 oz	33	75	58
Liver	3-1/2 oz	30	68	53
Beef	3-1/2 oz	30	68	53
Pork	3-1/2 oz	28	63	50
Lamb	3-1/2 oz	27	63	48
Frankfurter	2 med	13	29	23
Luncheon meat	2 oz	10	22	17
Turkey	3-1/2 oz	32	72	55
Chicken	3-1/2 oz	30	68	53
Fish	3-1/2 oz	26	59	46
Canned fish	1-3/4 oz	12	27	21
Egg	1 med	6	13	10
Dried beans or peas	3/4 cup	13	29	23
Peanut butter	2 T	8	18	14
Nuts	1/4 cup	5	11	9
Bread and Cereals				
Oatmeal	1/2 cup	2	4	3
Corn flakes	3/4 cup	2	4	3
Bread	1 slice	2	4	3
Fruits and Vegetables				
Potato, mashed w/milk added	1/2 cup	2	4	3
Carrots	1/2 cup	.5	1	.009
Peas, canned	1/2 cup	4	9	7
Broccoli	1 stalk	6	13	10
Oranges	1 med	1	2	1.5
Cantaloupe	1/2 med	2	4	3
Apple	1 med	tr.	–	–

*RDA of protein for women = 44 gm, for men = 56 gm.

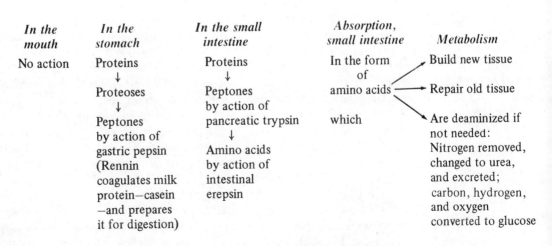

In the mouth	*In the stomach*	*In the small intestine*	*Absorption, small intestine*	*Metabolism*
No action	Proteins ↓ Proteoses ↓ Peptones by action of gastric pepsin (Rennin coagulates milk protein—casein—and prepares it for digestion)	Proteins ↓ Peptones by action of pancreatic trypsin ↓ Amino acids by action of intestinal erepsin	In the form of amino acids which	→ Build new tissue → Repair old tissue → Are deaminized if not needed: Nitrogen removed, changed to urea, and excreted; carbon, hydrogen, and oxygen converted to glucose

Figure 2–3. Digestion and Metabolism of Proteins.

TABLE 2–4. RDA For Protein*

	Age (years)	Weight (kg)	Weight (lb)	Height (cm)	Height (in)	Protein (gm)
Infants	0.0–0.5	6	13	60	24	kg × 2.2
	0.5–1.0	9	20	71	28	kg × 2.0
Children	1–3	13	29	90	35	23
	4–6	20	44	112	44	30
	7–10	28	62	132	52	34
Males	11–14	45	99	157	62	45
	15–18	66	145	176	69	56
	19–22	70	154	177	70	56
	23–50	70	154	178	70	56
	51+	70	154	178	70	56
Females	11–14	46	101	157	62	46
	15–18	55	120	163	64	46
	19–22	55	120	163	64	44
	23–50	55	120	163	64	44
	51+	55	120	163	64	44
Pregnant						+30
Lactating						+20

*From *Recommended Dietary Allowances*, 9th ed. National Academy of Sciences–National Research Council, Washington, D.C., 1980.

Study Questions and Activities

1. How do proteins differ from carbohydrates and fats?
2. What is the difference between a complete and incomplete protein?
3. Why is it possible for proteins to build and repair tissues in addition to furnishing energy?
4. Why is it uneconomical to use protein foods for energy?
5. How much protein do you require every day? See the RDA in Table 2–4.

Energy Requirements

WHAT IS THE MEANING OF "ENERGY," "KILOCALORIE," AND "METABOLISM"?

Energy is defined as the power to do work. Some energy (kilocalories, fuel, heat) is needed for even the slightest movements of the body. It is provided by the oxidation (burning) of the carbon-containing nutrients—carbohydrates, fats, and proteins. Without sufficient kilocalories in the food intake, the body burns its own tissues for needed energy.

A "kilocalorie" is simply a unit of measure to express the fuel value of these nutrients just as an inch measures length, an ounce weight, and so on. The large calorie (or kilocalorie, abbreviated as Kcal) used in nutrition represents the amount of heat necessary to raise the temperature of one kilogram (2.2 lb) of water 1 degree Centigrade.

Metabolism is a general term covering all changes food nutrients undergo after their absorption from the gastrointestinal tract and their utilization by the body cells. If the change is of a constructive nature building up new substances, it is called anabolism; if of a destructive or oxidative nature, it is called catabolism. Energy metabolism refers to the oxidation of nutrients within the body, with the release of heat and energy; protein metabolism refers to protein changes in the body.

WHAT ARE THE DAILY ENERGY NEEDS?

Food energy values and allowances are expressed in kilocalories. The accepted international unit of energy is the joule (J). The recommendations for energy represent the average needs of people in each age and sex category. Adjustments must be made for pregnancy and lactation.

Overweight individuals may require less energy than is recommended, because of a low activity level. For individuals who are already obese, energy intake should be reduced below the suggested levels as but one of several measures in a sound program of weight control that includes increased exercise. Increased activity is recommended for those who tend to gain excessive amounts of body fat while consuming daily energy apparently appropriate to their body weight, sex, age, and activity level. The reasons for this recommentation are:

1. Adequate energy intake is a requirement for efficient utilization of dietary protein for growth and maintenance.
2. It is difficult to have a nutritionally adequate diet if the calorie requirement is not met, because many essential nutrients are widely distributed in foods.
3. There is evidence that arterial disease and obesity and its many complications may be partly attributed to a sedentary life-style (WHO, 1969).[1]

The maintenance of desirable body weight by an individual throughout adult life is dependent on achieving a balance between energy intake and energy output.

The body needs energy for metabolic processes, including internal, involuntary activities of organs and tissues and oxidation within the tissues, circulation, respiration, digestion, elimination, maintenance of muscle tone, heart beat, and so on. All internal activities continue 24 hours a day, during sleeping and nonsleeping hours. The amount of energy required to sustain them alone is known as the **basal metabolism.** The basal metabolic rate is influenced by body composition, body size, and age. The more muscle tissue a person has, the more calories he or she needs. The basal metabolic rate varies from person to person, but on the average it amounts to approximately ½ Kcal per pound per hour, or 1,200–1,400 Kcal per day for women and 1,600–1,800 Kcal per day for men. This minimum calorie need usually accounts for more than half the total daily energy need of a moderately active adult and even more for less active adults.

A basal metabolism test is used for diagnostic purposes in disturbances affecting the metabolic rate and is taken in the morning before rising, usually prior to eating. It measures the body's expenditure of energy by recording its rate of oxygen intake and consumption.

Effect of Food Eaten

The body also needs energy for the stimulating effect (specific dynamic action, or SDA) each food exerts on basal metabolism after digestion and absorption. This raises the total energy needs about 10 per cent for a person eating a mixed diet.

External (Voluntary) Activities

Muscular movements, and other activities in moving about and carrying on daily activities and work, raise the energy requirement 30 to 100 per cent above basal needs, depending on the severity and extent of activity.

WHAT ARE ENERGY FOODS?

The body receives energy for basal metabolic processes, the SDA of food, and external activities by burning protein, fat, and carbohydrate. Carbohydrates and protein provide 4 kilocalories per gram and fat provides 9 kilocalories per gram. For example, 1 cup of whole milk contains:

12 gm carbohydrate	× 4	48 kilocalories
9 gm fat	× 9	81 kilocalories
8.5 gm protein	× 4	34 kilocalories
		163 kilocalories

HOW DOES THE BODY GET ENERGY FROM FOOD?

In some ways the body is like an engine. An engine needs fuel that can be burned for work. The body needs food (carbon-containing) which, after digestion and absorption into the blood stream, can be oxidized (burned) to do work. The body differs from a machine in several ways. First, an engine uses but one kind of fuel; the body can use three kinds interchangeably—carbohydrates, fats, and proteins. When an engine stops working, it requires no fuel. The body never stops working, as internal or involuntary activities continue even during sleep, so there is a 24-hour need for upkeep and repair.

HOW ARE ENERGY REQUIREMENTS DETERMINED?

The simplest method is to multiply the desirable weight in pounds by 18 (for a woman, by 21 for a man) for the approximate number of kilocalories needed by a moderately active adult. Add ¼ more calories if very active; subtract ¼ if sedentary.

Another method is to keep a record of the different activities undertaken during a representative 24-hour period, listing the time spent on each activity. With the help of Table 2–7 on p. 63, the energy expenditure and food kilocalories needed may be quickly determined for the period of time spent in each activity and the total figure obtained for 24 hours. You will be doing this problem for yourself when you complete Table 2–8.

WHAT DETERMINES ENERGY BALANCE?

A person's weight is a good index of energy balance, if one is at the desirable weight for height and age. If no weight gain or loss occurs over a period of time, it may be assumed that the number of calories eaten daily is sufficient or about equal to energy expenditure or needs. If fewer calories are eaten than the energy expended, some of the body tissues will be burned and there will be a weight loss. If more calories are eaten than calories expended, there will be a storage of fatty tissue and weight gain. "Energy balance" means that the kilocalories in the diet equal the calories expended by the body. If the same number of kilocalories are eaten and expended, but physical activity is increased, there will be a weight loss; weight gain will occur with decreased physical activity. Ten pounds can be gained in one year just by eating 100 kcalories more than needed daily, and 25 pounds by eating 250 kcalories more than needed daily.[5]

It takes about 3,500 extra calories to produce a pound of stored fat. For each pound to be lost, there must be 3,500 calories less in the diet than the body uses. A person who needs 2,400 calories a day to maintain his weight would cut down to 1,400 calories a day to lose 2 pounds a week. That means taking in 7,000 calories less each week than the body uses.[6] (See the Food Composition Table in the Appendix for the carbohydrate, fat, and protein content, and kilocalorie value of different foods.)

In general, foods high in kilocalories are rich in fat or low in water: fatty foods, cheese, nuts, dried legumes, and dried fruits. Foods moderate in calories are lean meats, cereals, and starchy vegetables. Kilocalories in the Four Food Groups are shown in Table 2–5.

TABLE 2–5. Kilocalories in Four Food Groups*

Milk Group		**Meat Group**	
Milk, whole, 1 cup	165	Meat, cooked, 4-oz ser.	
Milk, skim, 1 cup	90	Beef, veal	250–425
Buttermilk, 1 cup	90	Lamb	300–475
Cheese, Am. cheddar, 1 oz	115	Pork	375–450
Cheese, cottage, 1/2 cup	100	Note: variation depends on fat content	
Ice cream, vanilla, 2/3 cup	200	Poultry, cooked, 4-oz ser. (without added fat)	
Cream, light, 1/4 cup	125	Broiler-fryer	175
Cream, whipping, 1/4 cup	200	Roaster	225
Cereals–Bread		Hens	350
Bread, whole wheat or enriched,		Liver—1 tsp fat	235
Bakery, 1 slice	65	Heart	150
Homemade, 1 slice	100	Tongue	300
Breakfast cereals, whole-grain, 3/4 cup cooked	100	Fish	
Breakfast cereals, whole-grain, dry, 1 oz	100	Lean—broiled, baked, haddock, cod	125
Cornmeal, farina, spaghetti, macaroni, noodles, rice, 3/4 cup cooked	100	Fat—broiled, baked, halibut, salmon, tuna	225
Crackers, graham, 2 med	55	Shrimp	150
saltines, 3	50	Oysters, 1/2 cup	100
Flour, whole wheat or enriched,		Eggs, one	75
1 cup	400	Dry beans, peas, 1/2 cup cooked	100
1 Tbsp	25	Nuts, 1 Tbsp	50
		Peanut butter, 1 Tbsp	100

Vegetables–Fruits
1/2 cup servings

15 kcalories:	*25 kcalories:*	*50 kcalories:*	*75 kcalories:*
Asparagus, green	Broccoli	Grapefruit juice	Peas
Peppers, green	Carrots	Orange juice	Lima beans
Snap beans, green	Greens, cooked	Lemon juice	Sweet corn
Salad greens	Pumpkin	Strawberries	Apple, 1 med
Cabbage, raw	Squash, winter	Peach, 1 med	Apple juice
Peppers, raw	Tomato, 1 med	Pears, canned with water	Sweet potato, 1/2 med
Cantaloup	Tomato, canned or fresh cooked	Pineapple, raw	Banana, 1 med
Celery	Tomato juice	Onions	Pear, 1 med
Cucumbers	Beets	Parsnips	Apricots, dried
Eggplant	Brussels sprouts	Applesauce	Watermelon, 4″ wedge
Lettuce, head	Cabbage, cooked	Blackberries	Pineapple, canned or frozen
Radishes	Cauliflower	Blueberries	
Squash, summer	Rutabagas	Grapes	
	Turnips	Pineapple juice	
	Apricots, canned with water	Plums	
	Peaches, canned with water	Raspberries	

TABLE 2-5. Kilocalories in Four Food Groups* (*Continued*)

Miscellaneous			
Fats		*Sweets*	
Butter, 1 Tbsp	100	Sugar, 1 Tbsp	50
Margarine, fortified, 1 Tbsp	100	Molasses, 1 Tbsp	50
Cooking fats, salad oils, 1 Tbsp	125	Candy, 1 oz	100–150
Mayonnaise, 1 Tbsp	100	Jam or jelly, 1 Tbsp	50
Bacon, broiled, 2 strips	100	Pies, homemade	
		Fruit, 2 crust	500
		Single-crust pies	365
		Cakes	
		Angel or sponge, no icing, 2'' piece	100
		With fat, iced	400

*Adapted from a Cornell University extension bulletin.

Even though kilocalories are essential in the diet and we cannot live without an adequate number for our needs (undernutrition in many parts of the world is due to insufficient kilocalories), they are not the only dietary essential. They must be accompanied by "leader" nutrients—proteins (amino acids) fats (fatty acids)—and many different minerals and vitamins. Kilocalories in

TABLE 2-6. The Caloric Content of Various Snacks*

Item	Calories
Candy (except chocolate):	
Caramel, 1 medium	40
Gumdrop, 1 large	40
Jellybeans, 10	105
Peanut brittle, one 2-1/2 × 1-1/2 × 1-1/4-inch piece, 1 oz	120
Chocolate:	
Bar (sweetened milk chocolate with almonds), 1 oz	150
Cream, 2 or 3 pieces (35 per pound)	125
Fudge (milk chocolate), 1 piece, 1 to 1-1/2 inches square	115
Chocolate milkshake, 12-oz glass	515
Mint, 1 piece, 1-1/2 inches in diameter	35
Crackers:	
Graham, 2 medium	55
Saltines, 2 crackers, about 2 inches square	25
Doughnut, cake type, 3-1/4 inches in diameter	165
Popcorn, popped, 1 cup large kernels with added oil and salt	40
Potato chips, 5 medium	60
Pretzels, 5 sticks, about 3 inches long	10

*From *Food and Your Weight*, Home and Garden Bulletin No. 74, U.S. Department of Agriculture, Washington, D.C., 1977.

food unaccompanied by these other dietary essentials are frequently referred to as "empty calories" or "lone wolf kilocalories." Snack foods such as candy and other sweets are high in calories and contain little, if any, other nutrients. Table 2-6 shows the caloric content of various snack foods.

HOW MANY CALORIES ARE EXPENDED IN VARIOUS ACTIVITIES?[10]

The approximate number of calories per hour it takes to perform each of the five different types of activity is given in Table 2-7. These figures include the basal calorie need.

HOW MANY CALORIES DO YOU EXPEND DAILY?

Complete Table 2-8 to find your own energy requirement. Fill in the number of hours or part of hours you spend in each of the activities or similar ones for an average 24-hour period. Complete the table to obtain an approximate figure for your day's energy expenditures.

TABLE 2-7. Calories Expended Per Hour for Various Types of Activities*

Type of Activity	Cal/hour†	Type of Activity	Cal/hour
Sedentary activities: Reading, writing, eating, watching TV or movies, listening to radio; sewing; playing cards; typing, office work, and other activities done while sitting that require little or no arm movement.	80–100	*Moderate activities:* Making beds; mopping and scrubbing; sweeping; light polishing and waxing; laundering by machine; light gardening and carpentry work; walking moderately fast; other activities done while standing that require moderate arm movement; and activities done while sitting that require more vigorous arm movement.	170–240
Light activities: Preparing and cooking food; doing dishes; dusting; hand washing small articles of clothing; ironing; walking slowly; personal care; miscellaneous office work and other activities done while standing that require some arm movement; and rapid typing and other activities done while sitting that are more strenuous.	110–160	*Vigorous activities:* Heavy scrubbing and waxing; hand washing large articles of clothing; hanging out clothes; stripping beds; other heavy work; walking fast; bowling; golfing; gardening.	250–350
		Strenuous activities: Swimming; playing tennis; running; bicycling; dancing; skiing; playing football.	350 and more

*From *Food and Your Weight,* Home and Garden Bulletin No. 74, U.S. Department of Agriculture, Washington, D.C.

†A range of caloric values is given for each type of activity to allow for differences in activities and in persons. Of the sedentary activities, for example, typing uses more calories than watching TV. And some persons will use more calories in carrying out either activity than others; some persons are more efficient in their body actions than others. Values closer to the upper limit of a range will give a better picture of calorie expenditures for men and those near the lower limit a better picture for women.

TABLE 2-8. Energy Expenditure for Everyday Activities*

Activity†	No. hrs (or fraction of hr engaged in activity)	Kcal per lb per hr	Total for Period
Asleep		0.4	
Bicycling, moderate speed		1.7	
Cello playing		1.1	
Dancing, the "hustle"		2.4	
Dancing, waltz		2.0	
Dishwashing		1.0	
Dressing and undressing		0.9	
Driving an automobile		1.0	
Eating a meal		0.7	
Horseback riding, trot		2.6	
Ironing		1.0	
Laundry, light		1.1	
Lying still and awake		0.5	
Painting furniture		1.3	
Playing ping-pong		2.7	
Piano playing, moderate		1.2	
Reading aloud		0.7	
Running		4.0	
Sewing by hand		0.7	
Sewing, electric machine		0.7	
Sitting quietly, watching TV		0.6	
Skating		2.2	
Standing relaxed		0.8	
Sweeping, vacuum sweeper		1.9	
Swimming, 2 m.p.h.		4.5	
Tailoring		1.0	
Typing rapidly		1.0	
Walking, 3 m.p.h.		1.5	
Walking, 4 m.p.h.		2.2	
Writing	______	0.7	______
	24	Total per lb	______ ×
		Desirable wt. in lb	______
		Total number of kilocalories expended per day	______

*From C. M. Taylor, G. MacLeod, and M. S. Rose, *Foundations of Nutrition*, 5th ed. Macmillan Company, New York.

†For any one of your daily activities for which no figure is given above, use the figure for a similar activity.

HOW MANY CALORIES DO YOU CONSUME?

Keep a record below of *all* the food you eat for one day: at breakfast, during morning, at noon meal, during afternoon, at evening meal, at night. Do not forget "snack" foods! You will be referring to this food record as you progress with your study of nutrition, so keep it as accurately as possible. Determine the calorie and protein context of the foods on the food record. (Refer to food composition table, Appendix 6, pp. 331–341.)

Date: ______________________________

Meal	*Foods*	*Size of Serving*	*Calories*	*Protein (Gm)*

How does the kilocalorie content of the above food record compare with your calculated requirement?

How does the protein content compare with your protein requirement?

Study Questions and Activities

1. What factors affect the total number of kilocalories one needs daily? Which have the greatest effect?
2. Why does a child need more energy in proportion to size than an adult?
3. Two slices of whole wheat bread contain 22 grams carbohydrate, 2 grams fat, and 4 grams protein. How many kilocalories do the two slices contain?
4. How many kilocalories are needed daily by a woman weighing 125 pounds who is employed in a sedentary occupation? A man weighing 180 pounds who is engaged in very active employment?

Minerals and Water

WHAT ARE MINERALS?

Minerals are inorganic substances found in all body tissues and fluids. They exist in the form of salts such as sodium chloride or combine with organic compounds such as iron in hemoglobin. Some are in soluble form, giving certain properties to body fluids (lymph, blood plasma, fluids around cells and soft tissues). Others, in insoluble form, are found in the hard tissues of bones and teeth. They occur naturally in foods along with carbohydrates, proteins, and fats, and remain in the ash after foods are burned. They do not furnish energy. Minerals cannot be destroyed in food preparation.

Minerals compose approximately 4 per cent of body weight. See Table 2–9 for the mineral content of an adult male.

HOW DO MINERALS FUNCTION IN NUTRITION?

Minerals have both *building* functions, taking part in the structure of all body tissues, hard and soft, and *regulating* functions of a wide variety in body systems.

As *building material*, minerals enter into the formation of the following:

1. *Bony tissue:* Calcium and phosphorus in bones and teeth; fluorine in teeth
2. *Soft body tissue (muscles, nerves, glands):* All salts, especially phosphorus, potassium, sulfur and chloride
3. *Hair, nails, skin:* Sulfur

TABLE 2–9. Mineral Content of a 70-Kilogram Adult Man*

Water	41,400 gm	Magnesium	21 gm
Fat	12,600 gm	Chloride	85 gm
Protein	12,600 gm	Phosphorus	670 gm
Carbohydrate	300 gm	Sulfur	112 gm
Sodium	63 gm	Iron	3 gm
Potassium	150 gm	Iodine	0.014 gm
Calcium	1,160 gm		

*Modified from A. C. Guyton, *Textbook of Medical Physiology*, 6th ed. W. B. Saunders Co., Philadelphia, 1981.

4. *Blood:* All salts, especially iron for hemoglobin and copper for red blood cells

5. *Glandular secretions:* Chlorine in gastric juice; sodium in intestinal juice; iodine in thyroxine; manganese in endocrine secretions; and zinc in enzymes

As *regulators*, minerals play a role in:

1. *Fluid pressure:* All salts, especially sodium and potassium
2. *Muscle contraction and relaxation:* Calcium, potassium, sodium, phosphorus, chlorine
3. *Nerve responses:* All salts, with a balance between calcium and sodium
4. *Blood clotting:* Calcium
5. *Oxidation in tissue and blood:* Iron, iodine
6. *Acid-base balance:* Balance between acid compounds—chlorine, sulfur, phosphorus—and base compounds—calcium, sodium, potassium, magnesium

The amounts the body needs of certain essential minerals will vary widely with the mineral. Excesses as well as inadequate intakes of minerals can cause serious health problems. A mixed diet will provide essential minerals below toxic levels. The danger of toxicity arises when supplements are used in excess.

HOW ARE MINERALS CLASSIFIED?

Minerals are usually classified into two groups: *major minerals* and *trace minerals.* The major minerals (also referred to as macrominerals, macronutrient elements) are those present in amounts greater than 5 grams in the human body. The trace minerals (also referred to as microminerals or micronutrient elements) are found in the human body in amounts less than 5 grams.

MAJOR MINERALS

Calcium

Functions. As calcium phosphate, calcium is the major mineral constituent of the body. Ninety-nine per cent is found in bones (giving rigidity) and teeth, with the remainder in the blood, other body fluids, and soft tissues.

With the other minerals, calcium helps muscles to contract and relax normally, as well as taking part in the normal functioning of the nervous system and passage of materials in and out of cells.

Calcium also aids in blood coagulation and the functioning of some enzymes. It is needed daily throughout life. Vitamin D is required for proper absorption and utilization of dietary calcium.

Food sources. The best sources of calcium are milk and milk products, cheese (cheddar type), and ice cream. Other sources of calcium are green leafy vegetables (turnip, collard, and mustard greens, kale, and broccoli). The calcium in chard, beet greens, spinach, and rhubarb is not available to the body, as it forms an insoluble salt with the oxalic acid present.

The American diet is apt to be lacking in calcium. A good supply of dairy products, however, should insure adequate intake for everyone. The RDA for calcium can be found in Table 2–14. Each of the lists of foods in Table 2–10 supply the RDA for calcium in the adult (0.8 gm or 800 mg). As the amount of milk is decreased in each list, more of less calcium-rich foods must be added. These list show how difficult it is to get adequate calcium without milk or milk products in the diet. Table 2–11 shows the calcium

TABLE 2–10. Groups of Foods that Furnish the RDA for Calcium*

	Calcium (mg)		Calcium (mg)
(1)		(4)	
3 glasses milk (1-1/2 pints)	873	1/4 cup nonfat instant dry milk	202
(2)		3 oz pink salmon with bones	167
2 glasses milk (1 pint)	582	1 cup baked beans	95
1 inch cube cheddar cheese	124	2/3 cup turnip greens,	
3/4 cup ice cream	132	frozen, cooked	130
2/3 cup cut green beans,		2 eggs	56
frozen, cooked	36	4 dried prunes, extra large	14
2 slices white enriched bread	42	1 cup loose lettuce leaves	37
	916	3 Tbsp light cream	42
		2/3 cup dried apricots	58
			801
(3)			
1 glass milk (1/2 pint)	291		
1/2 cup creamed cottage cheese	67		
3 stalks broccoli, frozen, cooked	36		
1-1/2 cups orange juice, frozen,			
reconstituted	50		
4 slices whole wheat bread	96		
2/3 cup mustard greens	128		
1 tablespoon light molasses	33		
6 medium oysters	113		
	814		

*Calculated from *Nutritive Value of Foods*, Home and Garden Bulletin No. 72, U.S. Department of Agriculture, Washington, D.C., 1977.

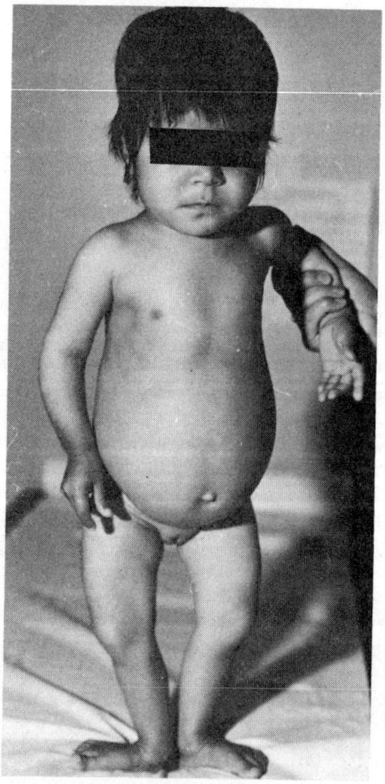

Figure 2–4. Rickets in young child. Chest and lower extremities are deformed. (From H. E. Harrison and H. C. Harrison, *Calcium and Phosphate Metabolism in Childhood and Adolescence*. W. B. Saunders Co., Philadelphia, 1979, p. 153.)

content of some basic four foods. It is also important to note that protein intake may affect calcium metabolism.

Deficiencies. Inadequate calcium in the diet leads to poor bone growth and tooth development, stunted growth, rickets in children (see Figure 2–4), osteomalacia and osteoporosis in adults (calcium supplements may relieve osteoporosis symptoms), thin fragile bones, and poor blood clotting.

Phosphorus

Functions. Phosphorus is second to calcium in amount in the body. The largest amount of phosphorus is with calcium in the bones; the remainder is in soft tissues and fluids. Phosphorus performs many functions in the body. It is involved in bone and tooth structure, is present in the nuclei of all cells, helps in oxidation of carbohydrates and fats, helps enzymes act in energy metabolism, and aids in maintaining the body's acid-base balance.

Food sources. Rich sources of phosphorus include milk, meat, eggs, cheese, dry beans, nuts, and whole-grain cereals. A diet adequate in protein and calcium will provide sufficient phosphorus for body needs. The RDA for phosphorus can be found in Table 2–14. It is equal to that for calcium for all age groups except the young infant.

TABLE 2–11. Calcium Content of Some Basic Four Foods

Food Group	Serving Size	Calcium (mg)*	% RDA†
Milk and Dairy			
Milk, whole	1 cup	291	36
Milk, skim	1 cup	303	38
Cheddar cheese	1 oz	211	26
Cottage cheese	1 cup	211	26
Yogurt (whole milk)	1 cup	275	34
Ice cream	1 cup	208	26
Meat and Alternates			
Beef, ground chuck, cooked	3-1/2 oz	11	1
Chicken, canned, boned	3-1/2 oz	14	2
Peanut butter	2 T	22	3
Egg	1	26	3
Kidney beans, cooked	1 cup	95	12
Salmon, canned with bones	3-1/2 oz	196	25
Breads and Cereals			
Bread, white	1 slice	19	2
Macaroni	1 cup	11	1
Rice, enriched, cooked	1 cup	15	2
Oatmeal, cooked	1 cup	21	3
Corn flakes	1 cup	2	0.2
Fruits and Vegetables			
Broccoli, cooked	2/3 cup	88	11
Sweet potato, cooked	1 small	40	5
Peas, cooked	2/3 cup	23	3
Orange	1 small	41	5
Grapefruit	1/2 medium	16	2
Peaches, canned	1/2 cup	4	0.5

*Calcium values from J. Pennington and H. Church, *Bowes and Church's Food Values of Portions Commonly Used*, 13th ed. J. B. Lippincott Co., Philadelphia, 1980.

†Based on adult requirement of 800 mg.

Deficiencies. A wide variation in the calcium:phosphorus ratio is tolerated in the adult diet with adequate vitamin D intake. A ratio of 1.5:1 is recommended in early infancy to prevent hypocalcemic tetany.

Magnesium

Functions. Along with the other minerals, magnesium is a component of bones and teeth. It activates many enzymes and participates in protein synthesis. It assists in the regulation of nerve and muscle tissue.

Food sources. The major food sources for magnesium are nuts, cereal grains, legumes, and green leafy vegetables. The RDA for magnesium can be found in Table 2–14.

Deficiencies. A diet inadequate in magnesium may lead to neuromuscular dysfunction.

Sulfur

Functions. Sulfur is a component of skin, hair, nails, cartilage, and some organ tissue. It is a component of all body proteins, as well as thiamin and biotin.

Food sources. Meat, eggs, poultry, and milk are all important food sources of sulfur. No RDA has been established, but diets adequate in protein provide liberal amounts of sulfur.

Deficiencies. No deficiency of sulfur has been documented in humans.

The other major minerals, sodium, potassium and chlorine, will be discussed under electrolytes, p. 74.

TRACE MINERALS

Iron

Functions. Very small amounts of iron in the body perform many very important functions in all cells. More than one-half of the 4 to 5 grams of iron in the body is in hemoglobin. About one-third is in the liver, spleen, and bone marrow; small amounts are found in muscle blood serum and oxidative enzymes in cells.

Hemoglobin facilitates tissue respiration by carrying oxygen from the lungs to the tissue cells and by carrying the carbon dioxide formed in oxidation away from cells.

Copper, adequate protein, and other substances are necessary for hemoglobin synthesis.

Food sources. Organ meats, i.e., liver, heart, and kidney, are excellent sources of iron. Other good food sources of iron include lean meat, oysters, egg yolk, dark-green leafy vegetables, potatoes, dried fruits, whole-grain and enriched cereals and bread, dried peas and beans, molasses, and raisins, if eaten in generous amounts.

Table 2–12 lists foods that will meet RDA for iron, and Table 2–13 shows the iron content of some basic four foods. The RDA for iron can be found in Table 2–14.

Deficiencies. Inadequate iron intake or poor iron absorption leads to iron-deficiency anemia. There is great variability in iron absorption per meal. It is enhanced by the presence of vitamin C and animal protein. Individuals deficient in iron will have an increase in absorption over nondeficient individuals. Populations at risk for iron deficiency include infants over 6 months of age, adolescents, females of child-bearing age, and pregnant females. These individuals need carefully planned diets to meet iron needs. Supplements are usually necessary to meet iron needs during pregnancy.

TABLE 2–12. Groups of Foods That Furnish Iron at Levels of 10 and 18 mg*

(1)	Iron (mg)	(2)	Iron (mg)
Hamburger, 1 average (85 gm)	3.0	Liver, lamb, broiled, 2 slices (75 gm)	13.4
Beet greens, 1/2 cup cooked	1.9	Beans, snap, 3/4 cup canned	1.5
Bread, whole-wheat, 3 slices	1.5	Milk, 1 pt	0.2
Egg, 1 medium large	1.2	Dried apricots or prunes, 1/2 cup, cooked	2.1
Potato, 1 medium	0.7	Bread, white, 2 slices	1.2
Beets, 2 small	0.5		18.4
Banana, 1 medium	0.7		
Orange, 1 medium	0.6		
Milk, 1 pint	0.2		
	10.3		

*From G. M. Briggs and D. H. Calloway, *Bogert's Nutrition and Physical Fitness*, 10th ed. CBS College Publishing, New York, 1979. Copyright 1979 by W. B. Saunders Company. Reprinted with permission of W. B. Saunders Company, CBS College Publishing.

TABLE 2–13. Iron Content of Some Basic Four Foods

Food Group	Serving Size	Iron (mg)*	% RDA† 10 mg	% RDA† 18 mg
Milk and Dairy				
Milk, whole	1 cup	.1	1	.05
Cheddar cheese	1 oz	.1	3	1.6
Cottage cheese	1 cup	.7	7	4
Meat and Alternates				
Beef, ground chuck	3-1/2 oz	3.3	33	18
Chicken	3-1/2 oz	1.7	17	9
Lamb, loin chop	1	1.4	14	8
Liver, calf	3-1/2 oz	14.2	142	79
Pork, loin chop	1	3.5	35	19
Egg	1 medium	1.2	12	7
Perch	3-1/2 oz	1.3	13	7
Baked beans, canned (with pork and molasses)	1/2 cup	2.9	29	16
Breads and Cereals				
Bread, white enriched	1 slice	.6	6	3
Corn Flakes, Kellogg's	1 cup	1.4	14	8
Noodles, enriched	1 cup	1.4	14	8
Rolled oats	1 cup	1.7	17	9
Cream of Wheat	1 cup	1.4	14	8
Fruits and Vegetables				
Potato, white	1 medium	1.0	10	6
Green beans	1/2 cup	.4	4	2
Spinach	1/2 cup	2.0	20	11
Raisins	1/4 cup	1.6	16	9
Banana	1 medium	1.0	10	6
Orange	1 medium	.6	6	3

*Iron values from J. Pennington and H. Church, *Bowes and Church's Food Values of Portions Commonly Used*, 13th ed. J. B. Lippincott Co., Philadelphia, 1980.

†RDA of iron for men = 10 mg, for women = 18 mg.

TABLE 2–14. RDA for Calcium, Phosphorus, Magnesium, Iron, Zinc, and Iodine*

	Age (years)	Weight (kg)	Weight (lb)	Calcium (mg)	Phosphorus (mg)	Magnesium (mg)	Iron (mg)	Zinc (mg)	Iodine (μg)
Infants	0.0–0.5	6	13	360	240	50	10	3	40
	0.5–1.0	9	20	540	360	70	15	5	50
Children	1–3	13	29	800	800	150	15	10	70
	4–6	20	44	800	800	200	10	10	90
	7–10	28	62	800	800	250	10	10	120
Males	11–14	45	99	1200	1200	350	18	15	150
	15–18	66	145	1200	1200	400	18	15	150
	19–22	70	154	800	800	350	10	15	150
	23–50	70	154	800	800	350	10	15	150
	51+	70	154	800	800	350	10	15	150
Females	11–14	46	101	1200	1200	300	18	15	150
	15–18	55	120	1200	1200	300	18	15	150
	19–22	55	120	800	800	300	18	15	150
	23–50	55	120	800	800	300	18	15	150
	51+	55	120	800	800	300	10	15	150
Pregnant				+400	+400	+150	†	+5	+25
Lactating				+400	+400	+150	†	+10	+50

*From *Recommended Dietary Allowances*, 9th ed. National Academy of Sciences–National Research Council, Washington, D.C., 1980.

†The increased requirement during pregnancy cannot be met by the iron content of habitual American diets nor by the existing stores of many women; therefore, the use of 30 to 60 mg of supplemental iron is recommended. Iron needs during lactation are not substantially different from those of nonpregnant women, but continued supplementation of the mother for 2 to 3 months after parturition is advisable in order to replenish stores depleted by pregnancy.

Iodine

Functions. Iodine is a constituent of the thyroid hormones thyroxine and thyroglobulin. As part of these hormones it helps regulate energy metabolism.

Food sources. Iodized salt and ocean or salt-water fish are the most common sources of iodine. The RDA for iodine can be found in Table 2–14.

Deficiencies. Inadequate iodine intake leads to goiter (Fig. 2–5).

Zinc

Functions. Zinc is a component of many enzymes. It participates in protein synthesis, has a role in taste sensitivity, and assists in regulation of cell growth.

Food sources. Oysters, liver, high-protein foods, and whole-grain cereals are good sources of zinc. The RDA for zinc are listed in Table 2–14.

Deficiencies. Inadequate zinc results in poor growth and impaired sense of taste.

Other Trace Minerals

The following minerals do not have established Recommended Daily Allowances at the present time but are essential to the body. Human requirements for these minerals are not known, but estimated safe and adequate intakes have been suggested until further data are available (see Table 2–15).

Copper. Copper aids in the absorption of iron from the intestinal tract

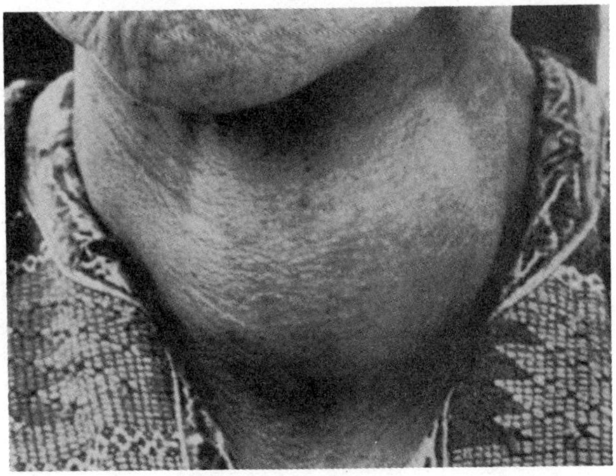

Figure 2–5. Goiter. (From A. E. Nizel, *Nutrition in Preventive Dentistry: Science and Practice,* 2nd ed. W. B. Saunders Co., Philadelphia, 1981, p. 248.)

and in the production and survival of red blood cells. The richest food sources are nuts, some shellfish, liver, kidneys, raisins, and dried legumes.

Manganese. Manganese is an essential mineral needed for normal bone structure, reproduction, and normal function of the central nervous system. It is a component of some enzymes. The best sources of manganese are nuts and grains.

Fluorine. Fluorine helps the formation of solid bones and teeth. It also helps reduce the incidence of dental caries. There is some evidence that it is related to the use of calcium in bone formation. The Food and Nutrition Board recommends fluoridation of public water supplies if natural fluoride levels are low. Fluorine, like other trace minerals, is toxic when consumed in an excessive amount.

Chromium. Chromium activates several enzymes. It plays a role in carbohydrate metabolism as a component of glucose tolerance factor (GTF), which enhances the removal of glucose from the blood. Good sources of chromium include brewer's yeast, beer, liver, whole-grain cereals, meat, and cheese.

TABLE 2–15. Trace Minerals — Estimated Safe and Adequate Daily Intake*

	Age (years)	Copper (mg)	Manganese (mg)	Fluorine (mg)	Chromium (mg)	Selenium (mg)	Molybdenum (mg)
Infants	0.0–0.5	0.5–0.7	0.1–0.5	0.1–0.5	0.01–0.04	0.01–0.04	0.03–0.06
	0.5–1.0	0.7–1.0	0.7–1.0	0.2–1.0	0.02–0.06	0.02–0.06	0.04–0.08
Children and adolescents	1–3	1.0–1.5	1.0–1.5	0.5–1.5	0.02–0.08	0.02–0.08	0.05–0.10
	4–6	1.5–2.0	1.5–2.0	1.0–2.5	0.03–0.12	0.03–0.12	0.06–0.15
	7–10	2.0–2.5	2.0–3.0	1.5–2.5	0.05–0.20	0.05–0.20	0.10–0.30
	11+	2.0–3.0	2.5–5.0	1.5–2.5	0.05–0.20	0.05–0.20	0.15–0.50
Adults		2.0–3.0	2.5–5.0	1.5–4.0	0.05–0.20	0.05–0.20	0.15–0.50

*From *Recommended Dietary Allowances,* 9th ed. National Academy of Sciences–National Research Council, Washington, D.C., 1980.

Since the toxic levels for many trace elements may be only several times usual intakes, the upper levels should not be habitually exceeded.

Selenium. This mineral functions as part of an enzyme system and as an antioxidant with vitamin E to protect the cell. The best sources of selenium include cereals, seafood, kidneys, and liver.

Molybdenum. This essential mineral is a component of an enzyme (xanthine oxidase). The best sources of molybdenum include organ meats, some cereals, and legumes.

There is no data for which an estimate of the human requirement of the following trace elements could be derived.

Cobalt. Cobalt is an essential component of vitamin B_{12}. Inadequate intake of cobalt results in pernicious anemia.

Nickel, Tin, Vanadium, and Silicone. Findings produced in experimental animal feeding suggest these elements are essential, but the implications for human nutrition are unknown.

ELECTROLYTES

An electrolyte is a compound that dissolved in water separates into charged particles (ions) capable of conducting an electric current. Within the body, electrolytes play an essential role in maintaining fluid and acid-base balance.

The chief electrolyte ions are sodium, potassium, calcium, magnesium, chloride, and phosphate. All body fluids contain electrolytes. The chief electrolytes outside the cell (extracellular) are sodium and chloride. Potassium, magnesium, and phosphate are found in large amounts inside the cell (intracellular).

Changes in the electrolyte composition of body fluids create electrical charges, which in turn are responsible for electrochemical reactions such as transmission of nerve impulses, contraction of muscles, and secretion of glandular cells.

Shifts in the electrolyte balance causing either an excess or a deficiency of electrolytes may occur as the result of various disease conditions. Careful monitoring of the blood levels of electrolytes is necessary. See Table 2–16 for the estimated safe and adequate daily intake of electrolytes.

TABLE 2–16. Electrolytes – Estimated Safe and Adequate Daily Intake*

	Age (years)	Sodium (mg)	Potassium (mg)	Chloride (mg)
Infants	0.0–0.5	115–350	350–925	275–700
Children and adolescents	0.5–1.0	250–750	425–1275	400–1200
	1–3	325–975	550–1650	500–1500
	4–6	450–1350	775–2325	700–2100
	7–10	600–1800	1000–3000	925–2775
	11+	900–2700	1525–4575	1400–4200
Adults		1100–3300	1875–5625	1700–5100

*From *Recommended Dietary Allowances*, 9th ed. National Academy of Sciences–National Research Council, Washington, D.C., 1980.

Sodium

Functions. Sodium is a key element in the maintenance of fluid and acid-base balances. It transmits nerve impulses, helps control muscle contractions, and regulates permeability of the cell membrane.

Food sources. Table salt, processed meats and other foods, and salt seasonings are primary sources of sodium.

For a more detailed discussion of sodium, see Chapter 8.

Potassium

Functions. Potassium also plays an important role in the maintenance of fluid and acid-base balances. It aids in the regulation of nerve impulses and muscle contractions and is necessary for enzyme reactions intracellularly as well as for the synthesis of proteins.

Food sources. Bananas, oranges, grapefruit, potatoes, whole-grain cereals, and meats are all good sources of potassium.

Chloride

Functions. Chloride is also involved in the maintenance of fluid and acid-base balances. It provides an acid medium for activation of gastric enzymes and aids in maintaining osmotic pressure. Its major food source is table salt.

HOW ARE MINERALS RELATED TO ACID-BASE BALANCE IN BODY?

The term *pH* is used to express the acidity, neutrality, or alkalinity of a solution (see Fig. 2–6). A neutral solution has a pH of 7; below 7 is acidic and above 7 is basic (alkaline). A neutral solution has an equal number of acid- and base-forming elements. An acid solution has a greater number of acid-forming elements and a basic solution has a greater number of base-forming elements.

The mineral content of a particular food will determine if it will be an acid-former or a base-former once the food has been metabolized by the body. In acid-forming foods, chlorine, sulfur, and phosphorus predominate. In base-forming foods, calcium, sodium, potassium, and magnesium predominate.

In an ordinary, mixed diet, a good balance exists between acid and basic elements, and this will help maintain the body's acid-base balance. Diet, however, will not cause disturbances in acid-base balance, since it is only a minor contributor of acid and basic elements.

Diet can have an effect on the pH of the urine. *Acid-ash* or *alkaline-ash* diets may sometimes be used along with medication to help dissolve kidney stones. See Table 2–17 for a list of these foods.

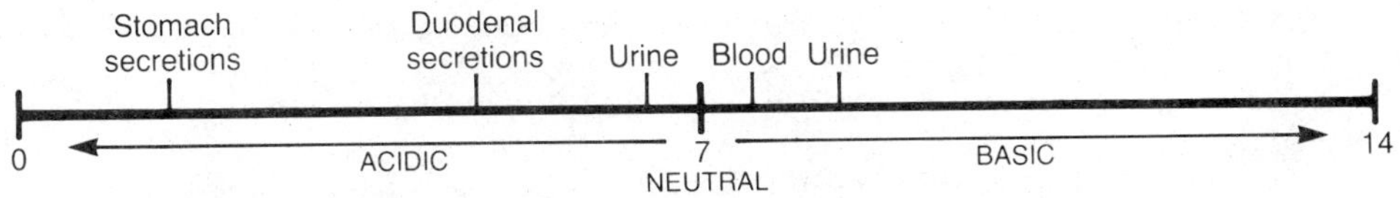

Figure 2–6. The pH of various body fluids.

TABLE 2-17. Foods Forming Alkaline-Ash and Acid-Ash

Base-Forming Foods (Alkaline-Ash)	Acid-Forming Foods (Acid-Ash)	Neutral Foods
Milk	Meat, fish, shellfish, eggs, poultry	Butter
Vegetables (except corn and lentils)	Cheese (all types)	Margarine
Fruits (except prunes, plums, cranberries, and some nuts), coconut, almonds, chestnuts	Cereals, crackers, cookies, cakes, breadstuffs	Lard, oils
Sweets—jams, jellies, honey	Prunes, plums, cranberries	Cornstarch
Molasses	Filberts, peanuts, walnuts, Brazil nuts	Tapioca, arrowroot
	Corn and lentils	Refined sugar
	Pastas—macaroni, noodles, spaghetti	Cooking fats
		Syrups
		Candy (plain)

WATER

Functions. Water is the principal constituent of the body. One-half to three-quarters of body weight is water. Most water is in cells (intracellular), the remainder is in blood, lymph, various secretions and excretions, and around cells (extracellular). Water helps every organ to function properly. It aids digestion, absorption, circulation, and excretion. It functions as a solvent for body constituents and a medium for all chemical changes in the body. As part of blood, it carries nutrients to and waste products from cells. It participates in the regulation of body temperature and the lubrication of the moving parts of the body, and is necessary for building and repair processes.

Sources. In addition to water as such, it can be found in varying quantities in foods (foods contain from 10 to 98 per cent water). It is also formed in the body's metabolic processes and is an end product of oxidation. The average diet with milk (87 per cent water) contains about 1,000 ml water daily.

Requirements. The adult requirement for water is 1 ml/Kcal and for infants is 1.5 ml/Kcal. Fluid balance is essential, and intake must balance output. Fluid requirements are closely related to salt requirements, and intake of increased amounts are needed under conditions of extreme heat or excessive sweating. Water is absorbed in the small intestine and colon with digested food. Since it is not stored, daily intake is necessary, and a total of 6 to 8 glasses (including that in foods) is recommended. Water requirements are increased for infants on high-protein formulas, comatose patients, those with fever, polyuria, or diarrhea, or those receiving high-protein diets. Water is normally lost through urine, in expired air, in feces, and from the skin.

Deficiency. Inadequate fluid intake will result in dehydration. If prolonged, death will result.

Study Questions

1. List several ways in which minerals play a role in regulating vital life processes.

2. Why is it difficult to get the right amount of calcium in the diet if milk and milk products are not consumed? What suggestions would you give to a person who cannot drink milk?

3. Why is an anemic person usually tired?

4. How does water function in the body? Why must there be a balance between intake and output?

5. Why are the requirements for calcium and iron increased during pregnancy and lactation?

6. How adequate is your mineral intake?

a. Using Table 2–14, jot down your RDA for minerals in the second column below.

		My RDA	*My diet record*
Calcium	mg	______	______
Phosphorus	mg	______	______
Iron	mg	______	______
Magnesium	mg	______	______
Iodine	μg	______	______
Zinc	mg	______	______

b. Determine the mineral content of one day's intake and write the totals under "My diet record." How do your results compare with the RDA? What improvements could you make to increase the mineral content of your diet?

Vitamins

WHAT ARE VITAMINS?

Long before the beginnings of nutrition science, it was a common observation that certain foods cured certain diseases. Lemons and limes added to the diet of sailors in the British navy on long voyages with limited rations prevented the scurvy so frequently encountered. Beriberi, the scourge of the Japanese navy, was prevented when the limited diet of polished rice and fish was supplemented. It is now thought that the potatoes and fruits eaten by New England and Pilgrim settlers curbed deaths from scurvy during those early days. The incidence of pellagra in the United States has decreased with dietary changes.

Only at the beginning of this century did it become evident that something was needed for good health in addition to carbohydrates, fats, proteins, and minerals. The term "vitamine," later changed to "vitamin," was coined to cover these new substances occurring in minute amounts in food and needed only in minute amounts. As each new vitamin, with specific functions, was discovered, an alphabetical designation was given. Five letters were originally used. The number of letters was extended as new vitamins were discovered. Some of the original letters were given subnumerical designations when a vitamin was found to be made up of several parts. A name indicating a "curative" property was frequently attached to each vitamin, as "antiscorbutic" for vitamin C, "antineuritic" for vitamin B_1, and so on.

When a vitamin could be isolated from a food, its chemical formula determined, and, in some instances, its synthesis accomplished, it was learned that each of these vitamins was a distinct chemical substance organic in nature with a chemical formula all its own and with specific nutritional functions. Names indicating chemical nature or coined names have now replaced the alphabetical designations for most of the vitamins. Some vitamins are groups of factors and are called complexes. Some vitamins are simple, some complex, and others have not yet been identified.

Solubility of vitamins in either fat or water provided an early basis for classification into fat-soluble and water-soluble groups. The classification continues in use for convenience in study, even though the vitamins in each group differ from one another in characteristics, functions, and sources.

Before beginning the study of vitamins, the following terms should be understood:

Avitaminosis ("without vitamins"): A deficiency state in which there is an insufficient amount of the vitamin to perform normal body functions. This can result in the development of a deficiency disease (see Fig. 2–7).

Hypervitaminosis: An excessive accumulation of a vitamin in the body that leads to toxicity. Fat-soluble vitamins A and D can accumulate in toxic amounts.

Precursor (or **provitamin**): Compounds that can be changed into the active form of the vitamin.

Vitamin antagonist (or **antivitamin**): Substances that interfere with the functioning of the vitamin. Certain drugs may be vitamin antagonists.

WHAT IS THE ROLE OF VITAMINS IN NUTRITION?

Vitamins are present in foods and needed by the body only in minute amounts, but proper growth and development and optimal health are impossible without them. Some may be synthesized in the body, but for the most part, they must be supplied in the daily diet of normal healthy persons. Vitamin supplements may be prescribed by a physician for therapeutic purposes. Vitamins, although organic in nature, do not provide energy, but they do help carbohydrates, fats, and proteins to be metabolized more efficiently. It is thought that vitamins act as catalysts. Early attention to the clear-cut manifest diseases caused by vitamin deficiencies (avitaminoses), which are seldom seen now, obscured for a time the very important function of vitamins in the promotion of optimal health. They are not, as advertising might lead us to believe, a cure-all for every ill, nor do they lessen the importance in the diet of the other essential nutrients such as proteins and minerals. Unlike minerals, vitamins are not a part of various body structures.

Vitamins are classified as *body regulators* because they:

1. Regulate the synthesis of many body compounds (bones, skin, glands, nerves, brain, and blood).
2. Participate in the metabolism of protein, carbohydrates, and fats.
3. Prevent nutritional deficiency diseases and allow for optimal health at all ages.

FAT-SOLUBLE VITAMINS

Each of the fat-soluble vitamins—A, D, E, and K—is a distinct chemical entity and performs specific functions in the body. These vitamins are absorbed along with dietary fats, requiring the same favorable conditions for

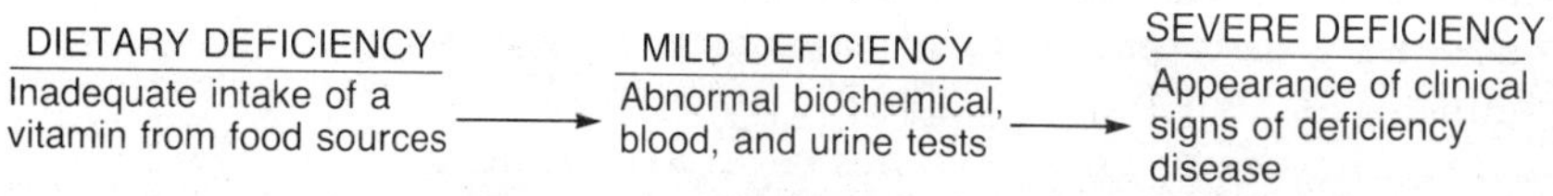

Figure 2–7. The progression of the development of vitamin deficiencies.

their intestinal absorption. Any condition or disease that results in malabsorption of fat will also result in poor absorption of these vitamins. Because these vitamins are, to some extent, stored in the body, deficiencies of these vitamins take longer to develop than those of water-soluble vitamins.

Vitamin A

History. Vitamin A was recognized in 1913, making it the first of the fat-soluble group to be discovered.

Nomenclature. Vitamin A activity is present in some animal and plant compounds. Preformed vitamin A is found in animal products containing *retinol, retinal,* or *retinoic acid.* These compounds possess more vitamin A activity than precursors of vitamin A that are found in plant products. Precursors, or provitamin A compounds, are *alpha, beta* and *gamma carotene.*

Functions. Vitamin A is important in maintaining epithelial cells and mucous membranes throughout the body. It is also a constituent of visual purple, which enables the eye to adapt to dim light. It is necessary for normal growth, development, and reproduction, and has a special role in maintaining the normal growth and development of bones and teeth.

Food sources. Animal food sources of vitamin A include liver, whole milk, butter, cream, fortified milk and milk products, and egg yolk. Plant sources are dark-green and yellow vegetables, and deep-yellow or orange fruits. Fortified margarine is also a source of vitamin A. As a food supplement, fish liver oils also contain vitamin A. Figure 2–8 lists the vitamin A content of some basic four foods.

RDA. The RDA for vitamin A is measured in retinol equivalents (R.E.) and international units (I.U.). The RDA for vitamin A can be found in Table 2-18.

Deficiency. Insufficient amounts of vitamin A may result in nyctalopia (night blindness), keratinized skin (rough, dry skin), dry mucous membranes, and xerophthalmia (an eye disease).

Toxicity. Hypervitaminosis A results from an intake of high daily doses (25,000 I.U. or more) over a period of several months. It occurs when the capacity of the liver to store the vitamin is exceeded. It is corrected by discontinuing the high doses. Symptoms of toxicity include loss of appetite, abnormal skin pigmentation, loss of hair, dry skin, bone and joint pain, and enlarged liver and spleen. It is important to note that carotene in large doses is not toxic, but usually causes yellow coloration of the skin.

Stability. Vitamin A is gradually destroyed by exposure to air, heat, and drying.

Vitamin D

History. Active research on the prevention of rickets began during World War I, although rickets in children had been known for centuries. In 1935, the pure form of the vitamin was first isolated by researchers.

Nomenclature. There are two major compounds with vitamin D activity: *cholecalciferol* (vitamin D_3) and *ergocalciferol* (vitamin D_2). Precursors of vitamin D are *ergosterol* in plants and *7-dehydrocholesterol* in skin.

Functions. Vitamin D aids in the absorption of calcium and phosphorus from the G.I. tract. It is necessary for the regulation of blood levels of calcium and promotes the mineralization of bones and teeth.

Sources. One of the main sources of vitamin D is ultraviolet light. It may also be found in small amounts in foods such as butter, egg yolk, liver, tuna, salmon, and sardines.

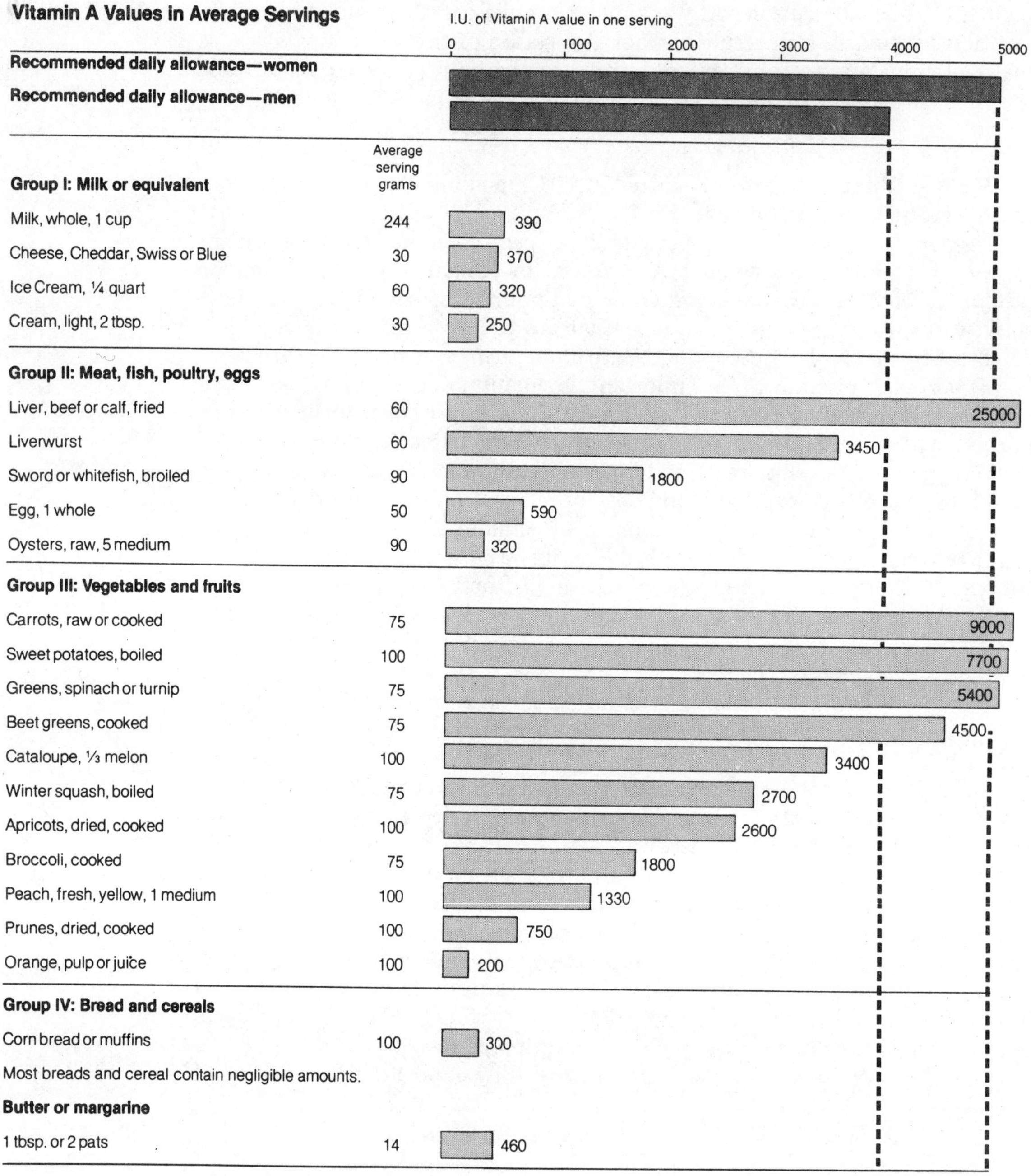

Figure 2–8. Vitamin A value in average servings of foods classified according to the four food groups. (From L. Anderson et al., *Nutrition in Health and Disease,* 17th ed. J. B. Lippincott Co., Philadelphia, 1982.)

RDA. The RDA for vitamin D is measured in micrograms (mcg) and I.U. (see Table 2–18). This requirement can be met by exposure to sunlight or ingestion of vitamin D in food sources or supplements. Ultraviolet light changes precursors of vitamin D in the skin into the active form of the vitamin. Ultraviolet light is cut off by fog, smoke, window glass, and clothing.

Deficiency. Inadequate vitamin D in children results in rickets, character-

TABLE 2–18. RDA for Vitamins A, D, and E*

	Age (years)	Weight (kg)	Weight (lb)	Vitamin A (R.E.)	Vitamin A (I.U.)	Vitamin D (mcg)	Vitamin D (I.U.)	Vitamin E (mg–T.E.)	Vitamin E (I.U.)
Infants	0.0–0.5	6	13	420	1400	10	400	3	4
	0.5–1.0	9	20	400	2000	10	400	4	6
Children	1–3	13	29	400	2000	10	400	5	7
	4–6	20	44	500	2500	10	400	6	9
	7–10	28	62	700	3300	10	400	7	10
Males	11–14	45	99	1000	5000	10	400	8	12
	15–18	66	145	1000	5000	10	400	10	15
	19–22	70	154	1000	5000	7.5	300	10	15
	23–50	70	154	1000	5000	5	200	10	15
	51+	70	154	1000	5000	5	200	10	15
Females	11–14	46	101	800	4000	10	400	8	12
	15–18	55	120	800	4000	10	400	8	12
	19–22	55	120	800	4000	7.5	300	8	12
	23–50	55	120	800	4000	5	200	8	12
	51+	55	120	800	4000	5	200	8	12
Pregnant				1000	5000	10	400	10	15
Lactating				1200	6000	10	400	11	16

*From *Recommended Dietary Allowances*, 9th ed. National Academy of Sciences–National Research Council, Washington, D.C., 1980.

ized by skeletal deformities, soft bones, poor teeth, bowed legs, and enlarged joints. In adults, vitamin D deficiency causes osteomalacia, or decalcified soft bones.

Toxicity. Hypervitaminosis D results from an intake of high daily doses of this vitamin (20,000 to 100,000 I.U.). These high doses manifest themselves in calcification of soft tissues, high blood levels of calcium, and kidney stones. Symptoms of hypervitaminosis D include loss of appetite, nausea, weight loss, growth failure, and fatigue. Mild toxicity can be seen with much lower amounts of vitamin D ingestion.

Stability. Vitamin D is resistant to heat, aging, and storage.

Vitamin E

History. In the 1920s, vitamin E was recognized as essential for reproduction in rats. Since the role of this vitamin is still not well defined today, it has become the target of many unscientific claims.

Nomenclature. Compounds possessing vitamin E activity are *tocopherols.*

Functions. As previously noted, the precise role of vitamin E is still not clearly defined. It is known, however, to prevent oxidative destruction of vitamin A in the intestine, to protect red blood cells from rupture (hemolysis), and to participate in the maintenance of normal cell membranes by reducing the oxidation of polyunsaturated fatty acids (PUFA).

Food sources. Vitamin E is widely distributed in common foods. Some of the best sources of vitamin E include wheat germ, leafy vegetables, vegetable oils, shortening, margarine, legumes, nuts, and whole-grain cereals.

RDA. Measurements are expressed as alpha-tocopherol equivalents (T.E.) or I.U. (see Table 2–18). The requirement is related to the intake of PUFA. Diets high in PUFA are also high in vitamin E.

Deficiency. There is no disease specific to vitamin E deficiency. The possibility of a deficiency is unlikely unless the diet is grossly inadequate in several nutrients.

Toxicity. Vitamin E has not been shown to be toxic with the ingestion of large amounts. However, there is no medical justification for the use of large doses. There are many claims about the benefits of vitamin E, but they are not scientifically proven at the present time.

Stability. Vitamin E is resistant to methods of processing and cooking. It is destroyed by oxidation and ultraviolet light.

Vitamin K

History. In 1935, vitamin K was first recognized as the antihemorrhagic factor.

Nomenclature. The two major compounds exhibiting vitamin K activity are: *menadione* and *phylloquinone.*

Functions. Vitamin K is necessary for the formation of prothrombin and other factors necessary to blood clotting.

Sources. Vitamin K is found in dark-green leafy vegetables and, in addition, is synthesized by intestinal bacteria.

RDA. The RDA for this vitamin is unknown.

Deficiency. Hemorrhage (excessive bleeding) will result if vitamin K synthesis and intake is low. Because newborn infants do not have the intestinal bacteria necessary for its production, some may have to be given vitamin K preparation to prevent hemorrhage. Deficiency of this vitamin is unlikely in the healthy person.

Antagonists of vitamin K, coumarin products, are used to treat circulatory diseases that form blood clots.

Stability. Vitamin K is resistant to heat and air. It is destroyed by sunlight, strong acids, and alkali.

WATER-SOLUBLE VITAMINS

The Vitamin B Complex

History. The term vitamin B complex refers to all water-soluble vitamins except ascorbic acid (vitamin C). Vitamin B was the first of this group to be discovered and was known as the "antiberiberi" or "antineuritic" vitamin or simply as vitamin B. Thiamine was the first to be obtained in pure form and is known as vitamin B_1. With further study, vitamin B proved to be not a single substance but a combination of a number of factors, each one of which was given a letter or a descriptive term or, later, a chemical designation as its chemical nature became known.

Nomenclature. Twelve factors in the vitamin B complex are recognized today. RDA have been established for six: thiamine (B_1), riboflavin (B_2—formerly G), niacin (nicotinic acid), B_6, B_{12}, and folacin (see Table 2–19). Important functions in the body have been assigned to biotin, choline, and pantothenic acid, but no definite daily allowances are established, although estimated safe and adequate intakes are now given. It is thought that the amount needed daily in each case will be met by the average daily diet.

Functions. All of the 12 substances now recognized in the vitamin B complex are essential to nutrition in one or more ways and must be supplied in the daily diet. Some are available in pure form. Several are components of one or more coenzyme systems which function as "catalysts" in the use of nutrients for energy and building and repair processes. All are closely interrelated.

TABLE 2–19. RDA for Water-Soluble Vitamins*

	Age (years)	Weight (kg)	Weight (lb)	Thiamine (mg)	Riboflavin (mg)	Niacin (mg)	Vitamin B_6 (mg)	Vitamin B_{12} (mcg)	Folacin (mcg)	Ascorbic Acid (mg)
Infants	0.0–0.5	6	13	0.3	0.4	6	0.3	0.5	30	35
	0.5–1.0	9	20	0.5	0.6	8	0.6	1.5	45	35
Children	1–3	13	29	0.7	0.8	9	0.9	2.0	100	45
	4–6	20	44	0.9	1.0	11	1.3	2.5	200	45
	7–10	28	62	1.2	1.2	16	1.6	3.0	300	45
Males	11–14	45	99	1.4	1.6	18	1.8	3.0	400	50
	15–18	66	145	1.4	1.7	18	2.0	3.0	400	60
	19–22	70	154	1.5	1.7	19	2.2	3.0	400	60
	23–50	70	154	1.4	1.6	18	2.2	3.0	400	60
	51+	70	154	1.2	1.4	16	2.2	3.0	400	60
Females	11–14	46	101	1.1	1.3	15	1.8	3.0	400	60
	15–18	55	120	1.1	1.3	14	2.0	3.0	400	60
	19–22	55	120	1.1	1.3	14	2.0	3.0	400	60
	23–50	55	120	1.0	1.2	13	2.0	3.0	400	60
	51+	55	120	1.0	1.2	13	2.0	3.0	400	60
Pregnant				+0.4	+0.3	+2	+0.6	+1.0	+400	+20
Lactating				+0.5	+0.5	+5	+0.5	+1.0	+100	+40

*From *Recommended Dietary Allowances*, 9th ed. National Academy of Sciences–National Research Council, Washington, D.C., 1980.

Deficiency. A lack of vitamins of the B complex is one of the widespread forms of malnutrition. Because of the similar distribution of the B vitamins in foods, a deficiency of several factors is observed more often than a deficiency of a single factor. The interrelationship of many of these vitamins in life processes means that signs of a deficiency are often similar when the diet lacks any one of several factors (see Fig. 2–9 A and B). Many physiological and pathological stresses influence the need for the B vitamins. Needs are increased during pregnancy and lactation, growth, fevers, hyperthyroidism, injury, and before and after surgery.

Stability. Thiamine is the most easily destroyed because of water solubility, dehydration, and cooking. Its destruction is speeded by the presence of alkali, copper, and iron and the release of enzymes by cutting raw foods. Foods cooked properly for thiamine retention retain other water-soluble vitamins. Riboflavin is light sensitive. Amounts of riboflavin eaten in excess of needs are eliminated in urine; there is very little body storage.

Thiamine (B_1)

The requirement for thiamine is small, but important, and is based on the Kcal requirement. The RDA is stated in milligrams and can be found in Table 2–19. A regular daily supply is needed, since the body stores little, and amounts eaten in excess of needs are eliminated in the urine.

Functions. Thiamine plays a role in carbohydrate metabolism. It promotes a good appetite and good functioning of the digestive tract. It helps

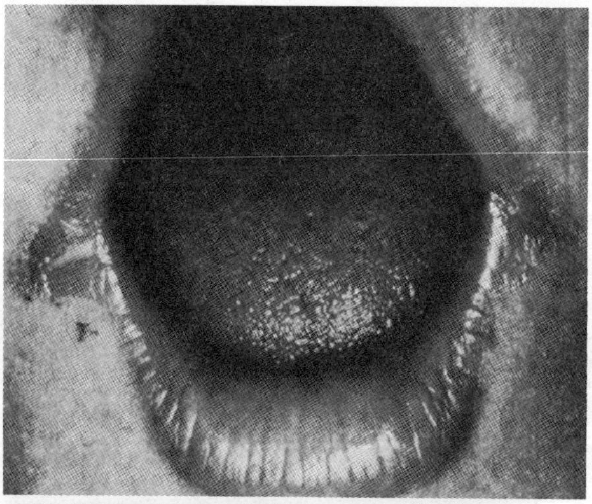

A

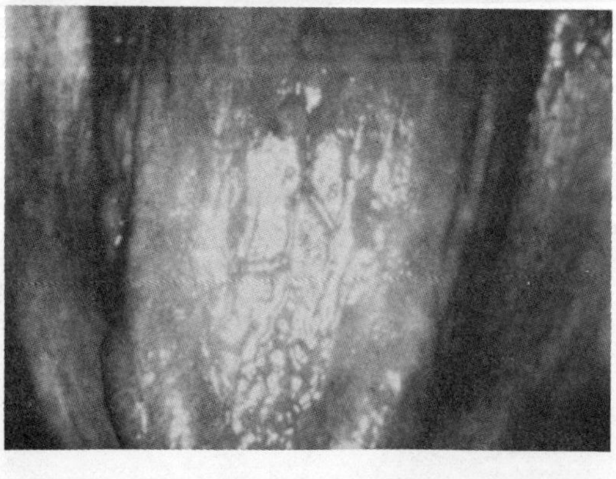

B

Figure 2–9. Vitamin B deficiencies. *A*, Angular cheilosis due to vitamin B-complex deficiency. *B*, Depapillation of the tongue from the same causation. (From H. A. Schneider et al., *Nutritional Support of Medical Practice.* Harper and Row Publishers, Inc., Hagerstown, Md., 1977.)

the nervous system, heart, and muscles function properly. It is needed throughout life for tissue functioning and in increased amounts during pregnancy and lactation.

Sources. Many foods contain small amounts of thiamine. It is found in whole-grain and enriched flour and bread, meats (especially organ meats), fish, and poultry. Pork contains three times as much thiamine as other meats. Dry beans and peas and peanuts also contain thiamine, and small amounts can be found in milk and eggs. Brewer's yeast and wheat germ are also sources of thiamine. Figure 2–10 lists the thiamine content of some basic four foods.

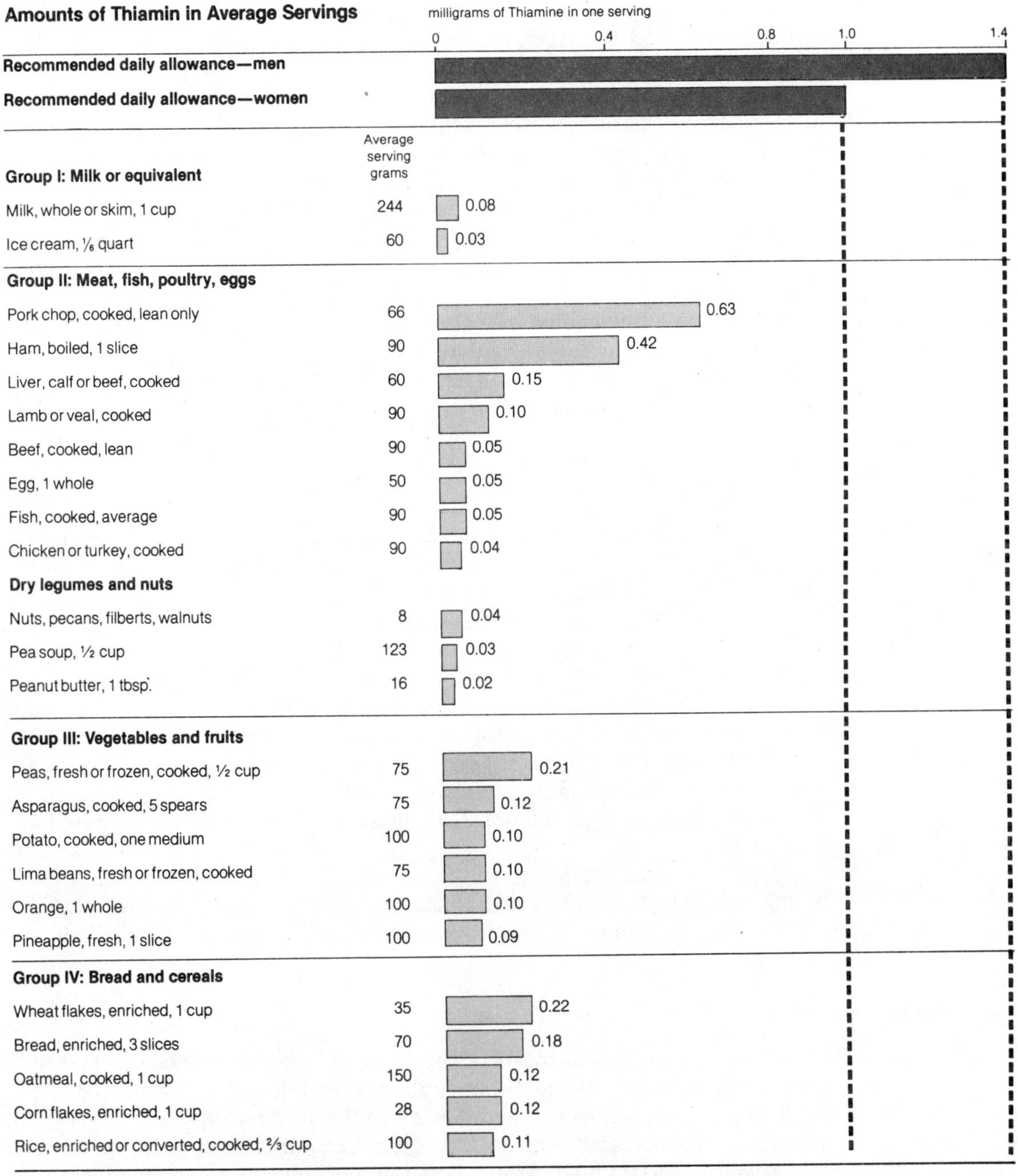

Figure 2–10. Thiamine in average servings of foods classified according to the four food groups. (From L. Anderson et al., *Nutrition in Health and Disease*, 17th ed. J. B. Lippincott Co., Philadelphia, 1982.)

Deficiency. Insufficient thiamine intake may result in polyneuritis, beriberi, fatigue, depression, poor appetite, poor functioning of the intestinal tract, and nervous instability.

Stability. Thiamine is lost in cooking unless the cooking water is retained and used. Alkali (baking soda), high temperatures, and long cooking all destroy thiamine.

Riboflavin (Vitamin B_2)

The requirement for riboflavin is also related to Kcal needs. It is stated in milligrams, and the RDA can be found in Table 2–19. The excess intake over needs is eliminated in the urine, and thus a regular supply is required.

Functions. Riboflavin is essential for certain enzyme systems that aid in metabolism of carbohydrates, proteins, and fats. It also promotes general well-being and is important for healthy eyes, skin, lips, and tongue.

Sources. Riboflavin can be found in milk, cheese, eggs, green leafy vegetables, organ meats (liver, kidney, and heart), dry yeast, peanuts and peanut butter. Adequate consumption of milk is important in maintaining an adequate intake of riboflavin. Figure 2–11 lists the riboflavin content of some basic four foods.

Deficiency. Inadequate riboflavin results in cheilosis (see Fig. 2–9A), tongue inflammation, scaling and burning skin, and sensitive eyes.

Stability. Riboflavin is resistant to heat, acid, and oxidation. Light, however, will destroy riboflavin.

Niacin (Nicotinic Acid)

Niacin requirements are related to caloric intake and are stated in milligrams (see Table 2–19). The excess intake over needs is eliminated in the urine, and thus a steady intake is required.

Functions. Niacin functions as part of two important enzymes that regulate energy metabolism. It promotes good physical and mental health and helps maintain the health of the skin, tongue, and digestive system.

Sources. Good food sources of niacin are organ meats (kidney, liver, and heart), other meats, poultry, fish, whole-grain and enriched cereal products, meat drippings, and brewer's yeast. Niacin can also be synthesized in the body from an amino acid, tryptophan, in protein. Precursors of niacin can be found in milk and eggs. Figure 2–12 lists the niacin content of some basic four foods.

Deficiency. Inadequate niacin intake can result in pellagra with skin and mouth manifestations, gastrointestinal disturbances, and mental disturbances.

Stability. Niacin is resistant to heat, oxidation, light, acid, and alkali.

Other B-Complex Vitamins

Vitamin B_6

Three interrelated substances—pyridoxine (plants), pyridoxal, and pyridoxamine (animal products)—are collectively known as vitamin B_6. The RDA is stated in milligrams and can be found in Table 2–19. The need for vitamin B_6 is increased with high-protein diets, pregnancy, certain tuberculosis therapy, certain medications, and some of the contraceptive pills.

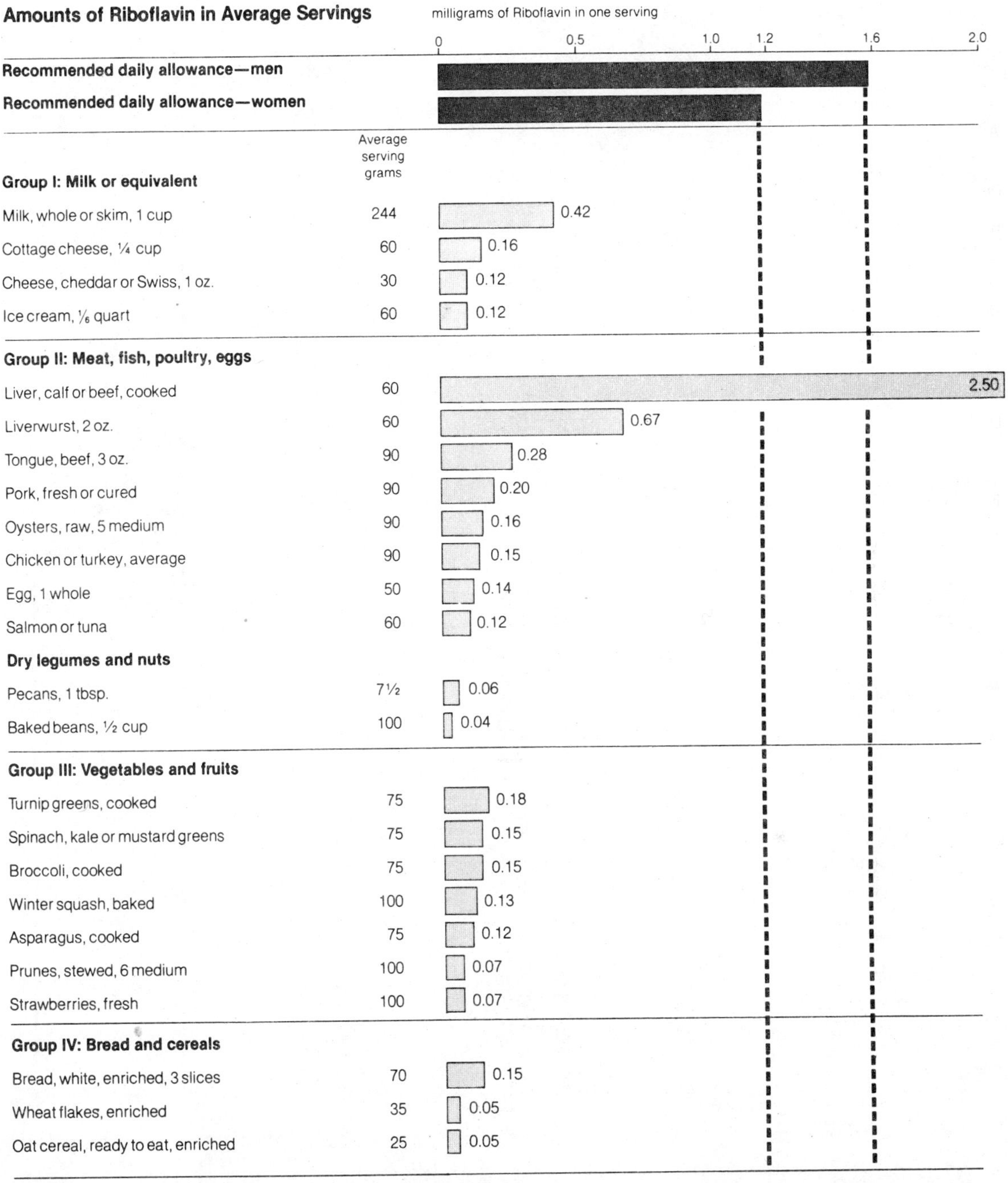
Amounts of Riboflavin in Average Servings
milligrams of Riboflavin in one serving
0
0.5
1.0
1.2
1.6
2.0
Recommended daily allowance—men
Recommended daily allowance—women
Average serving grams
Group I: Milk or equivalent
Milk, whole or skim, 1 cup
244
0.42
Cottage cheese, ¼ cup
60
0.16
Cheese, cheddar or Swiss, 1 oz.
30
0.12
Ice cream, ⅙ quart
60
0.12
Group II: Meat, fish, poultry, eggs
Liver, calf or beef, cooked
60
2.50
Liverwurst, 2 oz.
60
0.67
Tongue, beef, 3 oz.
90
0.28
Pork, fresh or cured
90
0.20
Oysters, raw, 5 medium
90
0.16
Chicken or turkey, average
90
0.15
Egg, 1 whole
50
0.14
Salmon or tuna
60
0.12
Dry legumes and nuts
Pecans, 1 tbsp.
7½
0.06
Baked beans, ½ cup
100
0.04
Group III: Vegetables and fruits
Turnip greens, cooked
75
0.18
Spinach, kale or mustard greens
75
0.15
Broccoli, cooked
75
0.15
Winter squash, baked
100
0.13
Asparagus, cooked
75
0.12
Prunes, stewed, 6 medium
100
0.07
Strawberries, fresh
100
0.07
Group IV: Bread and cereals
Bread, white, enriched, 3 slices
70
0.15
Wheat flakes, enriched
35
0.05
Oat cereal, ready to eat, enriched
25
0.05

Figure 2–11. Riboflavin in average servings of foods classified according to the four food groups. (From L. Anderson et al., *Nutrition in Health and Disease*, 17th ed., J. B. Lippincott Co., Philadelphia, 1982.)

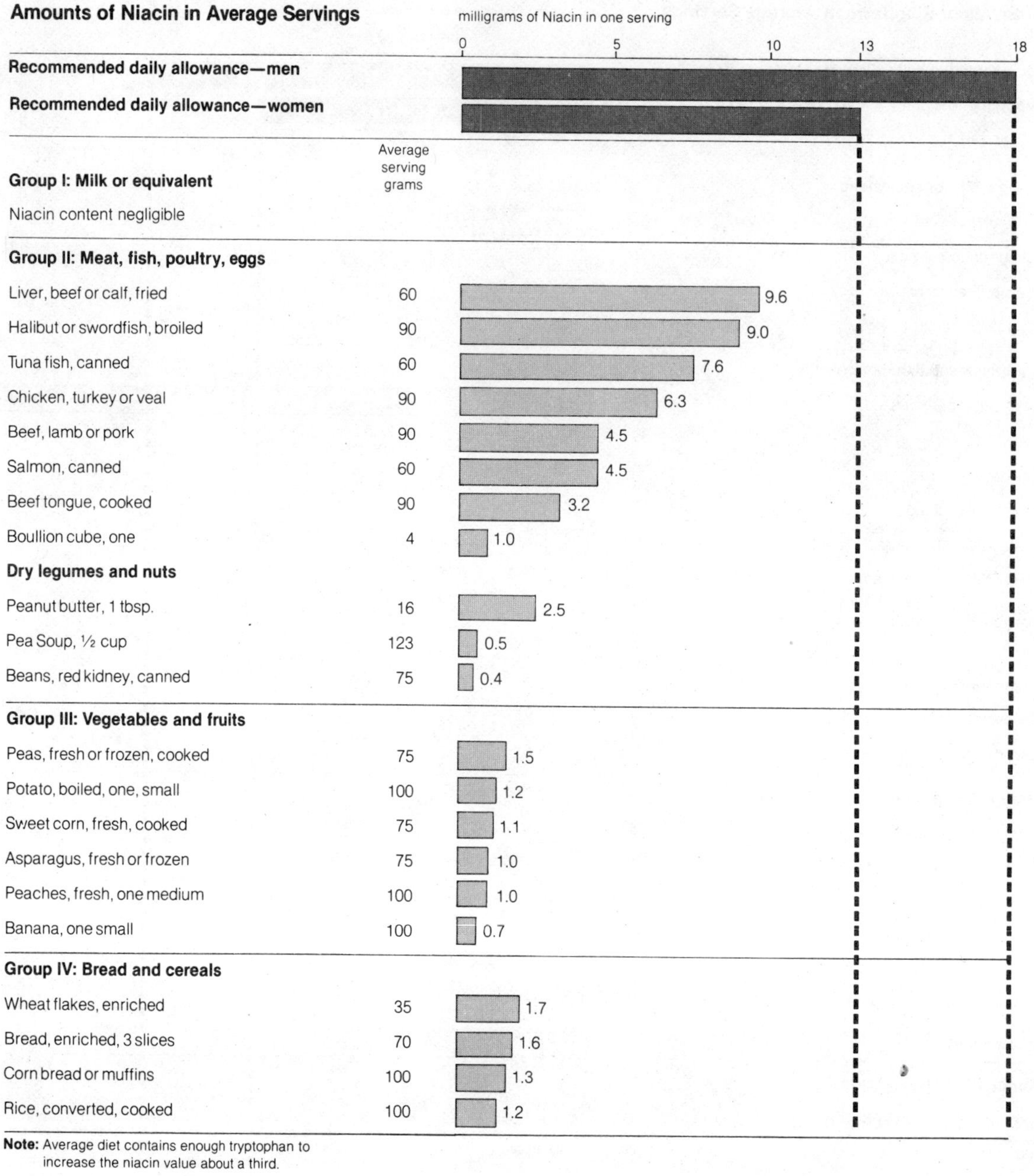
Amounts of Niacin in Average Servings
milligrams of Niacin in one serving
0
5
10
13
18
Recommended daily allowance—men
Recommended daily allowance—women
Average serving grams
Group I: Milk or equivalent
Niacin content negligible
Group II: Meat, fish, poultry, eggs
Liver, beef or calf, fried 60 9.6
Halibut or swordfish, broiled 90 9.0
Tuna fish, canned 60 7.6
Chicken, turkey or veal 90 6.3
Beef, lamb or pork 90 4.5
Salmon, canned 60 4.5
Beef tongue, cooked 90 3.2
Boullion cube, one 4 1.0
Dry legumes and nuts
Peanut butter, 1 tbsp. 16 2.5
Pea Soup, ½ cup 123 0.5
Beans, red kidney, canned 75 0.4
Group III: Vegetables and fruits
Peas, fresh or frozen, cooked 75 1.5
Potato, boiled, one, small 100 1.2
Sweet corn, fresh, cooked 75 1.1
Asparagus, fresh or frozen 75 1.0
Peaches, fresh, one medium 100 1.0
Banana, one small 100 0.7
Group IV: Bread and cereals
Wheat flakes, enriched 35 1.7
Bread, enriched, 3 slices 70 1.6
Corn bread or muffins 100 1.3
Rice, converted, cooked 100 1.2
Note: Average diet contains enough tryptophan to increase the niacin value about a third.

Figure 2–12. Niacin in average servings of foods classified according to the four food groups. (From L. Anderson et al., *Nutrition in Health and Disease*, 17th ed., J. B. Lippincott, Philadelphia, 1982.)

Functions. Its major function is in protein and amino acid metabolism, but it is also of importance in energy metabolism. It may also be of importance in red blood cell regeneration and normal nervous system functioning.

Sources. The three forms are present in varying amounts in different foods. A diet meeting the recommended amounts of food in the four food groups will meet the needs for vitamin B_6.

Stability. Vitamin B_6 is resistant to heat, light, and oxidation. High heat is likely to destroy it, however.

Vitamin B_{12} (Cobalamin)

Cobalt is an essential part of vitamin B_{12}. The RDA is stated in micrograms and can be found in Table 2–19.

Functions. Vitamin B_{12} is essential for normal function of all cells, particularly those of the bone marrow, the nervous system, and the gastrointestinal tract. It is important in energy metabolism, especially folic acid metabolism.

Sources. Vitamin B_{12} is present mostly in foods of animal origin, bound to protein. There is relatively little in vegetables. Kidneys and liver are high in B_{12}, with only moderate amounts in other meats. Milk, most cheeses, shellfish, most fish, whole egg, and egg yolk are all additional sources of vitamin B_{12}.

Deficiency. Pernicious anemia is caused by a lack of "intrinsic factor," a glycoprotein that attaches to vitamin B_{12} to aid its absorption.

Stability. Severe heating of meat and meat products is detrimental to vitamin B_{12} content.

Folacin

The active form of folacin is folic acid, which is formed from folacin by vitamin C. The RDA is stated in micrograms (see Table 2–19).

Functions. Folacin functions in the formation of red blood cells and in the normal gastrointestinal tract. It aids in the metabolism of protein and is readily absorbed by the gastrointestinal tract and stored primarily in the liver.

Sources. Folacin can be found in a wide variety of foods of animal and plant origin, particularly glandular meats, yeast, dark-green vegetables, dry beans, whole grains, peanuts, walnuts, and lentils.

Stability. Folacin is unstable to heat and oxidation.

Choline

Choline, another of the water-soluble B-complex vitamins, is a constituent of several compounds necessary in certain aspects of nerve function and lipid metabolism. No RDA has been established, and no deficiency disease has been demonstrated in humans. Mixed diets are estimated to provide adults with 400 to 900 mg of choline daily, and such diets are evidently adequate. In addition, the body can synthesize choline from methionine (an amino acid).

Pantothenic Acid

Pantothenic acid is a B vitamin that is an essential constituent of complex enzymes involved in fatty acid metabolism and synthesis of certain products. It is widely distributed in foods, occurring abundantly in animal sources, whole-grain cereals, and legumes. The estimated safe and adequate intake is 4 to 7 mg daily; the higher level is suggested for pregnant and lactating women. Dietary deficiencies are unlikely, but marginal deficiencies may exist in generally malnourished individuals, along with deficiency of other B-complex vitamins. The usual dietary intake is between 5 and 20 mg daily.

Biotin

This B-complex vitamin is essential for activity of many enzyme systems. It is widely distributed in nature, bound to protein in foods and tissues. It plays a central role in fatty acid synthesis as well as participating in several metabolic reactions. The estimated safe and adequate intake is 100 to 200 mcg daily for adults.

The body's requirements for these B-complex vitamins are increased by pregnancy, lactation, and other stressful conditions, including a variety of diseases and alcohol consumption. A deficiency of these vitamins causes certain types of anemias that result in a sore mouth and gastrointestinal disturbances that may, in turn, cause inadequate food intake, impaired absorption, excessive body demands, and metabolic abnormalities.

Vitamin C

History. Scurvy has been known to man since before the 19th century. Its relationship to vitamin C, however, was not recognized until the 20th century. On long sea voyages outbreaks of scurvy were frequent unless lemons, limes, or other fresh fruits and vegetables were included in the supplies. In 1932, vitamin C was first isolated in the pure crystalline form.

Nomenclature. Vitamin C occurs naturally in two forms: *ascorbic acid* and *dehydroascorbic acid.* Both are active forms of the vitamin.

Functions. Vitamin C performs a variety of functions. It aids in the formation and maintenance of intracellular cement substance of body tissue and is important for tooth dentin, bones, cartilage, connective tissue, and blood vessels. It is thought to protect the body against infections, and helps in wound healing and recovery following operations. It participates in the formation of red blood cells in the bone marrow, in changing folacin to folinic acid, and in the absorption of iron in the intestine.

Sources. Fruits and vegetables are the main sources of vitamin C. They contain more of the vitamin when they are fresh. Foremost among these are citrus fruits, tomatoes, strawberries, cantaloupes, and some of the green leafy vegetables. Additional sources of vitamin C are green peppers, broccoli, raw greens, cabbage, and newly harvested potatoes if cooked properly. Figure 2–13 lists the vitamin C content of some of the basic four foods.

RDA. The RDA for vitamin C has been set at levels that maintain normal plasma concentrations associated with normal health. Higher levels may be necessary during conditions of stress. Smoking as well as certain drugs will increase the excretion of vitamin C (see Table 2–19).

Deficiency. Inadequate vitamin C intake may eventually lead to scurvy, a disease characterized by swollen and bleeding gums, loose teeth, and ruptures of small blood vessels (see Fig. 2–14).

Toxicity. Vitamin C is not toxic in high doses. However, rebound scurvy

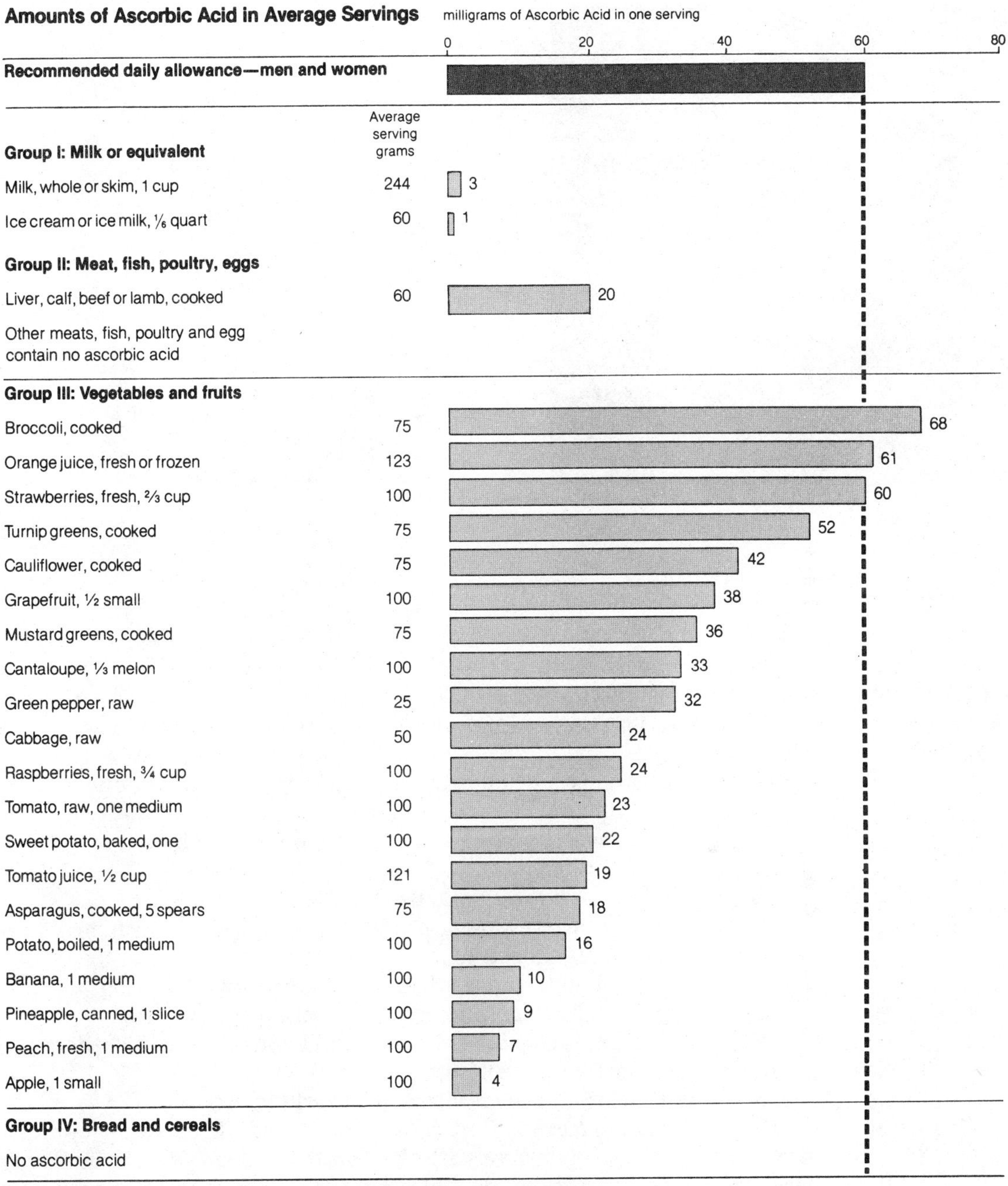

Amounts of Ascorbic Acid in Average Servings
milligrams of Ascorbic Acid in one serving
0
20
40
60
80
Recommended daily allowance—men and women
Average serving grams
Group I: Milk or equivalent
Milk, whole or skim, 1 cup
244
3
Ice cream or ice milk, ⅙ quart
60
1
Group II: Meat, fish, poultry, eggs
Liver, calf, beef or lamb, cooked
60
20
Other meats, fish, poultry and egg contain no ascorbic acid
Group III: Vegetables and fruits
Broccoli, cooked
75
68
Orange juice, fresh or frozen
123
61
Strawberries, fresh, ⅔ cup
100
60
Turnip greens, cooked
75
52
Cauliflower, cooked
75
42
Grapefruit, ½ small
100
38
Mustard greens, cooked
75
36
Cantaloupe, ⅓ melon
100
33
Green pepper, raw
25
32
Cabbage, raw
50
24
Raspberries, fresh, ¾ cup
100
24
Tomato, raw, one medium
100
23
Sweet potato, baked, one
100
22
Tomato juice, ½ cup
121
19
Asparagus, cooked, 5 spears
75
18
Potato, boiled, 1 medium
100
16
Banana, 1 medium
100
10
Pineapple, canned, 1 slice
100
9
Peach, fresh, 1 medium
100
7
Apple, 1 small
100
4
Group IV: Bread and cereals
No ascorbic acid

Figure 2–13. Ascorbic acid in average servings of foods classified according to the four food groups. (From L. Anderson et al., *Nutrition in Health and Disease*, 17th ed., J. B. Lippincott Co., Philadelphia, 1982.)

may occur if the body has been accustomed to high blood plasma levels and the dose is discontinued. Gradual decrease from high doses is recommended.

Much more research is needed in this area as well as with other vitamins. However, megadoses of vitamins are not seen at the present as having any substantial benefits.

Stability. Vitamin C is a very unstable vitamin. It is destroyed by high temperatures, long cooking times, oxygen and alkali.

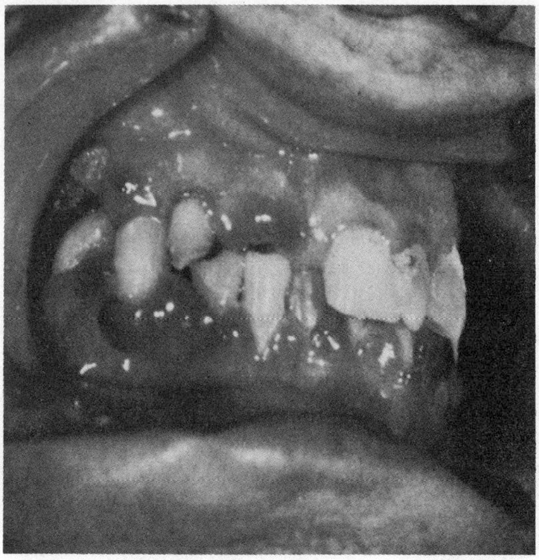

Figure 2–14. Scorbutic gingivitis. (From H. A. Schneider et al., *Nutritional Support of Medical Practice,* Harper and Row Publishers, Inc., Hagerstown, Md., 1977.)

WHAT FACTORS AFFECT VITAMIN VALUES OF FOODS?

There are many factors that affect both the quality and quantity of vitamins in food. The following are the most important.

1. The variety of food. Some foods have more or less of a certain vitamin.
2. Soil variations and climate. The same food grown in one area may have more or less vitamin value than the same food grown elsewhere.
3. Degree of maturity. Some foods have more of a vitamin when underripe; others when ripe.
4. Type of diet fed the animal used as food.
5. Storage after harvesting or production. Improper storage may have a destructive effect on vitamins.
6. Freezing. Some vitamins are lost in preliminary blanching.
7. Drying. Certain vitamin losses occur during this process.
8. Canning. Although some vitamins will be lost in canning, there is less loss in acid food than in nonacid food.
9. Cooking of food affects vitamins in various ways.
10. Antivitamin factors. Certain substances may inactivate vitamins, be antagonistic to them, interfere with their absorption and metabolism or synthesis in the body. Antibiotics and other drugs may kill intestinal bacteria which help in the synthesis. Oxidation may also be destructive.

On the other hand, there are favorable food handling practices that will enhance vitamin retention.

1. Store vegetables properly to avoid wilting and drying out, which cause loss of vitamin A.
2. Cook vegetables whole as often as possible. Cutting releases oxidative enzymes and increases cut surfaces where water-soluble vitamins leach out.
3. Use cooking water and canned food juices to conserve soluble nutrients.

4. Avoid use of baking soda in cooking vegetables, as it is destructive to thiamine and ascorbic acid. Also avoid long cooking for the same reason.
5. Store fats properly to prevent rancidity, a destructive factor for vitamin A.
6. Keep milk in glass containers away from light, which is destructive to riboflavin.
7. Use drippings when cooking meat to conserve thiamine and niacin.
8. Keep fruit juices covered and cold to prevent oxygen from destroying ascorbic acid.
9. Don't stir while cooking foods containing ascorbic acid as oxygen destroys vitamin C.
10. Cook vegetables covered, quickly, and just until fork-tender. Store leftovers covered and cold. Reheating causes further loss of vitamins.

IS IT NECESSARY TO USE VITAMIN SUPPLEMENTS?

Nutrition scientists and dietitians agree that if a healthy person chooses a diet from the four food groups, both an adequate supply of essential vitamins and also the right amounts of the other essential nutrients will be provided. Therefore it is not necessary to supplement a well-balanced diet with vitamin pills. Not only is it nutritionally advantageous to purchase one's vitamins in the foods from the supermarket rather than in the drug store, it is much more economical as well.

Vitamins are not a cure-all for the many ailments for which they are advertised: neither are they a substitute for good eating habits. Some vitamins taken in excess may be toxic. Others taken in excess are excreted, placing an added burden on the kidneys as well as being a waste of money for something not usable.

If for some reason the amount or quality of food must be restricted or if absorption from the intestinal tract is impaired, vitamin supplementation may be indicated. This is a medical problem, however, and should be treated by a physician.

If a person insists on taking a vitamin supplement for added nutritional "insurance," it should be one approximating the RDA.[7] Megadoses of vitamins are not recommended.

Study Questions

1. Name several reasons why vitamins are body regulators.
2. Why must foods containing vitamins be eaten daily? Which vitamins can be stored? Which ones cannot be stored?
3. What is meant by the vitamin B complex? What foods need to be included in the diet to insure an adequate amount of the B-complex vitamins?
4. List the foods in the Basic Four Food Groups with the correct servings that will help meet your vitamin requirements. Why is special emphasis placed on whole-grain or enriched cereals and breads, whole milk, meat, dark-green and yellow vegetables, and citrus fruits?
5. Name several procedures in food care, preparation, and cooking that will help retain the water-soluble vitamins.

Before beginning the study of nutrient utilization, refer to Table 2–20 for an overall summary of the major nutrients necessary for health. Each of these has been previously discussed in this chapter.

TABLE 2–20. Summary of Nutrients For Health

Nutrient	Important Sources of Nutrient	Some Major Physiological Functions		
		Provide Energy	*Build and Maintain Body Cells*	*Regulate Body Processes*
Protein	Meat, poultry, fish Dried beans and peas Egg Cheese Milk	Supplies 4 calories per gram.	Constitutes part of the structure of every cell, such as muscle, blood, and bone; supports growth and maintains healthy body cells.	Constitutes part of enzymes, some hormones and body fluids, and antibodies that increase resistance to infection.
Carbohydrate	Cereal Potatoes Dried beans Corn Bread Sugar	Supplies 4 calories per gram. Major source of energy for central nervous system.	Supplies energy so protein can be used for growth and maintenance of body cells.	Unrefined products supply fiber—complex carbohydrates in fruits, vegetables, and whole grains—for regular elimination. Assists in fat utilization.
Fat	Shortening, oil Butter, margarine Salad dressing Sausages	Supplies 9 calories per gram.	Constitutes part of the structure of every cell. Supplies essential fatty acids.	Provides and carries fat-soluble vitamins (A, D, E, and K).
Vitamin A (Retinol)	Liver Carrots Sweet potatoes Greens Butter, margarine		Assists formation and maintenance of skin and mucous membranes that line body cavities and tracts, such as nasal passages and intestinal tract, thus increasing resistance to infection.	Functions in visual processes and forms visual purple, thus promoting healthy eye tissues and eye adaptation in dim light.
Vitamin C (Ascorbic Acid)	Broccoli Orange Grapefruit Papaya Mango Strawberries		Forms cementing substances, such as collagen, that hold body cells together, thus strengthening blood vessels, hastening healing of wounds and bones, and increasing resistance to infection.	Aids utilization of iron.
Thiamin (B_1)	Lean pork Nuts Fortified cereal products	Aids in utilization of energy.		Functions as part of a coenzyme to promote the utilization of carbohydrate. Promotes normal appetite. Contributes to normal functioning of nervous system.

Riboflavin (B_2)	Liver Milk Yogurt Cottage cheese	Aids in utilization of energy.		Functions as part of a coenzyme in the production of energy within body cells. Promotes healthy skin, eyes, and clear vision.
Niacin	Liver Meat, poultry, fish Peanuts Fortified cereal products	Aids in utilization of energy.		Functions as part of coenzyme in fat synthesis, tissue respiration, and utilization of carbohydrate. Promotes healthy skin, nerves, and digestive tract. Aids digestion and fosters normal appetite.
Calcium	Milk, yogurt Cheese Sardines and salmon with bones Collard, kale, mustard, and turnip greens		Combines with other minerals within a protein framework to give structure and strength to bones and teeth.	Assists in blood clotting. Functions in normal muscle contraction and relaxation, and normal nerve transmission.
Iron	Enriched farina Prune juice Liver Dried beans and peas Red meat	Aids in utilization of energy.	Combines with protein to form hemoglobin, the red substance in blood that carries oxygen to and carbon dioxide from the cells. Prevents nutritional anemia and its accompanying fatigue. Increases resistance to infection.	Functions as part of enzymes involved in tissue respiration.

*From *Guide to Good Eating*, 4th ed. Courtesy of the National Dairy Council, Rosemont, Ill., 1978.

Utilization of Nutrients (Digestion, Absorption, Metabolism)

HOW ARE FOODS PREPARED FOR BODY USE?

Digestion. Digestion is the change of food from complex to simpler forms and from an insoluble to a soluble state in the digestive tract to facilitate absorption through intestinal walls into the circulation for eventual use by the body (Fig. 2–15).

The processes of digestion occur simultaneously:

1. *Physical* (mechanical). Breaks up food into small particles (chewing in mouth), mixes it with digestive juices (churning in the stomach action), and propels it through the digestive tract (peristaltic action).

2. *Chemical.* Enzymes in digestive juices change food nutrients—carbohydrates, fats, and proteins—into simple soluble forms that can be absorbed. Each enzyme has a specific action and optimal conditions under which it acts. The name of each group of enzymes ends in *-ase*: amylases act on starch; lipases on fat; proteases on protein. Other chemical substances such as hydrochloric acid (HCl) and mucin in the gastric secretion, bile from the liver excreted into the duodenum, and certain hormones assist in the physical and chemical processes.

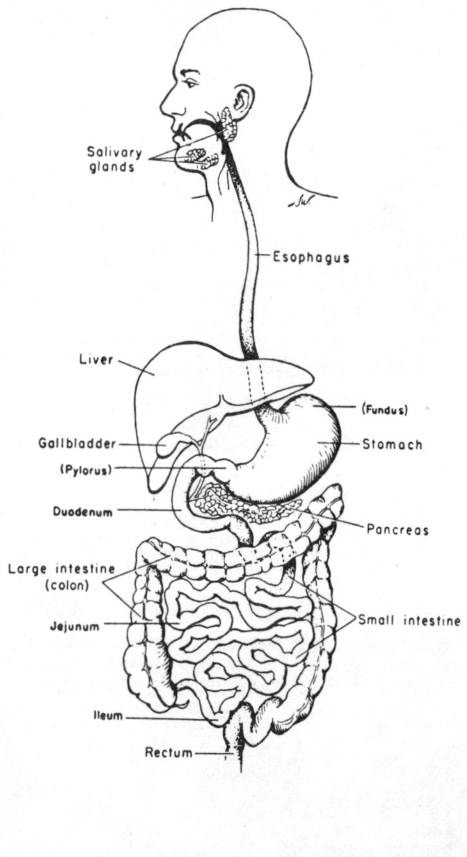

Figure 2–15. Alimentary Canal and Digestive Juices:

Mouth	Saliva
Stomach	Gastric, HCl
Intestine (small)	Intestinal juices
Liver	Bile (no enzymes)
Pancreas	Pancreatic

Pancreatic and intestinal juices and bile combine in intestinal tract.

3. *Results.* Carbohydrates are changed to simple sugars; fats to fatty acids and glycerol; and proteins to amino acids. Water, simple sugars, salts, and vitamins require no digestion.

Absorption. Absorption is the passage of soluble digested food materials through the intestinal walls into the blood, either directly or by way of the lymph, by means of osmosis. Absorbed materials are carried by blood to various organs and tissues to be used as needed. The greater part of absorption takes place in small intestine, lower duodenum and upper jejunum. Tiny fingerlike projections called villi, containing small capillaries and lacteals (part of the lymph circulation), line the intestinal wall. Simple sugars, amino acids, a few fatty acids, minerals, and water-soluble vitamins reach the general circulation through the capillaries. The rest of the fatty acids, certain fat molecules, and fat-soluble vitamins reach the lymph circulation through the lacteals. Absorbed materials are carried by blood to various organs and tissues to be used as needed. Water is also absorbed from the large intestine. The body is able to digest and absorb about 90 to 98 per cent of an average mixed diet.

Metabolism. Metabolism is the sum total of the physical and chemical processes that take place in the body using digested nutrients (simple sugars, amino acids, fatty acids, glycerol). Metabolism includes both anabolism, building of new tissue (constructive), and catabolism, breakdown of substances with the release of energy (destructive).

WHAT ROLE IS PLAYED BY EACH PART OF THE DIGESTIVE TRACT?

Mouth

Mechanical functions. Chewing reduces large food particles to smaller ones while saliva moistens food and prepares it for swallowing.

Chemical functions. Cooked starch is changed first to dextrin and then to maltose by the salivary enzyme, ptyalin (amylase), in the mouth.

Esophagus

Mechanical function. Peristaltic constrictions send food from the mouth into the fundus, or the storage portion of the stomach.

Stomach

Mechanical functions. The fundus of the stomach acts as a temporary storage place for food. It is kept in motion by the muscular walls of the stomach to bring it into contact with the gastric juice secreted by stomach cells. Once the food is reduced to a semiliquid state (chyme), it is passed from the stomach to the small intestine. The presence of food in the stomach stimulates functions of the digestive tract. The stomach empties in two to six hours after a meal.

Chemical functions. In the stomach, complex proteins are partially digested by the gastric juice enzyme pepsin (protease). Milk protein is coagulated by the gastric juice enzyme renin, and then partially digested by pepsin. Emulsified fats are digested to fatty acids and glycerol by the gastric juice enzyme lipase. Hydrochloric acid aids these digestive enzymes and increases the solubility of calcium and iron.

Small Intestine

The small intestine is made up of the duodenum, the jejunum, and the ileum. It is 20 feet long and the food mass from a meal remains in the intestine from three to eight hours.

Mechanical functions. In the small intestine chyme mixes with the digestive juices of the small intestine, with pancreatic and intestinal juices, and with bile, which is secreted by the liver and stored in the gallbladder. Digested food moves in peristaltic waves through the small intestine. Any unused food, waste materials, and water move to the large intestine.

Chemical functions. Alkaline juices neutralize chyme; and bile, excreted into the duodenum by the liver, prepares unemulsified fats for digestion. Digestion is then completed, with the pancreatic enzymes finishing starch digestion, digestion of fat, and partial digestion of protein. The intestinal enzymes complete protein and carbohydrate digestion.

Large Intestine

The large intestine consists of the cecum, the colon, the rectum, and the anal canal.

Mechanical functions. Water is absorbed from the contents of the large intestine to form solid feces. Waste, including indigestible residue, undigested food particles, meat fibers, and decomposition products, is eliminated.

Chemical functions. Since no enzymes are produced in the large intestine, no digestion takes place here.

Figure 2–16 provides a summary of digestion, absorption, and metabolism.

WHAT FACTORS AFFECT DIGESTIBILITY AND UTILIZATION OF FOODS?

The term "digestibility" of food refers to the rapidity and ease of digestion, as well as to its completeness. Thoroughly masticated solid foods and liquid foods are more rapidly digested than food left in large pieces. The amount and type of food eaten at one time also affects rapidity of digestion. Of the three organic nutrients, carbohydrates are digested and leave the stomach most rapidly, proteins less rapidly, and fats require the longest time for digestion. The flow of digestive juices is retarded by fatty food. Proteins or starches coated or mixed with fat require a longer time than either alone. Foods containing a large amount of cellulose are digested more slowly than the same foods with cellulose removed (seeds and tough fibers are not digested); a limited amount of cellulose or fiber is good, however.

Concentrated foods such as cheese require a long time to digest but are completely digested. Because of the completeness of digestion, cheese is often thought of as a constipating food. Serving cheese with fruit or vegetable or salad assures adequate fiber to go along with it.

No matter how digestible a food combination may be or how well the food has been prepared, mental factors may and do interfere, favorably or unfavorably, with proper digestion. Such factors as violent emotion, excitement, anger, excessive fatigue, fear, worry, or strain of any kind may slow down or even suspend it temporarily. Good digestion is also influenced by and depends upon regularity of meals, slow eating, thorough mastication, eating lightly at times, a cheerful frame of mind, and pleasant and happy conditions at mealtime. "Appetite juice," the so-called psychic secretion,

Carbohydrates

In the mouth	In the stomach	In the small intestine		Absorption small intestine	Fate in metabolism
Starch ↓ Dextrin ↓ Maltose by action of ptyalin	No action except continued action of ptyalin until destroyed by HCl	Starch ↓ Dextrin ↓ Maltose by action of pancreatic enzyme	Sucrose Lactose Maltose ↓ Glucose by action of sucrase lactase maltase	In the form of glucose →	Oxidized for energy to carbon dioxide and water Changed to glycogen and stored in liver Changed to fat and stored as fatty tissue

Fats

In the mouth	In the stomach	In the small intestine	Absorption, small intestine	Fate in metabolism
No action	*Emulsified fats* ↓ Fatty acids and Glycerol by action of gastric lipase	Fats after emulsification by bile ↓ Fatty acids and Glycerol by action of pancreatic and intestinal lipases	In the form of fatty acids and glycerol which are recombined into a new fat during absorption	New Fat ↓ oxidized for energy to carbon dioxide and water or stored as fatty tissue Some fat combines with phosphorus to form phospholipids

Proteins

In the mouth	In the stomach	In the small intestine	Absorption, small intestine	Fate in metabolism (of amino acids)
No action	Proteins ↓ Proteoses ↓ Peptones by action of gastric pepsin (needs acid medium)	Protein ↓ Peptones by action of pancreatic trypsin ↓ Amino acids by action of intestinal erepsin	In the form of amino acids which →	Build new tissue Repair old tissue Are deaminized if not needed: Nitrogen removed, changed to urea, and excreted. Carbon, hydrogen, and oxygen converted to glucose.

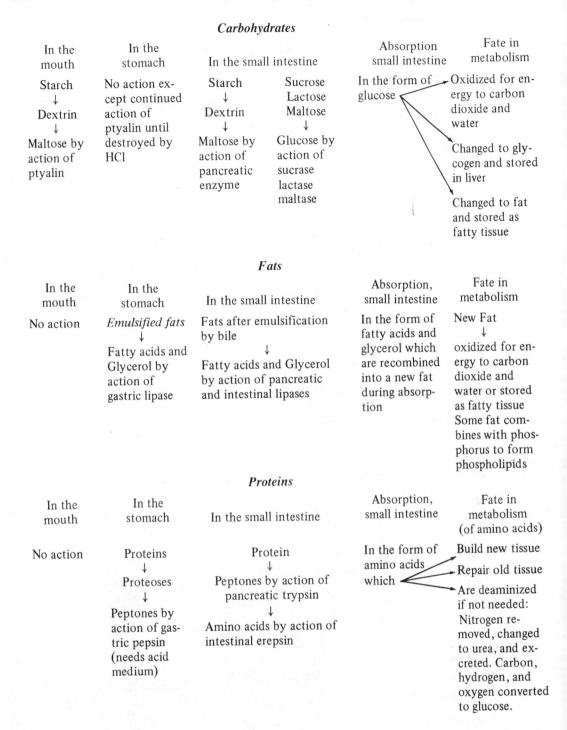

Figure 2–16. Summary of Digestion, Absorption, and Metabolism

also aids digestion. This juice is secreted at the thought, sight, smell, and taste of appetizing food, attractively served, and plays a considerable part in initiating the flow of true digestive juices. Certain of the vitamins influence appetite and proper functioning of the digestive tract.

Certain disorders of the digestive tract and hereditary disease characterized by the absence of digestive enzymes (discussed in Section Two) reduce completeness of digestion.

WHAT IS THE RELATIONSHIP OF DRUGS TO NUTRITION?

Drugs may affect the nutritional status of the patient. Some drugs may reduce appetite, cause nutrient malabsorption, or alter the metabolism of the nutrient. Food may also have an effect on drug absorption and metabolism.[8]

Some conditions, such as essential hypertension and cardiovascular diseases, often require lifelong drug therapy. Since chronic disorders as well as marginal intake of nutrients appear most frequently in the elderly population, this population is at greatest risk of drug-induced nutritional deficiencies.[9]

When reviewing a patient's medication profile one should consider (1) drug administration times and the effects of various foods upon the absorption of nutrients, (2) drugs that irritate the gastrointestinal tract, (3) drug-induced

TABLE 2–21. Nutritional Problems Due to Various Types of Medications*

Nutritional Problem	Medications
Stomatitis	Cancer chemotherapeutic agents Antibiotics
Hyperplasia of gums	Anticonvulsants
Nausea, vomiting, gastritis, gastric hemorrhage	Cancer chemotherapeutic agents Antibiotics Salicylates Steroids Potassium and other electrolytes Anticonvulsants
Malabsorption with diarrhea or steatorrhea	Cancer chemotherapeutic agents Antibiotics Laxatives Clofibrate and cholestyramine Antacids Alcohol
Constipation	Anticholinergics Hypnotics, sedatives
Nutrient Utilization	
Glucose	Steroids
Protein	Cancer chemotherapeutic agents Steroids
Lipids	Steroids
Vitamins and minerals	Cancer chemotherapeutic agents Anticoagulants Anticonvulsants Sedatives
Electrolytes	Diuretics, digitalis Steroids

*From L. Anderson, M. Dibble, P. Turkki, et al.: *Nutrition in Health and Disease*, 17th ed. J. B. Lippincott, Co., Philadelphia, 1982.

changes in body weight, appetite, and taste, (4) sodium, potassium, alcohol, and calorie content of medicinals, and (5) disorders and diseases precipitated by food and some drugs.[10]

An awareness of potential food-drug interactions will help prevent drug-induced malnutrition. The physician, dietitian, nurse, and pharmacist must work as a team in making sure drugs and nutrients are utilized for optimum patient benefit. See Table 2–21 for examples of food-drug interactions.

Study Questions

1. What is the purpose of digestion?
2. What is absorption? Where does it take place?
3. In what form are all carbohydrates absorbed? All fats? All proteins?
4. Why might taking baking soda for "indigestion" retard stomach digestion?
5. Why is well-prepared food, attractive in appearance and attractively served, important to good digestion?

REFERENCES

1. *Recommended Dietary Allowances*, 9th ed. National Academy of Sciences—National Research Council, Washington, D.C., 1980.
2. P. M. Randolph, "The Role of Diet and Nutrition in Dental Health and Disease," *Nutrition News*, Vol. 44, No. 1, Feb. 1981, pp. 1–2, National Dairy Council.
3. *Food for Health—The Carbohydrate Connection.* Leaflet, N.Y. State Cooperative Extension, Cornell University, Ithaca, New York, 1979.
4. H. B. Brown, *Current Focus on Fat in the Diet.* American Dietetic Association, Chicago, 1977, p. 7.
5. *Personalized Weight Control.* National Dairy Council, Rosemont, Ill., 1980.
6. *Food and Your Weight.* Home and Garden Bulletin No. 74, U.S. Department of Agriculture, Washington, D.C., 1977.
7. I. S. Scarpa, H. C. Kiefer, G. Garmon, and R. Tatum, eds., *Source Book on Food and Nutrition*, 2nd ed. Marquis Academic Media, Chicago, 1980.
8. D. A. Roe, "Drugs, Diet, and Nutrition," *Contemporary Nutrition*, Vol. 3, No. 6, June 1978.
9. B. Weiner, "Drug and Food Interactions," *RD*, Vol. 1, No. 5, 1981, p. 2.
10. C. J. Maslakowski, "Drug-Nutrient Interactions/Interrelationships, *Nutritional Support Services*, Vol. 1, No. 11, Nov. 1981, pp. 14, 17.

ADDITIONAL REFERENCES

A. E. Harper, "Recommended Dietary Allowances—1980, *Nutrition Reviews*, Vol. 38, No. 8, 1980, pp. 290–294.

3 Food Plans for Family Nutrition

CHAPTER OUTLINE

- FOOD BUDGETING
  - Guides for Budgeting
  - Food Cost Cutters
- MEAL PLANNING FOR THE FAMILY
  - Considerations for Planning Low-Cost Meals
  - Sample Menus
  - Buying and Management Pointers
  - Regional, Racial, and Religious Dietary Habits
  - Vegetarianism
  - Snacking
  - Fast Food
  - Junk Food

OBJECTIVES

- ☐ To learn the economics of family feeding through the use of food plans and budgets.
- ☐ To learn how to plan meals according to the family budget, food preferences, and needs of family members.

TERMS TO UNDERSTAND

Analogs
Enrichment
Fortification
Homogenized
Meat alternates
Modified skim milk
Organ or glandular meat
Pasteurization
Refined cereal
Restoration

Feeding a family well is a homemaker's major responsibility. To perform a task so vital to family health and important to happiness it is necessary to serve meals that are both nutritionally adequate and enjoyable, to practice thrift as necessary, and to save time and energy wherever possible. Planning and buying food for one's family presents a real challenge to the manager-homemaker. It takes knowledge, good judgment, and a sense of food values in relation to food costs to be able to shop well in today's supermarkets.

Food Budgeting

WHAT GUIDES ARE AVAILABLE FOR FAMILY BUDGETING FOR GOOD MEALS AND GOOD NUTRITION?

Following some plan is the only way a homemaker can be sure to provide each important kind of food and enough of it to see that the family is well fed. When families in this country are poorly fed, the foods they neglect most often are milk and milk products and vegetables and fruits—especially the leafy green and yellow vegetables and the citrus fruits. These foods need to be included in careful planning.

Four ready-made food plans (thrifty, low-cost, moderate-cost, and liberal-cost) that are workable and up-to-date guides to family food budgeting at different cost levels have been prepared by nutritionists in the U.S. Department of Agriculture to help in the choice of the right foods, in the right amounts and at the desired price level. These plans are also used by state and private institutions to plan food purchases and by lawyers to establish dependency rates. The thrifty food plan is presently being revised and is used as the basis for the coupon allotment for the Food Stamp Program.

The federal government authorized the Food Stamp Program in 1964, and ever since then millions of families with low incomes have participated in it. The stamps increase food purchasing power so that low-income households can receive nutritionally adequate diets even when the cost of living continues to rise. Dietary counseling is often necessary as well as important in encouraging families to accept this assistance and to help them learn to use food stamps wisely.

Each food plan specifies what amounts of food from the various food groups to buy to provide an adequate diet for men, women, and children of different ages (Tables 3–1, 3–2, and 3–3). To determine the quantity of food needed for a specific family, the amounts for individual family members can be totaled. Storage, preparation, affordability, and enjoyment are factors that should be considered when choosing a plan. Foods within any of the groups are of similar nutritive value, and the nutritional quality of the diet will be adequate as long as the family chooses a variety of foods. Most families will find the cost of one of the food plans similar to the amount they spend for food.

The revised 1983 food plans take into account new information concerning food prices, food composition, and nutritional needs as defined by the 1980 RDA. The number of food groups increased from 17 in the 1974–75 food plans to 31 in the 1983 food plans, taking into account new food composition data for several dietary substances: zinc, phosphorus, folacin, vitamin E, cholesterol, caloric sweeteners, and sodium. Additional food groups such as vegetable mixtures and meat and meat alternate mixtures were added, acknowledging the increased use of commerically prepared foods. Eating patterns for children under 1 year of age are quite different from other groups, and therefore food plans were not developed for this age group. Likewise, dietary standards for pregnant and lactating women were not developed, and food plans for that group were also discontinued. Categories for older men and women were changed from 55 years of age and over to 51 years of age, to conform to categories used in the RDA.

TABLE 3-1. Low-Cost Food Plan, 1983—Quantities of Food for a Week*

Food Group	Child 1–2 Years	3–5 Years	6–8 Years	9–11 Years	Male 12–14 Years	15–19 Years	20–50 Years	51 Years or More	Female† 12–19 Years	20–50 Years	51 Years or More	Totals
							Pounds‡					
Vegetables, fruit:												
Potatoes (fresh weight)	0.50	0.73	1.16	1.28	1.55	1.88	1.97	1.71	1.19	1.19	1.11	______
High-nutrient vegetables	.55	.50	.86	.98	1.30	1.34	1.91	2.00	1.19	1.86	2.17	______
Other vegetables	.82	.88	1.20	1.41	1.41	1.54	2.12	2.19	1.54	2.30	2.04	______
Mixtures, mostly vegetable; condiments	.06	.10	.14	.17	.18	.20	.29	.30	.15	.24	.15	______
Vitamin-C–rich fruit§	1.51	1.43	1.79	1.94	2.03	2.16	1.62	1.75	1.76	1.79	1.91	______
Other fruit§	1.97	1.58	2.30	2.44	2.07	1.45	1.98	2.21	1.81	1.53	2.19	______
Grain products:												
Whole-grain/high fiber breakfast cereals	.35‖	.27	.31	.35	.36	.28	.14	.22	.33	.21	.31	______
Other breakfast cereals	.38‖	.26	.33	.38	.39	.31	.16	.25	.36	.23	.22	______
Whole-grain/high-fiber flour, meal, rice, pasta	.11	.07	.08	.09	.10	.10	.11	.10	.09	.09	.12	______
Other flour, meal, rice, pasta	.86	.83	1.04	1.17	1.32	1.34	1.40	1.34	.95	1.01	.83	______
Whole-grain/high-fiber bread	.12	.17	.22	.26	.31	.39	.42	.30	.28	.30	.25	______
Other bread	.41	.79	1.08	1.28	1.52	1.95	2.08	1.45	1.19	1.24	.84	______
Bakery products, not bread	.09	.36	.62	.75	.96	.85	.86	.71	.44	.46	.19	______
Grain mixtures	.15	.20	.18	.30	.33	.34	.29	.13	.23	.22	.14	______
Milk, cheese, cream:												
Milk, yogurt (quarts)**	3.41	3.23	4.26	4.69	5.02	4.86	2.49	2.07	4.64	1.85	2.16	______
Cheese	.17	.17	.20	.19	.22	.30	.36	.28	.34	.34	.35	______
Cream, mixtures mostly milk	.13	.44	.57	.69	.67	.75	.51	.50	.65	.34	.55	______

Meat and alternates:												
Lower-cost red meats, variety meats	.71	.52	.60	.74	.99	1.23	1.65	1.23	1.13	1.57	1.67	———
Higher-cost red meats, variety meats	.37	.38	.47	.57	.79	.94	.86	1.04	.70	.95	1.21	———
Poultry	.42	.43	.63	.67	.85	.77	.94	.98	.83	.91	.95	———
Fish, shellfish	.09	.07	.14	.11	.16	.14	.25	.23	.17	.21	.19	———
Bacon, sausage, luncheon meats	.15	.39	.48	.51	.58	.57	.34	.58	.29	.41	.21	———
Eggs (number)	3.34	3.24	2.50	2.99	3.02	2.97	3.38	3.93	3.82	4.23	4.02	———
Dry beans, peas, lentils (dry weight)††	.22	.09	.12	.15	.20	.19	.27	.19	.24	.34	.14	———
Mixtures, mostly meat, poultry, fish, egg, legume	.08	.08	.11	.15	.19	.20	.22	.15	.16	.17	.16	———
Nuts, (shelled weight), peanut butter	.09	.20	.20	.22	.20	.22	.14	.08	.11	.07	.04	———
Other foods:‡‡												
Fats, oils	.09	.27	.43	.50	.55	.54	.68	.54	.25	.32	.26	———
Sugar, sweets	.15	.46	.57	.62	.74	.77	.84	.83	.43	.35	.43	———
Soft drinks, punches, ades (single-strength)	1.53	1.96	2.72	3.25	3.35	4.63	3.67	1.19	3.96	3.33	.96	———

*From *Family Economics Review*, No. 2. U.S. Department of Agriculture, Agriculture Research Service, Washington, D.C., 1983.

Quantities are for food as purchased or brought into the household from garden or farm. Food is for preparation of all meals and snacks for a week. About 10 per cent of the edible parts of food above quantities needed to meet caloric needs is included to allow for food assumed to be discarded as plate waste, spoilage, etc.

†Pregnant and lactating females usually require added nutrients and should consult a doctor for recommendations about diet and supplements.

‡Quantities in pounds, except milk, which is in quarts, and eggs, which are by number.

§Frozen concentrated juices are included as single-strength juice.

||Cereal fortified with iron is recommended.

**Quantities of dry and evaporated milk and yogurt included as their fluid whole milk equivalents in terms of calcium content.

††Count 1 pound of canned dry beans—pork and beans, kidney beans, etc.—as 0.33 pound.

‡‡Two small food groups—coffee and tea, and seasonings—are not shown. Their cost is a part of the estimated cost for the food plan.

TABLE 3-2. Moderate-Cost Food Plan, 1983—Quantities of Food for a Week*

Food Group	Child				Male				Female†			Totals
	1–2 Years	*3–5 Years*	*6–8 Years*	*9–11 Years*	*12–14 Years*	*15–19 Years*	*20–50 Years*	*51 Years or More*	*12–19 Years*	*20–50 Years*	*51 Years or More*	
							Pounds‡					
Vegetables, fruit:												
Potatoes (fresh weight)	0.68	0.81	1.34	1.90	1.69	2.17	2.11	1.81	1.31	1.31	1.03	
High-nutrient vegetables	.78	1.00	.88	1.48	1.33	1.55	2.22	2.17	1.56	2.51	2.76	
Other vegetables	1.06	.81	1.38	1.82	1.65	2.11	2.51	2.76	1.86	2.71	2.52	
Mixtures, mostly vegetable; condiments	.10	.12	.17	.22	.21	.26	.32	.34	.20	.29	.23	
Vitamin-C–rich fruit§	1.60	1.92	2.61	2.47	2.10	2.32	2.26	2.15	1.96	2.22	2.51	
Other fruit§	1.98	2.19	2.32	2.44	2.88	2.42	1.99	3.12	1.81	1.91	2.78	
Grain products:												
Whole-grain/high fiber breakfast cereals	.53‖	.24	.35	.42	.42	.38	.19	.22	.41	.23	.23	
Other breakfast cereals	.43‖	.26	.38	.47	.46	.43	.21	.25	.42	.24	.17	
Whole-grain/high-fiber flour, meal, rice, pasta	.07	.06	.07	.07	.09	.08	.11	.10	.06	.08	.11	
Other flour, meal, rice, pasta	.81	.81	.87	.86	1.19	1.03	1.53	1.38	.86	1.10	.85	
Whole-grain/high-fiber bread	.11	.19	.25	.31	.34	.50	.46	.34	.30	.32	.26	
Other bread	.41	.82	1.07	1.34	1.52	2.18	2.02	1.48	1.24	1.27	.87	
Bakery products, not bread	.21	.53	.76	.65	.78	.86	.93	.80	.59	.53	.31	
Grain mixtures	.14	.18	.26	.46	.43	.46	.30	.15	.32	.25	.18	
Milk, cheese, cream:												
Milk, yogurt (quarts)**	3.79	3.58	4.72	5.16	6.07	5.38	2.62	1.93	5.09	1.89	2.24	
Cheese	.18	.18	.29	.21	.26	.46	.39	.40	.38	.44	.40	
Cream, mixtures mostly milk	.28	.34	.71	.99	1.08	.75	.59	.61	.70	.25	.58	

Meat and alternates:												
Lower-cost red meats, variety meats	.51	.60	.85	1.11	1.36	1.19	1.48	1.37	1.12	1.60	1.58	———
Higher-cost red meats, variety meats	.46	.64	.90	1.17	1.43	1.35	1.60	1.46	1.04	1.35	1.50	———
Poultry	.57	.59	.82	1.00	1.15	.74	1.12	1.03	.94	1.06	1.03	———
Fish, shellfish	.10	.16	.22	.29	.40	.36	.41	.51	.41	.41	.56	———
Bacon, sausage, luncheon meats	.26	.42	.59	.50	.26	.72	.50	.43	.32	.24	.22	———
Eggs (number)	3.64	3.40	2.52	3.08	2.42	2.73	3.10	3.83	3.23	4.37	4.12	———
Dry beans, peas, lentils (dry weight)††	.10	.07	.16	.21	.20	.18	.23	.20	.24	.35	.19	———
Mixtures, mostly meat, poultry, fish, egg, legume	.08	.10	.14	.16	.17	.23	.29	.19	.17	.19	.17	———
Nuts, (shelled weight), peanut butter	.05	.13	.18	.15	.28	.13	.16	.04	.06	.03	.02	———
Other foods:‡‡												
Fats, oils	.11	.30	.31	.46	.52	.57	.65	.62	.28	.36	.29	———
Sugar, sweets	.17	.49	.60	.68	.79	.84	.92	.91	.42	.47	.44	———
Soft drinks, punches, ades (single-strength)	1.57	2.37	2.86	3.69	3.90	4.84	3.73	1.06	4.26	3.71	1.18	———

*From *Family Economics Review*, No. 2. U.S. Department of Agriculture, Agriculture Research Service, Washington, D.C., 1983.

Quantities are for food as purchased or brought into the household from garden or farm. Food is for preparation of all meals and snacks for a week. About 10 per cent of the edible parts of food above quantities needed to meet caloric needs is included to allow for food assumed to be discarded as plate waste, spoilage, etc.

†Pregnant and lactating females usually require added nutrients and should consult a doctor for recommendations about diet and supplements.

‡Quantities in pounds, except milk, which is in quarts, and eggs, which are by number.

§Frozen concentrated juices are included as single-strength juice.

‖Cereal fortified with iron is recommended.

**Quantities of dry and evaporated milk and yogurt included as their fluid whole milk equivalents in terms of calcium content.

††Count 1 pound of canned dry beans—pork and beans, kidney beans, etc.—as 0.33 pound.

‡‡Two small food groups—coffee and tea, and seasonings—are not shown. Their cost is a part of the estimated cost for the food plan.

TABLE 3-3. Liberal Food Plan, 1983—Quantities of Food for a Week*

Food Group	Child 1–2 Years	Child 3–5 Years	Child 6–8 Years	Child 9–11 Years	Male 12–14 Years	Male 15–19 Years	Male 20–50 Years	Male 51 Years or More	Female† 12–19 Years	Female† 20–50 Years	Female† 51 Years or More	Totals
							Pounds‡					
Vegetables, fruit:												
Potatoes (fresh weight)	0.70	0.78	1.13	1.48	1.57	2.44	2.06	1.74	1.20	1.18	1.10	______
High-nutrient vegetables	.78	.81	1.24	1.22	1.57	1.78	2.79	2.77	1.89	3.90	2.81	______
Other vegetables	1.03	.87	1.47	1.61	2.08	2.04	3.02	3.14	2.00	3.72	2.89	______
Mixtures, mostly vegetable; condiments	.10	.11	.18	.19	.24	.29	.49	.36	.19	.34	.28	______
Vitamin-C–rich fruit §	1.65	2.28	2.32	3.26	2.79	3.08	2.72	2.50	2.21	2.47	2.63	______
Other fruit §	3.24	2.47	2.68	3.38	2.54	2.29	2.44	3.02	2.09	2.15	3.13	______
Grain products:												
Whole-grain/high fiber breakfast cereals	.53‖	.25	.32	.37	.51	.48	.27	.19	.45	.20	.24	______
Other breakfast cereals	.54‖	.26	.34	.40	.56	.52	.30	.21	.46	.20	.17	______
Whole-grain/high-fiber flour, meal, rice, pasta	.05	.06	.09	.09	.08	.10	.11	.11	.07	.09	.09	______
Other flour, meal, rice, pasta	.85	.89	1.26	1.35	1.20	1.40	1.48	1.54	.93	1.22	.81	______
Whole-grain/high-fiber bread	.13	.20	.25	.33	.45	.52	.60	.43	.34	.21	.28	______
Other bread	.45	.76	.94	1.26	1.71	1.94	2.22	1.61	1.24	1.38	.86	______
Bakery products, not bread	.29	.62	.81	.64	.95	.98	.91	.97	.55	.56	.41	______
Grain mixtures	.23	.29	.34	.38	.46	.43	.35	.18	.42	.31	.15	______
Milk, cheese, cream:												
Milk, yogurt (quarts)**	4.14	3.64	5.05	5.13	6.12	5.30	2.46	1.87	5.44	2.05	2.42	______
Cheese	.23	.24	.41	.38	.34	.50	.45	.41	.43	.45	.45	______
Cream, mixtures mostly milk	.17	.57	.61	.77	.69	.33	.19	.68	.96	.15	.76	______

Meat and alternates:												
Lower-cost red meats, variety meats	.60	.54	.98	1.07	1.21	1.23	1.46	1.35	1.15	1.95	1.36	———
Higher-cost red meats, variety meats	.61	.73	1.13	1.44	1.66	1.65	2.00	1.80	1.42	1.64	1.69	———
Poultry	.38	.79	.89	1.18	1.06	1.05	1.17	1.20	.89	1.28	1.31	———
Fish, shellfish	.22	.26	.27	.36	.38	.34	.74	.77	.66	.91	.89	———
Bacon, sausage, luncheon meats	.18	.53	.51	.62	.68	.70	.36	.43	.27	.19	.22	———
Eggs (number)	3.51	2.72	2.48	3.73	2.87	3.11	3.55	3.84	3.86	3.90	4.27	———
Dry beans, peas, lentils (dry weight)††	.07	.13	.14	.20	.26	.17	.30	.20	.26	.27	.16	———
Mixtures, mostly meat, poultry, fish, egg, legume	.10	.13	.15	.19	.31	.26	.19	.21	.24	.28	.19	———
Nuts, (shelled weight), peanut butter	.03	.20	.26	.22	.21	.26	.21	.04	.03	.01	.06	———
Other foods:‡‡												
Fats, oils	.10	.25	.34	.48	.56	.65	.82	.68	.34	.43	.30	———
Sugar, sweets	.20	.47	.71	.84	.89	.94	1.06	1.01	.43	.48	.67	———
Soft drinks, punches, ades (single-strength)	1.65	3.20	3.14	4.10	4.84	5.95	4.46	1.46	5.07	3.83	1.28	———

*From *Family Economics Review*, No. 2. U.S. Department of Agriculture, Agriculture Research Service, Washington, D.C., 1983.

Quantities are for food as purchased or brought into the household from garden or farm. Food is for preparation of all meals and snacks for a week. About 10 per cent of the edible parts of food above quantities needed to meet caloric needs is included to allow for food assumed to be discarded as plate waste, spoilage, etc.

†Pregnant and lactating females usually require added nutrients and should consult a doctor for recommendations about diet and supplements.

‡Quantities in pounds, except milk, which is in quarts, and eggs, which are by number.

§Frozen concentrated juices are included as single-strength juice.

‖Cereal fortified with iron is recommended.

**Quantities of dry and evaporated milk and yogurt included as their fluid whole milk equivalents in terms of calcium content.

††Count 1 pound of canned dry beans—pork and beans, kidney beans, etc.—as 0.33 pound.

‡‡Two small food groups—coffee and tea, and seasonings—are not shown. Their cost is a part of the estimated cost for the food plan.

HOW DO THE FOOD PLANS DIFFER?

As the cost of the plan increases, quantities of vegetables and fruits and foods in the meat, poultry, and fish groups generally increase and quantities of grain products, dry beans and peas, nuts, and eggs generally decrease.

The low-cost plan relies more heavily than the other food plans on the food groups that are the most economical sources of nutrients. In addition, users of the low-cost plan are expected to select the lower cost foods within food groups more often—for example, to choose ground beef rather than steak. On the other hand, more expensive choices within the food groups account for much of the greater cost of the liberal plan.

Table 3–4 shows the average cost of food at home estimated for food plans at the four cost levels for one week as compiled in January 1983. Allowance is made for larger families, who can buy food more economically. The cost of food varies from season to season, and families with the same income have been found to spend different amounts for food. In general, as income increases, the amount spent for food increases.

WHAT ARE THE STEPS IN FOLLOWING A FOOD PLAN?[1]

1. The first step is to select the plan (thrifty, basic low-cost, moderate cost, or liberal) which fits your family situation and the amount you are able to spend for food weekly.

2. Write down the name of each person who eats at your table at the top of the appropriate age-group column.

3. Circle the quantities of food under each name, taking each family member in turn, then add across. This will result in a total for each line on the food plan. This could serve as a shopping list. These plans provide for 3 meals a day, 21 meals a week for each family member, including any lunchbox meals. If any member regularly eats one of the day's meals away from home, you will buy that much less.

4. The quantities of foods for adults are based on the needs of "moderately active" persons. If your activities or those of your family are more or less than those specified, food quantities may need to be increased or decreased accordingly. Adjustments in the quantities of fats and oils and in sugars and sweets are easily made to take care of minor variations in activity.

5. Keep records of foods used from each group. Remember that the weight or measure of food you record is as it was purchased, not after it has been prepared for serving.

6. Compare quantities and costs of foods used with the food plan that you have chosen. If quantities are similar and cost is much more or less than estimated, the cost difference may be due to:
   a. Choices of foods within the groups that are more or less expensive than the average assumed for the plans.
   b. Local food prices that are higher or lower than estimated in plans.
   c. Use of large amounts of home-produced foods for which you assumed no cost.
   d. Changes in cost of food since January 1983.
   e. Inclusion of non-food items in food bill. You should remember to subtract such items from the supermarket sales slip.

If the quantities of any food group are much less than in the plan or if any group is left out entirely, your family's meals may be inadequate. Meals are

TABLE 3-4. Cost of Food at Home Estimated for Food Plans at Four Cost Levels, January 1983, U.S. Average*

Sex-Age Group	Cost for 1 Week				Cost for 1 Month			
	Thrifty Plan†	*Low-Cost Plan*	*Moderate-Cost Plan*	*Liberal Plan*	*Thrifty Plan*	*Low-Cost Plan*	*Moderate-Cost Plan*	*Liberal Plan*
Families								
Family of 2:‡								
20–54 years	$33.90	$43.80	$54.80	$65.60	$146.60	$189.40	$237.20	$283.80
55 years and over	30.40	39.00	48.30	57.50	131.90	169.00	209.20	249.20
Family of 4:								
Couple, 20–54 years and children—								
1–2 and 3–5 years	48.10	61.40	76.50	91.50	208.00	265.90	331.30	396.00
6–8 and 9–11 years	58.00	74.30	93.00	111.20	251.10	321.60	402.90	481.70
Individuals §								
Child:								
7 months to 1 year	6.90	8.30	10.20	12.00	29.90	36.10	44.10	52.00
1–2 years	7.80	9.80	12.10	14.40	33.70	42.70	52.60	62.30
3–5 years	9.50	11.80	14.60	17.50	41.00	51.00	63.10	75.70
6–8 years	12.10	15.30	19.20	22.90	52.20	66.40	83.10	99.30
9–11 years	15.10	19.20	24.00	28.70	65.60	83.00	104.20	124.40
Male:								
12–14 years	16.10	20.30	25.40	30.40	69.80	88.10	110.30	131.60
15–19 years	17.70	22.40	28.10	33.70	76.50	97.20	121.70	146.00
20–54 years	17.00	22.00	27.70	33.30	73.50	95.30	120.00	144.10
55 years and over	15.10	19.40	24.10	28.90	65.50	84.00	104.40	125.00
Female:								
12–19 years	14.30	18.20	22.50	26.70	61.90	78.70	97.40	115.90
20–54 years	13.80	17.80	22.10	26.30	59.80	76.90	95.60	113.90
55 years and over	12.50	16.10	19.80	23.40	54.40	69.60	85.80	101.50
Pregnant	17.30	22.00	27.00	32.10	74.80	95.10	117.10	138.90
Nursing	18.30	23.30	29.00	34.40	79.50	100.90	125.50	148.90

*From *Family Economics Review*, No. 2. U.S. Department of Agriculture, Agriculture Research Service, Washington, D.C., 1983.

Assumes that food for all meals and snacks is purchased at the store and prepared at home. Estimates for each plan were computed from quantities of foods published in the Winter 1976 (thrifty plan) and Winter 1975 (low-cost, moderate-cost, and liberal plans) issues of *Family Economics Review*. The costs of the food plans were first estimated using prices paid in 1965–66 by households from USDA's Household Food Consumption Survey with food costs at four selected levels. USDA updates these survey prices to estimate the current costs for the food plans using information from the Bureau of Labor Statistics: "Estimated Retail Food Prices by Cities" from 1965–66 to 1977 and "CPI Detailed Report," tables 3 and 9, after 1977.

†Coupon allotment in the Food Stamp Program based on this food plan.

‡Ten per cent added for family size adjustment. See following footnote.

§The costs given are for individuals in 4-person families. For individuals in other size families, the following adjustments are suggested: 1-person—add 20 per cent; 2-person—add 10 per cent; 3-person—add 5 per cent; 5- or 6-person—subtract 5 per cent; 7-person or more—subtract 10 per cent.

likely to be unbalanced if the neglected food groups are milk, cheese, ice cream; dark-green, deep-yellow vegetables; citrus fruits and tomatoes; or flour, cereals, baked goods, enriched or whole grain.

This may be made an individual class activity, with students determining the weekly food needs of their family according to the chosen cost plan. Or it may be used as a class problem for a family chosen by the class with the desired number of family members or a real family known to the whole class.

HOW CAN FOOD COSTS BE CUT?[1]

No matter what one's budget, it is always a challenge to cut food costs and at the same time plan nutritious meals. A few points will be helpful to the conscientious food shopper.

1. Use one of the less expensive food plans.
2. Check newspaper advertisements for food store specials.
3. Compare costs, keeping family preferences in mind, as well as the time and skill needed for preparation of each food.
4. Accurately estimate quantities of food needed to feed the family.
5. Study unit pricing to determine the best buy per pound, ounce, or pint. Be sure, however, that larger items can be properly stored and used without waste.
6. Foods packaged in individual servings are more expensive than when bought in bulk.
7. Check the date on perishable items such as milk. Be sure you can use all of it before it spoils.
8. When buying meat, consider the amount of fat in the cut. Leaner meats often mean less waste. Poultry and fish are often better buys when compared with meats.
9. Use smaller servings of meat, fish, and poultry and supplement with complex carbohydrates, which are more economical. Also, sometimes substitute eggs, dry beans, and peanut butter for meat.
10. Use nonfat dry milk rather than fluid milk in cooking.
11. Purchase milk in as large a container as is convenient at a food or dairy store.
12. Buy fruits and vegetables in season, when they are more abundant and at their peak quality.
13. Try lower priced or "generic" store brands, which may be similar in quality to more expensive ones.
14. Get your money's worth in nutrients by using whole grains, including bran for fiber, and enriched flour, bread, and cereal in some form at each meal.
15. Ready-to-eat or instant cereals are more expensive than cooked cereals. Buy the larger boxes.
16. Compare the cost and quality of a homemade product to a convenience food. The choice may depend on the amount of time expended and on how much enjoyment is received from cooking the product.
17. Study labels and nutritional panels on packages to compare prices, net contents, and ingredient lists to see if the cost is justified in your estimation.
18. Shop for low-cost foods within each food group.

19. Check your grocery choices at home critically.

20. Compare amounts purchased with one of the food plans you have chosen.

Meal Planning for the Family

WHY IS SOME PLAN FOR DAILY MEALS DESIRABLE?

Without some kind of plan for choosing and combining into meals the foods needed daily for good nutrition, the meals of many families may be found wanting in both nutrition and satisfaction. Any plan needs to be flexible enough to take advantage of sales and other specials in the market, seasonal foods, family tastes and desires, holidays, special family occasions, and guests. A plan will also prove to be a time, work, and money saver and a good way to avoid uninviting, unpalatable, and unsatisfying meals. A plan is especially important when the food allowance is low, to insure sufficient and nutritionally adequate food.

The Four Food Groups of the *Guide to a Better Diet* (see Chapter 1) provide a framework for the daily meals. The foods on this guide fit easily into our three-meals-a-day way of eating, safeguard the nutritional quality of the diet, and permit the addition of other foods as desired (if consistent with maintenance of normal weight) to supplement the basic foods.

The same basic foods are needed by every person in the family; the amount depends upon the age, activity, physical condition, and special needs of the individual. Except for milk, children will require less of foods than adults — smaller helpings rather than fewer foods — and sometimes food that is prepared differently. Variety in the type of servings helps in the establishment of good eating habits. Even weight watchers in the family need the same basic foods, with calories being cut by substituting skim and buttermilk for whole milk, skim milk cheese for whole milk cheese, and uncreamed cottage cheese for creamed type; using only meat trimmed of fat; using broiled and roasted instead of fried meats, vegetables without butter or cream sauce, and fruits without sugar and cream; and avoiding sweets. See Table 3–5 for approximate amounts of foods eaten by various family members for one day.

WHAT ARE ADDITIONAL CONSIDERATIONS IN MEAL PLANNING?

Good meal planning is both a science and an art. *Science* dictates what foods should be included in meals to *nourish our bodies*, and *art* is involved in the combination of the needed foods into meals that are *attractive, appetizing*, and *satisfying* in all ways. Many factors affect our acceptance of food— individual and family attitudes toward food; individual tastes and preferences; racial, regional, and religious customs; and very importantly, how foods look and taste.

Appearance of Food

Color. Food colors should be attractive and appealing. Natural colors are the most attractive, and there should be no predominance of white, neutral, or a single color. Colorful combinations and avoidance of too intense colors (or of too much artificial color, if used) contribute to the attractive appearance of foods.

TABLE 3-5. A Pattern for Planning Meals and Snacks*

The Food Groups		A Day's Meals/Snacks	*1 to 3 Year-Old*	*Girl 11–14†*	*Boy 15–18†*	*Man 23–50†*	*Woman 23–50†*	*Pregnant Woman 23–50*
			Approximate Amounts Eaten by Various Family Members					
		A Breakfast Plan						
Meat	1	Egg‡ (hard-cooked as snack)	1 egg	1 egg	1 egg	1 egg	1 egg	1 egg
Fruit-Vegetable	1	Tomato juice‡	¼ cup	½ cup	½ cup	½ cup	½ cup	½ cup
Grain	2	Enriched instant farina	½ cup	½ cup	¾ cup	¾ cup	½ cup	¾ cup
		Toast (enriched bread)	½ slice	1 slice	1 slice	1 slice	1 slice	1 slice
Milk	1	Milk (to drink, on cereal)	¾ cup	1 cup	1 cup	1 cup	1 cup	1 cup
Others		Butter	½ tsp	1 tsp	1 tsp	1 tsp	1 tsp	1 tsp
		Jelly	—	2 tbsp	2 tbsp	2 tbsp	1 tbsp	1 tbsp
		Coffee or tea	—	—	—	2 cups	2 cups	2 cups
		A Lunch or Supper Plan						
Meat	1	Peanut butter sandwich‡	1 tbsp	2 tbsp	4 tbsp	4 tbsp	2 tbsp	2 tbsp
Fruit-Vegetable	2	Vegetable soup	½ cup	1 cup	1 cup	1 cup	1 cup	1 cup
		Banana (for dessert)	½ medium	1 medium	1 medium	1 medium	1 medium	1 medium
Grain	3	Enriched bread (for sandwich)	1 slice	2 slices	2 slices	2 slices	2 slices	2 slices
		Saltine crackers (with soup)	2 squares	5 squares	5 squares	5 squares	5 squares	5 squares
Milk	1	Milk‡	¾ cup	1 cup	1 cup	—	—	1 cup
Others		Butter for sandwich	—	—	—	—	2 tsp	2 tsp
		Coffee or tea	—	—	—	1 cup	1 cup	1 cup

		A Dinner Plan						
Meat	1	Meat loaf	1½ ounces	3 ounces	3 ounces	3 ounces	3 ounces	3 ounces
Fruit-		Baked potato	½ medium	1 medium	2 medium	2 medium	1 medium	1 medium
Vegetable	3	Buttered cabbage	¼ cup	½ cup	½ cup	½ cup	½ cup	½ cup
		Tossed salad	¼ cup	¾ cup	1 cup	1 cup	¾ cup	¾ cup
Grain	1	Whole wheat bread	½ slice	1 slice	2 slices	2 slices	1 slice	1 slice
Milk	1	Strawberry yogurt‡	¼ cup	1 cup	1 cup	1 cup	1 cup	1 cup
Others		Catsup	—	1 tbsp	2 tbsp	2 tbsp	1 tbsp	1 tbsp
		French dressing	½ tbsp	1 tbsp	1 tbsp	1 tbsp	1 tbsp	1 tbsp
		Butter for bread, on vegetables	1 tsp	1 tbsp	2 tbsp	2 tbsp	2 tsp	2 tsp
		Coffee or tea	—	—	—	1 cup	1 cup	1 cup
		Extra Snacks						
Milk	½–1	Milk	½ cup	1 cup	1 cup	—	—	¾ cup
Fruit-		Raisins,	2 tbsp		4½ tbsp	4½ tbsp		
Vegetable		Pear	½ medium	—	—	1	1	1
Grain		Graham crackers	2		4	4		
Totals: Meat	2+		1300	2430	3022	2689	2003	2300 Calories
Fr.-Veg.	4+							
Grain	4+							
Milk	2–4							

*From *Nutrition Source Book*. National Dairy Council, Rosemont, Ill., 1980.
†These amounts supply 100 per cent or more of the U.S. RDA for eight key nutrients. Amounts for all age/sex groups also exceed the 1974 RDA.
‡These foods may be eaten with or between meals as nutrient-plus snacks.

Contrast. Different *shapes*, forms and sizes (slices, strips, wedges, diced, round), and *types* of food (concentrated and bulky, with neither predominating) help make food attractive. A pleasant balance between simple and richer dishes and variation in *texture*, assortment among hard and soft, moist and dry, without overcooked or mushy foods also contribute to an attractive plate.

Arrangement of Foods

The way food is arranged on a dining table to be served or on plates as served should also be taken into consideration. The food should be uncrowded and suitably garnished. Simple but attractive table appointments complement food as well. It is important to keep the serving area free from disagreeable odors.

Taste and Flavor

Contrast. There should be a pleasing balance between bland and sharp, sweet and sour, distinct and mild, with none predominating.

Method of Preparation. There should be a balance between creamed, fried, and baked without repetition of same method.

Seasoning. Spices and seasonings should be used with care.

Variety. There should not be the same food or a preponderance of one type of food in a meal.

Temperature. Some hot and some cold food in each meal is desirable. Food should be served at the appropriate temperature.

Food Costs

See the discussion of cost cutting on p. 112.

Racial, Regional, and Religious Food Tastes and Customs

Cultural influences on dietary habits are discussed on p. 120.

Time and Effort Involved in Preparation

Planning meals ahead with the help of the "Guide to a Better Diet" (page 24) and the Daily Meal Pattern (page 114), from which shopping lists may be made, can be a real timesaver in shopping (with more food for every food dollar) and in meal preparation (with better use of storage and equipment facilities and more efficient work habits), as well as in better meals for the family.

Familiarity with basic recipes and standard proportions and the use of standardized recipes and accepted methods of food preparation can produce high-quality foods with ease and efficiency. Adequate equipment for meal preparation, with a supply of basic foods and emergency items on kitchen shelves and in refrigerator and freezer, aids in shopping and quick food preparation.

Start meal planning with the main dish and then choose appropriate accompaniments. Plan the salad (or appetizer or both) and dessert next to avoid repetition of the same foods and flavors in a meal; certain salads may serve as both salad and dessert. Serve a light dessert with a heavy main course, a heavier dessert with a lighter main course. Try to have meat, poultry, fish, eggs, cheese, or milk at each meal. Fruit may sometimes be used in place of a vegetable.

WHAT ARE SPECIAL CONSIDERATIONS IN PLANNING LOW-COST MEALS?

An easy to make, hearty, and economical main dish is the core around which the rest of the meal is built — usually it is the main source of protein. The average family in the United States spends well over a third of each food dollar for foods commonly used in main dishes — meat, poultry, fish — and other foods such as eggs, cheese, dry beans, and dry peas.

The main dish should provide about one-fourth of the day's need for protein. If it furnishes less, additional protein foods should be included in the meal. Or the amount of protein-rich food may be increased in the main dish. The rest of the protein for the day will come from milk as a beverage and from cereals, bread, and other foods eaten as part of the day's meals.

To supply one-fourth of the day's protein requirement, a main dish for a family of four must contain about 2 ounces of protein (average 1/2 ounce or 15 grams per person, more for men and teen-age boys and girls, and less for women and younger children). Table 3–6 lists amounts of foods that provide about 15 grams of protein.

The best proteins (other nutrients, also) come from animal sources, such as meat, poultry, fish, eggs, cheese, and milk. It is good to include some in each meal.

The next best proteins are from soybeans, nuts, and dry beans and peas. When these or grain products are featured in main dishes, try to combine them with a little top-rated protein foods — animal proteins.

No one food is exactly like any other food and no food is complete in all nutrients, so use a variety of main dishes and a wide choice of other foods to complete the meal.[2]

Table 3–7 provides sample menus to use with the various food plans.

TABLE 3–6. Foods Providing 15 Grams of Protein

1/5 to 1/2 pound meat, poultry, fish (depending on bone, gristle, fat)	Four 1-inch cubes or two 1-ounce slices American or Swiss cheese
2-1/2 frankfurters	1/2 cup creamed cottage cheese
Four 1-ounce slices bologna	1/3 cup dry or 1 cup canned or cooked dry beans or peas
6 to 8 slices bacon	4 tablespoons peanut butter
2-1/2 large eggs	8 slices bread or 1-1/3 cups dry crumbs
1-3/4 cups fluid whole or skim milk	1 cup dry or 2 cups cooked macaroni, spaghetti, noodles
Scant 2/3 cup nonfat dry instant milk	
Less than 1/2 cup compact instant milk	
Scant cup evaporated milk	

TABLE 3–7. Sample Menus for a Day*

Meal Pattern	Thrifty Plan	Low-Cost Plan	Moderate-Cost Plan	Liberal Plan
Breakfast:				
Fruit or juice	Orange juice (canned)	Sliced banana	Grapefruit sections (fresh)	Strawberries (fresh or frozen)
Main dish and/or cereal	Oatmeal with milk	Ready-to-eat cereal with milk	Omelet	Bacon and egg
Bread	Cinnamon toast	Corn muffin (from mix)	Toast	English muffin
Beverage	Coffee for adults	Coffee for adults	Milk (fresh) or coffee	Milk (fresh) or coffee
Lunch:				
Main dish	Peanut butter and jelly sandwich	Split-pea soup	Sloppy Joe sandwich	Chicken, lettuce, and tomato sandwich
Vegetable or fruit	Banana	Celery	Waldorf salad	Asparagus (frozen)
Bread	White bread (in sandwich)	Rye toast	Whole-wheat bun (in sandwich)	Seeded roll (in sandwich)
Beverage	Milk (nonfat dry)	Milk (nonfat dry)	Milk (fresh)	Milk (fresh)
Other	Cookies (homemade)	Rice pudding	Potato chips	Sherbet
Snack:				
Fruit, cookies, etc.	Cereal party snack	Orange	Ice milk, cookie	Cheese and crackers, peanuts
Beverage	As desired	As desired	As desired	As desired
Dinner:				
Main dish	Hamburger stroganoff	Fried chicken	Baked ham	Beef steak
Vegetable, pasta, or rice	Noodles	Mashed potatoes (fresh)	Sweet potatoes	Corn on cob (fresh or frozen)
Vegetable and/or salad	Carrot-raisin salad (fresh)	Spinach (frozen)	Green beans (frozen)	Broccoli with butter sauce (frozen)
Bread	Bread, white enriched	Bread, white enriched	Biscuit (ready-to-bake)	Dinner roll (bakery)
Dessert	Cookies (homemade)	Spiced cake (from mix)	Fruit gelatin	German chocolate cake (frozen)
Beverage	Milk (nonfat dry) or coffee	Milk (fresh) or coffee	Milk (fresh) or coffee	Milk (fresh) or coffee

*From *Family Food Budgeting for Good Meals and Good Nutrition.* Home and Garden Bulletin No. 94, U.S. Department of Agriculture, Washington, D.C., 1976, p. 11.

Note: Milk for everyone at least once daily, and for children, teenagers, and pregnant and nursing women, more often. Spreads for bread and sugar for cereal and coffee may be added, if desired.

WHAT ARE SOME BUYING AND MANAGEMENT POINTERS FOR LOW-COST MEALS?

Buying Pointers

1. The amount of bone, gristle, and fat on a cut of meat affects the cost of a serving. Less tender cuts of beef such as chuck, heel of round, brisket, and short ribs usually provide protein for less money than some of the more tender cuts.

2. The less tender *Good* grade of meat (3rd grade) provides more lean meat than higher grades and costs less per pound.

3. Chicken and turkey are low-cost protein sources compared with some cuts and types of meats.

4. Larger well-fleshed birds are often better buys than smaller ones. When sold whole, the price is less per pound than when halved, quartered, or cut up.

5. Whole ready-to-cook turkey provides more meat for the money than a boned, rolled turkey roast.

6. Medium and small eggs are a better buy than large ones at certain seasons.

7. Cheaper, grade B eggs are as good as grade A for combination dishes and baked foods.

8. Grade B and C fishery products are as nutritious as higher grades for dishes in which appearance is unimportant.

9. "Light meat" tuna costs less than "white meat" tuna and flaked or grated tuna less than solid or chunk. Pink or chum salmon is less expensive than red or king.

10. Dry beans and peas are among the least costly sources of protein.

11. Cheese wedges cost less than sliced, cubed, or grated cheese. Mild natural cheese costs less than aged sharp cheese, and domestic less than imported. Home-flavored cottage cheese is less than similar flavored purchased products.

12. Nonfat dry and evaporated milk costs less than whole fluid for cooking and baking. Store-bought milk is more economical than home delivered; and large containers (1/2 or 1 gallon) are less expensive than quart containers.

Management Pointers

Money-saving Ideas

1. Use less tender cuts of meat made tender by cooking slowly with moisture; grinding, cubing, pounding, or scoring; marinating with acid ingredients; or using commercial tenderizers.

2. Make the most of flavor and food value from meat, poultry, and fish by using small pieces in casseroles, sandwiches, and salads. "Meaty" bones are good in soups and stews and for seasoning vegetables. Use broth in gravies, sauces, soups, stews, and other combination dishes and drippings in gravies, sauces, pan frying, and seasoning vegetables.

3. Extend meat, poultry, and fish by combining with mild-flavored foods such as dry beans or peas, macaroni products, rice, or potatoes in casseroles, stews, and soups; use breads or cereals as stuffings in meat, poultry, or fish loaves, patties, and balls.

4. Replace the meat in some meals with less expensive protein sources, e.g., dry beans and peas, lentils; peanut butter; eggs; American or Swiss-type cheese; cottage cheese.

5. Make good use of leftovers.

Time-saving Ideas

1. Prepare larger amounts of main dishes than needed for one meal—use some, freeze the rest. Freeze in meal-size packs; roasts, meat sauce; combination dishes; and lunchbox sandwiches.

2. Use previously partly or fully prepared items for sauces and toppings for casseroles, for added flavor with little preparation time.

3. Prepare a major part of the meal in the oven. Use a pressure cooker to shorten the cooking time for pot roasts, swiss steaks, meat sauces, and dry beans and peas.[2]

HOW DO FOOD AND DIETARY PATTERNS DEVELOP?

Our food selection patterns are habits which have been acquired in many different ways over our lifetime. Cultural influences, religious beliefs, and geographical location are some of the factors that mold our food selection patterns. Dietary patterns are developed not only by one's ethnic group practices but by society in general and the society's access to food.

Customs within individual family groups are influential in the development of likes and dislikes, "accepted" or "rejected" foods, and certain eating habits. Many dietary habits in the individual can be traced to an early association, pleasant or otherwise, of food with people, places, or events of one kind or another.

More recently recognized as powerful influences in our food choices and habits are emotional and psychological needs. Our physiological needs as a source of dietary habits are probably the least influential in the establishment of patterns. Unfortunately, lacks in our daily diet do not immediately show up in effects on the body, so we do not immediately become aware of the significance of food. Also, the food faddist and self-styled "nutrition specialist" (with very little or, more frequently, no knowledge of nutrition but with a product or idea to sell) influence food choice for far too many persons.

Improvement in food selection patterns (for bettering one's health) frequently means changing habits of long standing. This is a slow, step-by-step, almost never-ending process for which a real desire to change, a deep conviction that change is important (due to good teaching), and the willingness to substitute desirable food habits for undesirable ones are necessary. Persons dealing with nutrition improvement, while primarily concerned with the metabolic role of food in health, must also have some understanding of the circumstances under which diet habits are acquired and the various meanings food may have for different individuals (its nonmetabolic significance). This is especially true in dealing with patients whose disorder or disease imposes drastic changes in dietary habits if a cure is to be effected.

Since there appears to be no doubt that many nutritional deficiencies are due to poor dietary habits, the establishment of correct habits early in life and adherence to such throughout life is of extreme importance. A good diet insures good nutrition. The nurse or dietitian has a unique opportunity to foster good food habits.

WHY IS IT IMPORTANT TO UNDERSTAND REGIONAL, RACIAL, AND RELIGIOUS DIETARY HABITS IN STUDYING NUTRITION AND MEAL PLANNING?

A surprisingly large number of foreign-born people are included in the population of the United States. Coming, as they do, from all parts of the world, they have brought with them, and tend to retain, habits of eating and food tastes very different from those we think of as American. These tastes and habits, some of which are poor in terms of present-day nutrition standards, have been fixed for generations and are not too easily changed.

One-sided diets have been brought from some countries where limited food production has restricted the diet to a few types of foods. Persons coming from such countries need to learn better food habits here, and how to incorporate in their native dishes the nutrients necessary for good nutrition. More adequate diets have been brought from other countries. However, foods familiar in these countries may be rare and expensive in America, and consequently they may be omitted from the diet. If a racial group does give up some of its own food habits and adopt those of the new country, it frequently chooses the poorest of the new country's nutritional habits, such as the liking for excessive sweets and breadstuffs.

If the general level of nutrition in the United States is to be improved, the education of the various racial groups in the best ways to supplement the good features of their racial diets is an important starting point in a nutrition education program. In most cases, the answer lies in the greater use of milk, fruits, and vegetables in their cheaper forms and prepared in dishes that are accepted and enjoyed. Some assistance in planning the expenditure of food money to permit the purchase of the needed supplemental foods, and also some help in combining these foods into dishes and meals that the family will eat, are also frequently needed. The problem becomes more difficult when religious restrictions are applied to the family diet.

Just as food tastes and habits differ among different racial groups, so do they differ also from region to region in the United States. From the Far West to the East Coast and New England by way of the Southwest and South or the North Central states, differences are apparent in the special regional dishes, the types of meals served, and the ways food is prepared, to say nothing of the food patterns and habits encountered in the metropolitan areas across the country and in less accessible areas.

Table 3–8 shows how the Basic Four Food Groups are incorporated in different types of eating patterns. A typical day's diet for any racial, regional, or religious group may be evaluated nutritionally by checking it against an acceptable diet plan such as the "Guide to a Better Diet" (p. 24).

VEGETARIANISM

Who Follows Vegetarian Diets?

The number of vegetarians has increased rapidly over the last few years. Two religious groups that forego meat and other animal product consumption are the Seventh Day Adventists and Catholic Trappist Monks. Others follow vegetarian diets for health, political, cultural, and/or economic reasons. Many college students find vegetarianism appealing because it inspires creative cooking as well as a means to have a more natural life-style by using organically grown foods.[3]

How Do Vegetarian Diets Differ?

There are three main classifications of vegetarian diets:

1. *Lacto-ovo vegetarian.* Plant foods are supplemented with dairy products and eggs. This is probably the most common type of vegetarian diet.
2. *Lacto-vegetarian.* Dairy products are included, but not eggs.
3. *Total vegetarian (vegan).* Animal food sources (including both eggs and dairy products) are completely excluded. This diet is low or inadequate in iodine, vitamin B_{12}, iron, calcium, zinc, riboflavin, and vitamin D for this reason.[3]

How Should One Plan a Vegetarian Diet?

The Four Food Groups Plan, including a wide variety of plant foods, should be the basis of an adequate vegetarian diet. Meat is replaced with an increased intake of legumes, nuts, meat analogs, and nonfat or low-fat milk products. Total vegetarians must replace the nutrients in the milk group, possibly by supplementation with B_{12} and calcium.

The use of whole grains should be increased and the use of "empty calorie" foods minimized. Caloric intake must be maintained at an appropriate level for the individual.[4]

TABLE 3–8. Ethnic, Regional, and Racial Food Patterns According to the "Basic Four" Food Groups

Ethnic Group	Bread and Cereal	Eggs, Meat, Fish, Poultry	Dairy Products	Fruits and Vegetables	Seasonings, etc.
Italian	Crusty white bread Cornmeal and rice—Northern Italy Pasta—Southern Italy	Beef Chicken Eggs Fish	Milk in coffee Cheese	Broccoli, zucchini, other squash, eggplant, artichokes, string beans, tomatoes, peppers, asparagus, fresh fruit	Olive oil, vinegar, salt, pepper, garlic
Puerto Rican	Rice, beans, noodles, spaghetti, oatmeal, cornmeal	Dry salted codfish, meat, salt pork, sausage, chicken, beef	Coffee with hot milk	Starchy root vegetables, green bananas, plantain, legumes, tomatoes, green pepper, onion, pineapple, papaya, citrus fruits	Lard, herbs, oil, vinegar
Near Eastern	Bulgur (wheat)	Lamb Mutton Chicken Fish, eggs	Fermented milk Sour cream Yogurt Cheese	Nuts, grape leaves	Sheep's butter, olive oil
Greek	Plain wheat bread	Lamb Fresh fruit Pork Poultry Eggs Organ meats	Yogurt Cheese Butter	Onions, tomatoes, legumes	Olive oil, parsley, lemon, vinegar
Mexican	Lime-treated corn	Little meat (ground beef or pork) Poultry Fish	Cheese Evaporated milk as beverage for infants	Pinto beans, tomatoes, potatoes, onions, lettuce	Chili pepper, salt, garlic

Chinese	Rice Wheat Millet Corn Noodles	Little meat and no beef Fish, including raw fish Eggs of hen, duck, and pigeon	Water buffalo milk occasionally Soybean milk Cheese	Soybeans, soy bean sprouts, bamboo sprouts, soy curd cooked in lime water, radish leaves, legumes, vegetables, fruits	Sesame seeds, ginger, almonds, soy sauce
American Black	Hot breads Cookies Pastries Cakes Cereals White rice	Chicken Salt pork, ham, bacon, sausage Salted salmon, salt herring	Milk and milk products Little cheese	Kale, mustard, turnip greens Cabbage Hominy grits	Molasses
Jewish	Noodles Crusty white seed rolls Rye bread Pumpernickel bread	Koshered meat (from forequarters and organs from beef, lamb, veal) Milk not eaten at same meal Fish	Milk and milk products	Vegetables—usually cooked with meat Fruits	

Sources of Important Nutrients in Vegetarian Diets[5]

Soy protein, a legume high in protein and unsaturated fat, is particularly useful in vegetarian diets because it contains all eight essential amino acids in abundance. Soybeans must be cooked or roasted before processing.

The addition of dairy products, with or without eggs, to a selection of legumes and whole grains will, along with the use of vegetable oils that provide polyunsaturated fatty acids, constitute a nutritious diet. Legumes contribute fiber as well as B vitamins and iron, and whole grains provide carbohydrates, protein, thiamine, and iron, and are a good source of trace minerals.[4, 5]

Table 3–9 lists a variety of "non-meat" food sources for important nutrients. Table 3–10 lists food sources for calcium for those following a vegetarian diet that excludes milk but includes fish sources.

By combining different foods in vegetarian diets, complete proteins can be formed from the available amino acids. For example, the following combinations are recommended for nutritious menu items.[6]

1. Grains and legumes: e.g., corn tortillas and beans: chili and beans, served with cornbread; split-pea soup and whole wheat crackers; or baked beans and brown bread
2. Grains and milk products: e.g., oatmeal with milk, rice and cheese casserole, grilled cheese sandwich, macaroni and cheese, or rice pudding
3. Seeds and legumes: e.g., soybean casserole with sesame seeds, Waldorf salad with peanuts and sunflower seeds, or cashew chili

SNACKING

The traditional meal pattern of having only three meals a day is becoming less common with today's busy life-styles. Many people find it more convenient to eat when they can, and "snacking" has become part of our culture. The daily coffee break is a popular custom for people in all walks of life.

When one eats does not matter. Rather, it is more important to consider *what* is eaten, and *how much.* Three meals a day may be satisfactory for some people, but others find the best way to receive adequate calories and nutrients is to eat more often. Snacking can be beneficial to children and adults alike, especially if appetites are small in relation to physical needs. As a general rule, snacks should not replace breakfast, which is a very important meal, nutritionally speaking.

TABLE 3–9. Food Sources for Important Nutrients in the Vegetarian Diet

Nutrient	Sources
Calcium*	Milk and milk products, particularly cheese and yogurt; fortified soy milk; dark-green leafy vegetables such as parsley, kale, spinach, and mustard, dandelion, and collard greens
Iron	Legumes, green leafy and other vegetables, whole-grain or enriched cereals or breads, some nuts, and dried fruits. However, there are many factors that may affect absorption of this nutrient.
Riboflavin (vitamin B_2)	Milk, legumes, whole grains, and vegetables.
Vitamin B_{12}	Milk and eggs, fortified soybean milk, and fortified soya meats.
Zinc	Nuts, beans, wheat germ, and cheese.

*See also Table 3–10.

TABLE 3-10. Sources of Calcium in the Vegetarian Diet*

Food Source	Calcium (mg)
1 cup oysters	226
3 oz salmon	167
3 oz sardines	372
1 cup almonds	352
1 cup Brazil nuts	260
1 cup peanuts	107
1 cup pork and beans	138
1 cup greens	200 (average)
1 cup dried apricots	100
1 cup cranberry sauce	104
1 cup dates	130
1 tbsp blackstrap molasses	137

*Diet excludes milk and includes fish. From U. D. Register and L. M. Sonnenberg, "Principles of the Vegetarian Diet." *Nutrition and the M.D.*, Vol. 1, No. 5, 1975.

How Should Snacks Be Chosen?

There is no one perfect snack, but some are more nutritious than others, and careful selection is necessary in order to avoid potential problems. Snacks should be planned according to the needs of each member of the family. A homemaker who nibbles food during food preparation or clean-up may find that an easy way to put on unwanted pounds and cause failure of any weight reduction plan. On the other hand, planned snacking can be an effective means for meeting the energy and nutrient needs of a growing and very active child.[7]

Many snack foods are high in energy value but contain little protein, vitamins, or minerals. Hunger can be satisfied by many foods other than candy, potato chips, and soda pop. The traditional carrot and celery sticks or apple and banana are always wise choices, but other fruits and vegetables are equally nutritious. Snacks that contribute vitamins and minerals as well as kilocalories are listed in Table 3-11. Snacks lowest in energy value are listed first.[8]

Snacks should be chosen from the Four Food Groups. This will help reduce the desire for "empty calorie" foods such as sticky sweets, which have been found to increase the susceptibility to tooth decay. Several small wholesome meals a day can be beneficial to teenagers. Pizza, hamburgers, and similar "fast foods" are considered to be nutritious snacks (see also Table 2-6).

FAST FOODS

What Is the Definition of Fast Foods?

"Fast food" is relatively low-cost food purchased at an outlet featuring quick service and convenience.[9] "Fast-food service" would be a more accurate term, because it is the speed and style of service, rather than the food itself, which distinguishes fast-food restaurants from others.

How Nutritious Are Fast Foods?

It is unfortunate that fast foods are often referred to as "junk food." The Basic Four Food Groups concept can easily be applied to fast food. To illustrate, a cheeseburger with lettuce, tomato, and onion, a serving of french

TABLE 3-11. Selected Nutritious Snacks*

Food	Calories	Nutrients Provided†
1/2 cup cabbage	8	C
1 carrot	30	A, C
1/2 grapefruit	45	C
1/2 cup fresh pineapple	45	C
1 cup tomato juice	45	Fe, A, C
1 orange	65	C
1 oz cheddar cheese	70	C, A, P
1 medium apple	80	C
1 cup skim milk	85	P, Ca, A
10 dried apricot halves	91	Fe, A
1 banana	100	C
1/4 cup raisins	105	Fe
1 cup apple juice	120	Fe
1 cup grape juice	135	C
8 oz plain yogurt	145	P, Ca
1 cup whole milk	150	P, Ca, A
8 oz fruit-flavored yogurt	230	P, Ca
1/7 pumpkin pie	275	A

*Modified from *Food for Health: The Carbohydrate Connection—The Knack of Snacking.* Cornell Cooperative Extension, Division of Nutritional Sciences, Cornell University, Ithaca, New York, 1979.

†Contains 10 per cent or more of the U.S. RDA for the listed nutrient. C = vitamin C; A = vitamin A; Fe = iron; Ca = calcium; P = protein.

fries, and a shake represent four food groups; a taco is composed of a cereal shell, ground beef, shredded cheese, and shredded lettuce and tomato; pizza has a cereal crust, tomato sauce, cheese, and various vegetable and meat toppings; a typical fried chicken dinner with mashed potato, coleslaw, a roll and a glass of milk also represents all four food groups.

Fast foods can also meet the nutrient density criteria required by the USDA for Type A school lunches by providing one-third of the RDA for selected nutrients.[10]

The fast-food industry has achieved high standards of production for maximum nutrient retention. Registered dietitians have helped in directing its nutrition education programs.

NUTRIENTS IN FAST FOODS

Protein. Animal products such as fish, chicken, beef, cheese, and milk are excellent protein sources and are available in all fast-food restaurants. It is possible to fulfill 60 to 100 per cent of one's protein RDA with a single fast-food meal.

Fat. Some of the major components of fast foods (beef, cheese, mayonnaise, and deep-fat frying) are rich sources of fat. Since fat is high in calories, eating in a fast-food restaurant can be a problem, especially for those who need to limit their caloric intake.

Carbohydrate and Fiber. Carbohydrate is found in enriched rolls, french fries, shakes, soft drinks, and desserts. Fast-food menu items are generally low in fiber, except for salads and coleslaw, which are recent additions to many menus.[9]

Calories. Menus include many high-calorie items but with calorie counts available, weight-conscious people can incorporate fast foods in their diets.

Vitamins. Most fast-food meals provide adequate amounts of thiamin, riboflavin, niacin, pyridoxine, and cobalamin. Vitamin C is found in orange juice, coleslaw, potatoes, and the increasingly common salads. Vitamin A is low in hamburger or chicken fast-food meals, but Mexican-style foods and pizza provide some vitamin A from the tomato and cheese. Salads are also good sources of vitamin A if raw carrots, tomatoes, and dark-green leafy vegetables are included.

Minerals. Shakes and milk are high in calcium and phosphorus. Hamburgers are high in iron, and rolls, if made with enriched flour, are a fair source of this mineral. Beef and dairy products, which are used in many entrees, are good sources of zinc. Sodium can be a problem for those advised by physicians to lower their intake of that element, because many fast foods are relatively high in sodium in the form of salt (sodium chloride).[9]

A nutritional drawback of fast foods, particularly for frequent consumers, is the lack of variety on many fast-food restaurant menus. Therefore, it is best to incorporate meals eaten at fast-service restaurants into a varied diet that includes many other food choices. This will aid in assuring an adequate nutrient intake. The variety of menu items has increased, however, from the original hot dog/hamburger/fried chicken meals to include pizza, Mexican foods, roast-beef sandwiches, seafood, and other items.

How Popular Are Fast Foods?

According to the American Council on Science and Health, the fast-food industry has grown tremendously over the last 25 years.[9] There are over 140,000 fast-food outlets in the United States. Sales from fast foods increased to 23 billion dollars annually in 1980. A consumer survey in 1978 showed that 90 per cent of Americans ate in a fast-food restaurant at least once that year; 10 per cent were found to eat at fast-food restaurants more than five times weekly.

At the present time, price and convenience are more important to consumers than nutritional quality in choosing fast food. An entire fast-food meal including entree, fries, soft drink or shake, and dessert will usually cost twice as much as the same meal prepared at home but only about half as much as eating in a conventional restaurant.

JUNK FOOD

The term "junk food" implies worthlessness, but this generalization is not necessarily justified. Some people characterize foods as "junk" simply because they are high in sugar or fat or lacking in some nutrient. Whether the food is nutritious or junk depends on its effect on the diet as a whole.

Study Questions and Activities

1. Explain what is meant by the following statement: "Good meal planning is both a science and an art."

2. Below are shown some poor breakfasts, poor lunches, and poor dinners. How would you change each of the meals to make them more attractive and appealing and at the same time improve nutritive value?

		Poor Meals	*Good Meals*
Breakfast		Orange juice Buttered toast	
Lunch	(1)	Hamburger on buttered bun French-fried potatoes Fruit gelatin	
	(2)	Macaroni and cheese Muffin and butter Soft drink	
Lunch, carried	(3)	Luncheon meat sandwich Vanilla wafers Soft drink	
Dinner	(1)	Meat and vegetable stew Rolls and butter Frosted layer cake	
	(2)	Roast chicken Parsley potato Rolls and butter Jam Apple pie	

3. Using the menu form (Table 3–12), plan menus for five days for *your* family which will include the foods in the Four Food Groups and also illustrate other important considerations in meal planning. Note that each time you use a food, you are to indicate the food group to which it belongs.

4. Become familiar with the racial, religious, or regional diet assigned you by the instructor and summarize information about it to present to the class. Be prepared to discuss this racial diet in terms of the Four Food Groups you have studied previously. What are the good points? How could the diet be improved?

Each student in the class will then use the following chart to record important information about each diet presented in class.

TABLE 3–12. Suggested Family Meals for Five Days*

Basic Plan for the Three Daily Meals	Menu 1	Food Group	Menu 2	Food Group	Menu 3	Food Group	Menu 4	Food Group	Menu 5	Food Group
Breakfast										
Fruit or fruit juice										
Cereal in some form and/or egg										
Cereal in some form and/or meat										
Bread in some form										
Milk										
Hot beverage for adults										
Dinner										
Meat, fish, poultry										
Potatoes										
A vegetable										
A vegetable or fruit salad or vegetable relish										
Bread and butter if extra energy food is needed										
Dessert—light or heavy depending on meal										
Milk										
Beverage for adults										
Lunch or Supper										
Heavy main dish										
Salad or relish										
Bread and butter if extra energy food is needed										
Dessert—light or heavy depending on meal										
Milk										

*Form from a Cornell Extension Bulletin.

RACIAL DIETARY HABITS

Regional or racial diet (list foods used)	*Characteristics and main dish*	*Good nutritional features*	*Desirable nutritional improvements*

5. Students with foreign backgrounds might tell about their food customs and dietary habits and possibly demonstrate the main dishes popular in their family meals. Markets in foreign sections of a city and foreign restaurants afford good opportunities for learning about foods used by families with different racial backgrounds. The class might prepare a foreign meal for the teachers and students.

WHAT HAS HAPPENED TO YOUR FOOD HABITS AND NUTRITION ATTITUDES AS YOU HAVE STUDIED ABOUT NUTRIENTS AND FOODS FOR GOOD NUTRITION?

Now is a good time for you to check your food habits once more.

1. Keep a record of your food intake (at meals and between meals) for one week.
2. Score your diet for each day, using the Food Selection Score Card on page 30, and determine your average score for the week.
3. What is your average score for the week? How does this score compare with the score you obtained for your weekly food record when you started the course? See page 30.
4. Analyze and comment on your last food selection score in the space provided below.
5. Why are good food habits important? How are they formed? How can they be improved?
6. What are five good food habits for *you* to acquire and follow daily?

Food Groups	*Perfect Score*	*My Score*	*Comments*
Milk Group			
Meat Group			
Vegetable-Fruit Group			
Bread-Cereal Group			
Water	________	________	
	100		

What improvements have you made in your food selection habits thus far?

What further improvements do you think it desirable to make?

What thought have you given to the principles of meal planning as you have selected the necessary foods for your various meals? See Score Card for Meals, page 30.

Note to Instructor: It is suggested that each student keep and score a week's food intake at least *once more* (*preferably twice*) before the end of the course.

REFERENCES

1. *Family Food Budgeting for Good Meals and Good Nutrition*, Home and Garden Bulletin No. 94. U.S. Department of Agriculture, Washington, D.C., 1976.
2. "Money-saving Main Dishes," Home and Garden Bulletin No. 43. U.S. Department of Agriculture, Washington, D.C.
3. J. H. Price, "Vegetarianism—Food Faddism or Nutritious Alternative?" *Journal of Nursing Care*, June 1980.
4. U. D. Register and L. M. Sonnenberg, "Principles of the Vegetarian Diet," *Nutrition and the M.D.*, Vol. 1, No. 5, 1975.
5. I. B. Vyhmeister, U. D. Register, and L. M. Sonnenberg, "Safe Vegetarian Diets for Children," *Pediatrics Clinics of North America*, Vol. 24, No. 1, Feb. 1977.
6. F. M. Lappe, *Diet for a Small Planet.* Ballantine Books, New York, 1971, rev. 1975, pp. 152–153.
7. *Food and Your Weight*, Home and Garden Bulletin No. 74. U.S. Department of Agri-Culture, Washington, D.C.
8. *Food for Health—The Carbohydrate Connection.* N.Y. State Cooperative Extension, Cornell University, Ithaca, New York, 1978.
9. American Council on Science and Health, "Fast Food and the American Diet," report, Nov. 1981.
10. H. Appledorf, "How Good Are Fast Foods," *The Professional Nutritionist*, Winter 1982, pp. 2–4.

Nutrition in the Life Cycle

4

CHAPTER OUTLINE

NUTRITION IN PREGNANCY AND LACTATION
- Nutrient Needs
- Meal Planning
- Clinical Problems
- Nutrition Counseling

NUTRITION OF INFANTS
- Nutrient Needs
- Feeding Formulas
- Formula Preparation
- Introduction of Solid Foods

NUTRITION IN CHILDHOOD AND ADOLESCENCE
- Growth and Development
- Nutrient Needs
- Feeding Considerations
- Meal Planning

GERIATRIC NUTRITION
- Physiological, Economic, Social Changes
- Nutrient Needs
- Nutrition Programs
- Meal Planning

NUTRITION AND THE ATHLETE
- Nutritional Guidelines
- Meal Planning
- Pre- and Post-Game Meals
- Fluid Requirements

OBJECTIVES

To understand
- ☐ The nutritional needs during various stages of the life cycle.
- ☐ The nutritional needs imposed by athletic training and competition.

To apply
- ☐ Knowledge of these nutrient needs to meal planning that meets the RDA.

TERMS TO UNDERSTAND

Aging	Gerontology	Marasmus
Development	Glycogen loading	Meals-on-Wheels
Efficient body weight	Growth	Pica
Fetus	Heat exhaustion	Prenatal
Geriatrics	Kwashiorkor	Toxemia

Nutrition in Pregnancy and Lactation

WHAT IS THE IMPORTANCE OF NUTRITION DURING PREGNANCY AND LACTATION?

The nutritional status and the nutritional intake of the mother during pregnancy has a profound effect on the growth of the fetus. If the mother's intake of nutrients is not sufficient or there is a problem with the placenta that limits the supply of nutrients to the fetus, this can lead to "fetal malnutrition."[1]

"Stillborn, low birthweight, premature and congenitally defective infants are more frequently born to mothers who have had an inadequate diet prior to and during pregnancy."[2]

An adequate supply of nutrients during pregnancy also helps to assure an adequate supply of good quality breast milk during lactation.

WHAT ARE SPECIFIC NUTRIENT NEEDS DURING PREGNANCY?

Energy. Energy needs are increased during pregnancy to allow for the building of maternal tissue (breast tissue, uterus, placenta, fat, increased fluids and blood volume) and for the development of the enlarging fetus.

There is an approximate increase of 15 per cent over nonpregnancy energy needs. This represents an increase of approximately 300 Kcal per day. Total weight gain during pregnancy should average approximately 24 pounds (11 kg).

Weight gain during pregnancy should be gradual and steady. First trimester weight gain is usually 1.5 to 3 lb (0.7 to 1.3 kg); thereafter, a gain of .8 lb (0.35 kg) per week is suggested as a guideline.

Protein. Additional protein is needed during pregnancy for synthesis of maternal and fetal tissue. The current RDA is 30 gm per day in addition to the basic allowance. This is 1.3 gm/kg/day in females 19 years of age or older, 1.5 gm/kg/day in females 15 to 18 years of age, and 1.7 gm/kg/day in females under 15 years of age.

Adequate calorie intake is necessary for maximum utilization of protein for tissue synthesis. Energy intake should not fall below 36 Kcal/kg/day.[1]

Iron and Folacin. During pregnancy there is an increased need for iron to allow for (1) increased blood volume production and (2) the transfer of iron to the fetus's liver for storage and use during the first six months of life, when a diet of milk provides little iron. Because of this increased demand for iron, which cannot be met by food alone, and because many women enter pregnancy with insufficient iron stores, iron supplementation is recommended. The Food and Nutrition Board recommends a supplement in the range of 30 mg to 60 mg per day.

Folacin is needed in increased amounts because of rapid red blood cell production as well as being needed as a coenzyme by rapidly growing tissues. Therefore the RDA for folacin is doubled during pregnancy, from 400 mcg to 800 mcg. An oral supplement is suggested to meet this demand and reduce the risk of folacin deficiency.

Calcium, Phosphorus, and Vitamin D. Calcium and phosphorus needs during pregnancy reflect the mother's own needs, as well as the need for calcification of the fetal skeleton and formation of teeth. Therefore the RDA for these minerals is increased by 400 mg per day. These needs can easily be met by consumption of an additional 1½ cups of milk.

Vitamin D needs increase to facilitate greater calcium and phosphorus absorption. Active forms of vitamin D cross the placenta and participate in calcium metabolism in the fetus.[1] An additional allowance of 5 mcg (200 I.U.) is recommended. This can be met by the consumption of vitamin D-fortified milk or increased exposure to the sun.

Other Nutrients. The RDA for most nutrients are increased during pregnancy (see Table 4-1). The increased needs for these nutrients can generally be met by the increased consumption of foods without the addition of a vitamin or mineral supplement (except folacin and iron). See Table 4-2 for changes in the Basic Four Food Groups to meet nutrient needs during pregnancy, and Table 4-3 for sample menu plans.

Meals and Snacks. Part of the day's food may be taken in the form of snacks between meals and at bedtimes. Some doctors may recommend five small meals a day instead of three large ones (as in Table 4-3). Smaller amounts of food at more frequent intervals helps prevent hunger between meals and may prevent nausea, and the hot drink at night may help sleep. Avoid extras—food treats high in kilocalories. If snacks are needed between meals, milk, fruits, and raw vegetables are best.

Fluids. Physician may recommend as much as two quarts fluid daily, some of which is furnished by milk, soup, fruit juices, and other beverages in addition to water.

TABLE 4-1. RDA During Pregnancy and Lactation*

	Nonpregnant Women				
	15-18 Yr.	*19-22 Yr.*	*23-50 Yr.*	**Pregnancy**	**Lactation**
Calories (kcal)	2100	2100	2000	+300	+500
Protein (gm)	46	44	44	+30	+20
Vitamin A (R.E.)	800	800	800	+200	+400
Vitamin D (mcg)	10	7.5	5	+5	+5
Vitamin E (mg T.E.)	8	8	8	+2	+3
Ascorbic acid (mg)	60	60	60	+20	+40
Folacin (mcg)	400	400	400	+400	+100
Niacin (mg)	14	14	13	+2	+5
Riboflavin (mg)	1.3	1.3	1.2	+0.3	+0.5
Thiamine (mg)	1.1	1.1	1.0	+0.4	+0.5
Vitamin B_{12} (mcg)	3.0	3.0	3.0	+1.0	+1.0
Calcium (mg)	1200	1200	800	+400	+400
Phosphorus (mg)	1200	1200	800	+400	+400
Iodine (mcg)	150	150	150	+25	+50
Iron (mg)	18	18	18	Supplemental Iron	
Magnesium (mg)	300	300	300	+150	+150
Zinc (mg)	15	15	15	+5	+10

*From *Recommended Dietary Allowances*, 9th ed. National Academy of Sciences—National Research Council, Washington, D.C., 1980.

TABLE 4–2. Changes in Basic Four During Pregnancy and Lactation*

Basic Four†	Nonpregnant	Pregnant (2nd half)	Lactating
Milk			
Adult	2 or more cups	3 or more cups	4 or more cups
Adolescent	4 or more cups	5 or more cups	5 or more cups
Vegetable-fruit			
Citrus or substitute	1 serving	2 servings	2–3 servings
Dark-green or deep-yellow vegetable	1 serving at least every other day	1 serving daily	1–2 servings daily
Other fruits or vegetables, including potatoes	2 servings	2 servings	2 servings
Meat or alternate	2 or more servings	3 or more servings (6 oz cooked) Include liver or heart every week.	
Cereal-bread	4 or more servings	4 or more servings	4 or more servings
		If fortified milk is not used, obtain physician's instructions for vitamin D supplementation. Use iodized salt. Use water or other beverages—at least 6 to 8 cups daily.	

*From P. S. Howe, *Basic Nutrition in Health and Disease*, 7th ed. W. B. Saunders Co., Philadelphia, 1981, p. 177.

†Additional servings of these or any other food may be added as needed to provide the necessary calories and palatability.

WHAT ARE SOME OF THE CLINICAL PROBLEMS DURING PREGNANCY?

Nausea. Nausea may sometimes occur in the first trimester. Eating high-carbohydrate foods such as dry toast or crackers before arising may alleviate the problem. Fried foods and other high-fat foods are a common cause of nausea and should be avoided. Fluids should be taken between meals. Increasing food intake gradually during the late afternoon and evening will help replace nutrients.

Anemia. Anemia due to iron deficiency may occur during pregnancy because iron intake and stores do not meet the demand. This is preventable and treatable by supplements of 30 to 60 mg of ferrous salts.

Anemia due to folacin deficiency may occur if intake of food and nutrients is poor. A supplement of 400 mcg of folacin as well as improvement in eating habits will correct the anemia.

Toxemia. This is a condition which may occur during the third trimester of pregnancy. It is characterized by proteinuria, elevated blood pressure, and rapid weight gain due to edema. Toxemia is also sometimes referred to as pre-eclampsia. The exact cause of toxemia is not known. Theories involving malnutrition as a factor in its etiology have been advanced. Its incidence is lower among women who have good diets and increased in underweight and overweight women.[3]

TABLE 4–3. Sample Meal Plans for Pregnancy

	Pregnant Woman	Pregnant Adolescent
		(more kilocalories, protein, calcium)
Breakfast	Orange juice, 1 cup Shredded wheat Scrambled egg Toast, 1 slice Milk, 1 cup Decaffeinated coffee	Orange juice, 1 cup Shredded wheat Scrambled egg Toast, 2 slices Butter or margarine Marmalade Milk, 1 cup
Lunch	Meat sandwich Carrot and green pepper sticks Oatmeal cookies Milk, 1 cup	Meat sandwich on whole-wheat bread Carrot and green pepper sticks Cheese cubes Oatmeal cookies Fresh fruit Milk, 1 cup
Midafternoon	Milk, 1 cup	Chicken sandwich Milk, 1 cup
Dinner	Broiled beef liver Steamed broccoli Baked potato Tomato salad with French dressing Baked apple	Broiled beef liver with bacon and onion Steamed broccoli Baked potato with sour cream Vegetable salad with French dressing Baked apple with raisins Milk, 1 cup
Bedtime	Hot milk or cocoa, 1 cup	Milk or cocoa, 1 cup

In the past, altering dietary components to prevent toxemia has not been successful. Sodium restrictions are no longer recommended and may actually be harmful, since sodium needs are increased during pregnancy.[4]

Overweight. For obese women, a weight reduction regimen should not be initiated at any time during pregnancy. They should observe the same principles of prenatal nutrition as normal-weight women. Weight reduction should begin after pregnancy has terminated.

Pica. Pica is an abnormal craving for nonfood substances. Laundry starch, clay, and chalk are the most common cravings during pregnancy. When intake of these substances interferes with consumption of adequate nutrients, it should be corrected to ensure optimal fetal development.

WHAT ARE THE NUTRIENT NEEDS DURING LACTATION?

To meet the needs of both mother and baby during lactation an additional 500 calories and 20 grams of protein, as well as increases in vitamins and minerals (see Table 4–1), are necessary. This will allow for the production of an adequate milk supply (550 to 850 ml) of high-quality breast milk. Additional servings from the Basic Four Food Groups (see Table 4–2) will meet these requirements.

When lactation is terminated, food intake should return to normal to prevent excess weight gain.

NUTRITION COUNSELING

Nutrition counseling is likely to be well accepted by the prospective mother who is anxious to do everything she can to have a healthy baby. Such advice must be individualized to meet the woman's own particular food preferences, customs, and budget.

For the pregnant teenager, nutrition counseling to provide for optimum nutrients for the demands of her maturing body as well as for the developing fetus will help decrease the risks of pregnancy complications, low birth weight infants, and infant mortality.

The mother-to-be must be taught what changes are necessary to meet their nutrient needs and how to modify their current food habits to accommodate these necessary changes.

Study Questions and Activities

1. What benefits may the mother-to-be expect if she is well nourished? How will the baby benefit?
2. Why should the pregnant teenager be sure she receives adequate calories as well as sufficient amounts of all important nutrients?
3. Why are protein and calcium key nutrients in the diet during pregnancy? How are the additional demands for these nutrients met in the diet of the pregnant woman?
4. How and why do the foods needed in the daily diet during pregnancy and lactation differ from those needed by nonpregnant women?
5. Name several different ways for the pregnant woman to incorporate milk in the diet if she does not find it possible to drink the desired amount.

Nutrition of Infants: Birth to One Year

HOW DOES AN INFANT GROW AND DEVELOP?

The greatest growth and development during a lifetime takes place during the first year. At birth the average weight is 7 pounds (boys weigh a little more than girls), and the average length is 18 to 24 inches. For the first five months, the average weekly gain in weight is 5 to 8 ounces (about 1½ to 2 lb per month), resulting in a doubling of birth weight at about 5 months. From 6 to 12 months, the average weekly weight gain is 4 to 5 ounces (about 1 pound per month), with the birth weight tripled at 10 to 12 months.

During the first year, the average gain in height is 9 to 10 inches, with rapid growth of the arms and legs, which are short in proportion at birth.

At birth the stomach capacity is 1 ounce, or 2 tablespoons. At two weeks of age this has increased to 2 ounces, or 4 tablespoons, and by three months is up to 4½ ounces, or 9 tablespoons.

Even the infant's digestive ability increases within the first year. At birth, infants are able to digest protein, simple carbohydrates, and emulsified fats. Later, digestive enzymes develop for digestion of starch and some fat.

A well-nourished infant will show steady gain in weight and height (with some fluctuations from week to week), is happy and vigorous, sleeps well, has firm muscles, will have some tooth eruption at about 5 to 6 months, with about 6 to 12 teeth erupted by 12 months, has good elimination characteristic of the type of feeding — breast or formula. Each infant has an indi-

TABLE 4-4. RDA for Infants – Birth to 1 Year*

	0 – 6 Months	6 – 12 Months
Energy (kcal)	Wt. in kg × 115	Wt. in kg × 105
Protein (g)	Wt. in kg × 2.2	Wt. in kg × 2.0
Vitamin C	35 mg	35 mg
Folacin	30 mcg	45 mcg
Niacin	6 mg	8 mg
Riboflavin	0.4 mg	0.6 mg
Thiamine	0.3 mg	0.5 mg
Vitamin B_6	0.3 mg	0.6 mg
Vitamin B_{12}	0.5 mcg	1.5 mcg
Vitamin A	420 mcg of R.E.	400 mcg of R.E.
Vitamin D	10 mcg	10 mcg
Vitamin E	3 mg of T.E.	4 mg of T.E.
Calcium	360 mg	540 mg
Phosphorus	240 mg	360 mg
Iodine	40 mcg	50 mcg
Iron	10 mg	15 mg
Magnesium	50 mg	70 mg
Zinc	3 mg	5 mg

*Adapted from *Recommended Dietary Allowances*, 9th ed. National Academy of Sciences—National Research Council, Washington, D.C., 1980.

vidual rate of growth, but all grow faster in weight than in height. A steady weight gain is more important than a large amount gained.

HOW ARE THE INFANT'S NUTRITIONAL NEEDS MET?

Infants require more kilocalories, protein, minerals, and vitamins in proportion to weight than adults (see RDA, Table 4-4). Because of growth, more active tissue, and activity, fluid requirements are also high (see Table 4-5).

To meet this demand for nutrients, the mother is faced with the decision to breast- or bottle-feed her infant. The decision should be made only after the mother has been well educated on the advantages and disadvantages of each method.

TABLE 4-5. Fluid Requirements of Infants – Birth to 1 Year*

Age	Amount of Water (ml/kg/day)
1 week	80–100
2 weeks	125–150
3 months	140–160
6 months	130–155
9 months	125–145
1 year	120–135

*Adapted from V. C. Vaughan, R. J. McKay, and R. E. Behrman, eds., *Nelson Textbook of Pediatrics*, 11th ed. W. B. Saunders Co., Philadelphia, 1979.

Breast Feeding. This is generally agreed by experts to be the preferred method of feeding if feasible for the mother. Human milk is species-specific and therefore perfectly suited to supply all the infant's nutritional needs for the beginning of life.

Breast milk is free from contamination, is the proper temperature, requires no preparation, is more economical than bottle feeding, and contains helpful antibodies that fight infection. It is easier for the infant to digest and absorb, since human milk forms finer, softer curds in the infant's stomach.

If the mother is chronically ill, unable to produce adequate amounts of milk, or is taking certain drugs, breast-feeding is contraindicated. Premature infants or infants with cleft palate or lip may be fed breast milk using bottles with special nipples.

Bottle Feeding. This may be the more practical method of feeding for the working mother, since it allows other persons to feed the baby when the mother is not present. It is more expensive than breast-feeding, since the formula, bottles, nipples, and utensils for sterilization must be purchased.

Whether the mother chooses to bottle- or breast-feed, feeding time should enhance the mother-child relationship. Touch is important in establishing a firm bond. If bottle feeding is chosen, the baby should be cradled in the mother's arms instead of propping the bottle (see Fig. 4–1). The mother should be relaxed.

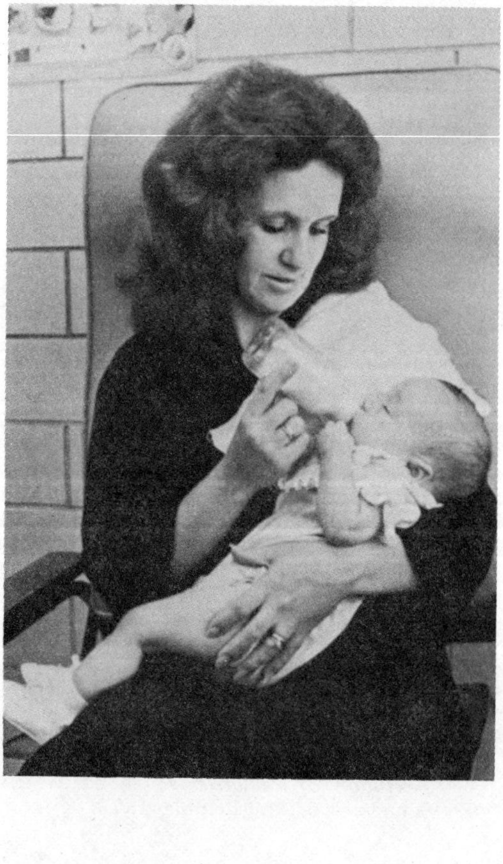

Figure 4–1. Correct position for bottle feeding. Photo from Arkansas Children's Hospital. (From B. Alford and M. Bogle, *Nutrition During the Life Cycle.* Prentice-Hall, Inc., Englewood Cliffs, N.J., 1982.)

Feeding Schedule

Feeding "on demand" is preferred to a rigid schedule, since it permits the baby to obtain food when he or she is hungry. The mother will soon learn to recognize when the baby is hungry or satisfied. This will help avoid overfeeding. "For small infants a rigid schedule may be necessary as infants tend to sleep excessively without 'demanding' feedings frequently enough to meet their growth needs."[5] As the infant establishes an individual feeding schedule a rigid feeding schedule may be compromised.

Table 4-6 provides a suggested feeding schedule. It should be regarded as only a guide, since each infant may vary greatly in appetite and capacity.[5]

WHAT TYPES OF INFANT FORMULAS ARE USED?

Cow's Milk Formula. A formula containing cow's whole, canned evaporated, or dried milk fortified with vitamins A and D, a source of carbohydrate, and water constitutes an alternative to breast-feeding. The milk is diluted with water to reduce its protein content to resemble that of human milk. It is heated to make the curd more digestible and free of bacteria. Corn syrup, granulated sugar, or Dextri-Maltose is added to increase the carbohydrate calories. (It is important to note that canned evaporated milk should *not* be confused with sweetened condensed milk.)

Commercial Formulas. These formulas are formulated to closely approximate human milk. They are available in powder, liquid concentrated, and ready-to-feed types. Powdered forms are more economical but require mixing and careful measuring. Liquid concentrated formulas require proper dilution before using. These formulas are fortified to meet all the vitamin and mineral requirements of the infant. If the infant requires iron supplements, formulas containing iron are available.

Examples of commercial formulas are Enfamil, Similac, SMA, and Advance.

Soybean-based Formulas. Soybean-based formulas are used if the infant shows signs of allergy to cow's milk or when the parents are strict vegetarians (vegans). These commercially prepared formulas are fortified with vitamins and minerals.

Examples of soybean-based formulas are ProSobee, Neo-Mull-Soy, Isomil, and CHO-Free.

TABLE 4-6. Suggested Feeding Schedule*

Age of Infant	Number of Feedings	Volume per Feeding	Total Volume
0 to 2 weeks	6–10	60–90 ml (2–3 oz)	600–700 ml
2 weeks–1 month	6–8	90–120 ml (3–4 oz)	700–750 ml
1–3 months	5–6	150–180 ml (5–6 oz)	750–850 ml
3–7 months	4–5	180–210 ml (6–7 oz)	900–1000 ml
7–12 months	3–4	210–240 ml (7–8 oz)	950–1000 ml

*From B. Alford and M. Bogle, *Nutrition During the Life Cycle.* Prentice-Hall, Inc., Englewood Cliffs, N.J., 1982, p. 29.

This schedule may apply to both breast- and formula-fed infants.

Special Formulas. Special formulas may be necessary for digestive disturbances, allergy, or inborn errors of metabolism. Examples of these formulas are Portagen, Pregestimil, Lonalac, and Lofenalac.

See Table 4–7 for a more complete breakdown of some of these formulas.

HOW IS AN INFANT'S FORMULA PREPARED?

It is important that the baby's formula be as sterile as possible. Either of the two sterilization methods below may be used.

Fresh Milk Formula – Traditional Method

Method 1: Sterilizing utensils and formula together (terminal). A prepared mixture, ordered by a physician, is poured into washed and rinsed nursing bottles, then the bottles and mixture are boiled. This method eliminates possible contamination and is easy to use. It is recommended by the American Hospital Association.

1. Measure exact amounts of sugar, water, and milk, as ordered by doctor, in a clean quart measure (or use measuring cup and sauce pan). Stir well to dissolve and blend ingredients.
2. Pour correct amount of formula into each clean bottle.
3. Cap bottles with clean nipples (inverted if using certain types of screw tops); cover with clean discs and screw caps, or with clean nipple covers. Do not screw cap on tightly, or press down covers. They should be loose enough for steam to circulate.
4. Place bottles in rack in deep pan. Put 2 to 3 inches of hot water into pan, cover tightly, and bring water to boil. Boil 25 minutes.
5. Turn off heat and let bottles cool in covered pan until lukewarm. Tighten screw tops, or press down covers. Refrigerate bottles at once.

Method 2: Sterilizing utensils and formula separately (sterile or aseptic). A prepared mixture is boiled for 3 minutes (counting from the time it comes to a boil), then poured into sterilized nursing bottles. This is the traditional method.

1. Sterile utensils: Put clean nursing bottles, funnel, strainer, and tongs in rack in pan that holds 2 to 3 inches of hot water. (Keep tong handles out of hot water.) Cover and boil 10 minutes. Boil clean nipples and all parts of bottle caps or nipple covers 3 minutes in small covered pan. Drain off water and keep nipples and caps in the sterile pan. Take utensils from sterilizing pan with sterile tongs. Put sterile funnel and strainer on inverted lid of bottle sterilizer. Do not let hands touch any part of sterile utensils which the formula will touch.
2. Follow step 1 under Method 1, using enamel sauce pan.
3. Heat quickly to boiling, boil 3 minutes. Stir continuously.
4. Strain hot formula into the sterile bottles using sterilized strainer and funnel. Fill each bottle with exact amount of formula for each feeding.
5. Put on sterile nipple and cap. Do not touch nipple with hands.
6. Cool bottles at room temperature until lukewarm. Refrigerate bottles at once.

Complete Commercial Formulas

Equipment Needed:

1. Six to 8 oz nursing bottles with caps (boilable, plastic).
2. Nipples, one for each bottle and a few spares. The ones made of silicone will last longer.
3. A bottle and nipple brush.

TABLE 4–7. Composition of Infant Formulas per Liter*

Milk or Formula	Kcal	Protein (gm)	Fat (gm)	CHO (gm)	Calcium (mg)	Phosphorus (mg)	Sodium (mg)	Potassium (mg)	Iron (mg)	Protein Source	Fat Source	CHO Source	Comments
Human Milk	750	11	45	68	340	140	161	507	0.2	Lactalbumin, casein	Human	Lactose	Protein readily digested, adequate in all vitamins and minerals except possibly C and D.
Similac	680	15.5	36	72	510	390	220	700	tr.†	Casein	Soy, coconut and corn oils	Lactose	Vitamins and minerals added.
Enfamil	670	15	37	69	550	460	280	700	1.4	Casein	Soy and coconut oils	Lactose	Vitamins and minerals added.
Evaporated Cow's Milk Formula‡	660	28	32	69	1027	827	498	1212	2	Casein	Butterfat	Lactose	Inadequate in iron, vitamin C, and possibly fluoride.
ProSobee	680	25	34	68	790	530	420	740	12.6	Soy protein	Soy oil	Sucrose, corn syrup solids	Vitamins and minerals added. For infants allergic to cow's milk.
Isomil	680	20	36	68	700	500	300	710	12	Soy protein	Coconut and soy oils	Sucrose and corn syrup solids	Vitamins and minerals added. For infants allergic to cow's milk.
Pregestimil	670	22	28	88	630	470	315	680	12.6	Casein hydrolysate	MCT oil, corn oil	Dextrose, modified tapioca	Protein and fat easily digested, nonallergenic protein. Used in malabsorption.
Lofenalac	670	22	27	87	470	470	483	1053	12.7	Casein hydrolysate	Corn oil	Corn syrup solids	Low in phenylalanine. Used in phenylketonuria (PKU). Vitamins added.

*Adapted from M. Krause and L. Mahan, *Food, Nutrition and Diet Therapy*, 6th ed., W. B. Saunders Co., Philadelphia, 1979, p. 302.
†Available with iron supplement (12 to 13 mg/l)
‡Formula (25 oz): 10 oz evaporated milk, 1 oz corn syrup, and 14 oz water.

Procedure:

1. Use a concentrated prepared infant formula containing vitamins and iron.

2. Use bottles, caps, and nipples that have been washed in clean water and dishwashing soap or detergent (wash them first when you do the family dishes). Use a bottle brush.

3. Squeeze water through the nipple holes to be sure they are open. Rinse them well so that all soap or detergent is gone and let them stand in a rack to dry.

4. Clean the top of the formula can with soap and water and rinse.

5. Open the formula can with a clean punch-type opener and pour out the necessary amount. Cover the can with fresh foil or plastic wrap and put it in the refrigerator.

6. Pour formula directly into the feeding bottle. Use the markings on the bottle to measure just one-half as much formula concentrate as the total amount of formula you want in the bottle.

7. Add an equal amount of fresh water directly from the tap. Put on the nipple and cap.

Special Instructions

If you use water from a well or pump or from a water supply that is not regularly inspected, boil each day's supply of water for 20 minutes, pour the boiling water into a clean jar, and keep it covered in the refrigerator for use in making formula. Wash and clean the water jar daily.

If you do not have a reliable refrigerator, use powdered formula containing vitamins and iron. This formula is prepared by pouring safe tap water or boiled water into the nursing bottle and adding one level tablespoon of powdered formula for each two ounces of water. Put on the cap and nipple and shake the bottle well until the powder is dissolved. The can of powdered formula should be covered but need not be refrigerated.

If you are breast-feeding and need only an occasional formula feeding, the above method using powdered formula is especially convenient and inexpensive.

What Not To Do

1. Do not use formula that has been left standing at room temperature for more than 30 or 40 minutes or in the refrigerator for more than three days.

2. Do not use any formula unless you have read the instructions on the can or bottle.

3. Do not give added vitamins or iron if you are using a prepared infant formula that contains added vitamins and iron.

WHAT ADDITIONAL FOODS ARE GIVEN DURING THE FIRST YEAR?

Neither breast milk nor a milk formula will furnish adequate amounts of all nutrients required by the infant during the first year. One important reason for introducing some solid foods into the infant's diet is to replenish the depleting stores of iron during the early months of life.

The suggested age at which solid or semisolid foods should be introduced, as well as their sequence, varies widely among pediatricians. Some infants may acquire the necessary physiological skills that enable an earlier introduction of these foods. However, semisolid foods are usually not introduced before three months. A possible feeding schedule for introduction of these foods is found in Table 4–8.

Mealtime should be a pleasant experience for the infant. Semisolid foods should be introduced only one food at a time and in small amounts. If the baby does not like the food the first time, it should be tried again later. New foods should be given at the beginning of the meal, when the baby is hungriest. It is important that the mother show a positive reaction to the food even if it is not one of her favorites, since babies quickly reflect the food preferences of those feeding them.[6]

The mother should not expect the baby to consume all the food at every meal. Forcing an infant to eat when he or she is not hungry may lead to overfeeding.

By the end of the first year, the baby will be getting mashed and chopped foods instead of strained and finely ground foods. The infant will have developed the skills necessary for self-feeding, and will usually be consuming three meals a day, with snacks of those foods not consumed at meals. A sample pattern might be:

Breakfast: Cereal, egg, milk
Midmorning: Orange juice
Lunch: Meat, milk, vegetable
Midafternoon: Milk, crackers
Dinner: Cereal, milk, fruit

TABLE 4–8. Suggested Guide for the Introduction of Foods During the First Year of Life

Age	Food	Rationale	Amount
2–3 weeks	Orange juice	Provides vitamin C if not supplied in formula.	Start 1 tsp orange juice and 1 tsp water, gradually add more juice. At 6 months, infant should be receiving 4 oz to continue through 1 yr.
3–4 months	Iron-fortified cereal	Provides iron as stores in liver decrease, thiamine	Start 1 tsp one time a day, mixed with formula. Gradually increase to 5 Tbsp by 6 months, ½ cup at 1 year.
4–5 months	Strained vegetable	Provides vitamins A and C	Start with 1 tsp. Gradually increase to 3–4 Tbsp at 1 year.
5–6 months	Strained fruit	Provides vitamins A and C	Start with 1 tsp. Gradually increase to 3–4 Tbsp at 1 year.
6–7 months	Strained meats	Provides protein, iron, vitamin B complex	Start with 1 tsp. Gradually increase to 2 Tbsp.
7–9 months	Egg yolk	Provides iron	Start with ¼ tsp, adding a small amount until whole egg yolk is consumed at about 11 months. At 1 year, whole egg is given.

Study Questions and Activities

1. Name the characteristics of a well-nourished infant.
2. What are advantages of breast-feeding? Why is breast milk so suitable for the infant?
3. What nutrients are supplied in the infant's diet by cereals? By fruits? By a green or yellow vegetable? By egg yolks? By meat?
4. What is the difference between the sterile and terminal techniques for preparing a baby's formula? Which is considered more desirable? Why?
5. List some ways to encourage good food habits in children as soon as they begin to get foods in addition to breast milk or formula.

Nutrition in Childhood and Adolescence

WHAT IS THE IMPORTANCE OF NUTRITION TO HEALTHY GROWTH AND DEVELOPMENT?

Without a supply of adequate nutrients, optimal growth and development of the infant to adulthood would not be possible. Nutrients supplied by the food the child consumes provide energy and the necessary building blocks for synthesis of new tissues.

"The nutritional requirements of the child vary with the chronological age, growth rate, maturation stage, physical activity, and the efficiency of absorption and utilization of nutrients."[7]

The RDA for children were designed in amounts that will maintain a satisfactory rate of growth (see Table 4–9). They are not a precise requirement for each child.

WHAT IS MEANT BY GROWTH AND DEVELOPMENT?

Growth is the increase in weight and height with age, or "size" as it is popularly designated, that comes about as a result of the multiplication of cells and their differentiation for many different functions in the body. Height is the more significant factor as the type of body build and amount of fatty tissue cause weight variation. Growth is a continuous but not uniform process from conception to full maturity. During fetal life and infancy, the rate of growth is very rapid. This period is followed by one of slower growth during early and middle childhood. Another period of very rapid growth occurs during adolescence, followed by a tapering off until the growth period ends.

Development refers to the increasing ability of body parts to function. Factors affecting the rate of growth and development include heredity, or inborn capacity to grow, and various environmental factors, an extremely important one of which is nutrition. Better diets, which accompany improved economic conditions, and advances in medical care and health services are credited for the taller stature of children and adults in the United States today as compared with children and adults of similar ages some decades ago. It has also been noted that in the technologically advanced countries the average height and weight of children of any given age have increased over the last 100 years. There is accumulating evidence that well-nourished

TABLE 4–9. Recommended Dietary Allowances for Children*

Age (years)	Weight (kg)	Weight (lbs)	Height (cm)	Height (in)	Energy (kcal)	Protein (gm)	Vitamin A Activity (RE)	Vitamin A Activity (IU)	Vitamin D Activity (μg)	Vitamin D Activity (IU)
1–3	13	29	90	35	1300	23	400	2000	10	400
4–6	20	44	112	44	1800	30	500	2500	10	400
7–10	28	62	132	52	2400	34	700	3300	10	400

Vitamin E Activity (mg T.E.)	Ascorbic Acid (mg)	Folacin (μg)	Niacin (mg)	Riboflavin (mg)	Thiamine (mg)	Vitamin B_6 (mg)
5	45	100	9	.8	.7	.9
6	45	200	11	1.0	.9	1.3
7	45	300	16	1.4	1.2	1.6

Vitamin B_{12} (μg)	Calcium (mg)	Phosphorus (mg)	Iodine (μg)	Iron (mg)	Magnesium (mg)	Zinc (mg)
2.0	800	800	70	15	150	10
2.5	800	800	90	10	200	10
3.0	800	800	120	10	250	10

*From *Recommended Dietary Allowances*, 9th ed. National Academy of Sciences—National Research Council, Washington, D.C., 1980.

children reach the potential set by their heredity, not only in physical growth but also in mental development.

WHAT ARE THE EFFECTS OF MALNUTRITION ON GROWTH AND DEVELOPMENT, LEARNING, AND BEHAVIOR?

As many as half of the world's children may suffer some degree of malnutrition, from temporary to permanent, that causes mental and physical development problems. Children who do not get enough to eat and are malnourished tend to be smaller and sick more often. They also may be less able to learn.

To the extent that malnutrition occurs in the United States, children will not be able to achieve their full potential and realize a healthy and satisfying adult life. For developing nations worldwide, where children may constitute a large percentage of the population, malnutrition may constrain the country's future social and economic development.

A prolonged lack of one or more nutrients retards physical development or causes specific clinical conditions to appear. For example, anemia, goiter, and rickets constitute a state of malnutrition. Severe malnutrition, characterized by clinical manifestations, is of two basic types: *kwashiorkor* (protein deficiency) (see Fig. 4–2) and *marasmus* (overall deficit of food, especially kilocalories) (see Fig. 4–3). Infantile marasmus is frequently the result of early cessation of breast-feeding, overdilution of bottle-fed formula, or gastrointestinal infection early in life and is accompanied by wasting away of tissues and extreme growth retardation. Kwashiorkor generally occurs at or after weaning, when milk high in protein is replaced by a starchy staple food providing insufficient protein. A child with this type of malnutrition is usually stunted in growth and has edema, skin sores, and discoloration of dark hair to red or blond.

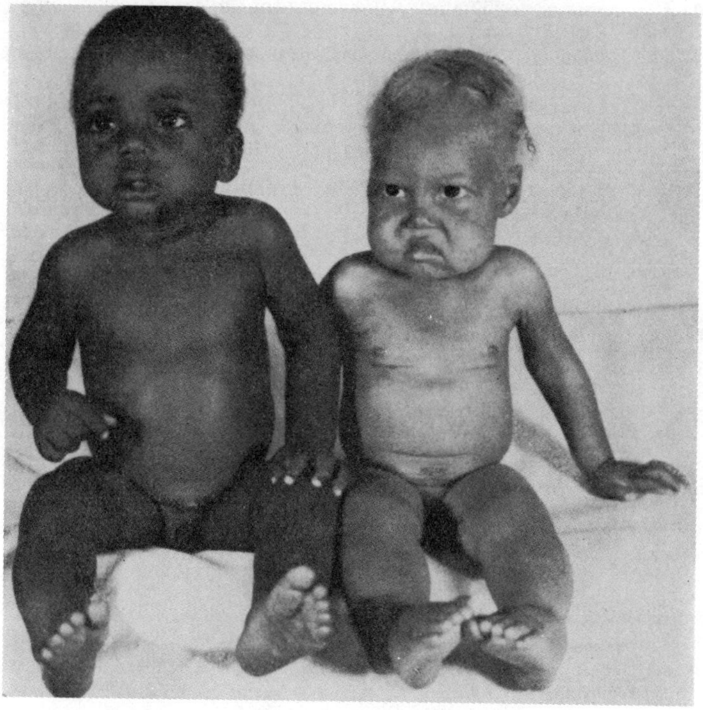

Figure 4–2. *Right*, Infant with "sugar baby" kwashiorkor, commonly seen in Jamaica and attributed to a high-sugar, low-protein diet. Infant has stunted growth, edema of the feet and hands, fatty liver, moon face, and dyspigmentation of the skin and hair. *Left*, normal infant. (From D. B. Jelliffe, Hypochromotrichia and malnutrition in Jamaican infants. *Journal of Tropical Pediatrics*, Vol. 1, 1955, p. 25.)

Undernourished children are identified most often by biochemical and clinical signs of malnutrition, but the values of these signs are limited to extremely inadequate diet. Chronic long-term undernutrition generally results in stunting of growth, and the degree of malnutrition is often proportional to the degree to which the child is subnormal in height or weight (see Fig. 4–4). Therefore, anthropometric measures (height, weight, and fatness) are the most commonly used indices of undernutrition (see Appendix A–3 for physical growth charts).

Types of moderate malnutrition include (1) that caused by chronic food reduction (manifested by growth retardation) and (2) that which results from vitamin or mineral deficiency and is accompanied by clinical symptoms such as rickets or pellagra. Malnutrition is most often associated with poverty. Exact determination of effects on the individual is difficult, since other factors influence human growth and behavioral development, including an individual innate potential, health status, and environment.

In the world, malnutrition is mankind's most pervasive health problem; more than half of the children in developing countries are moderately or severely undernourished. Kilocalorie deprivation (food quantity shortage), not necessarily protein lack, seems to be the world's primary problem.

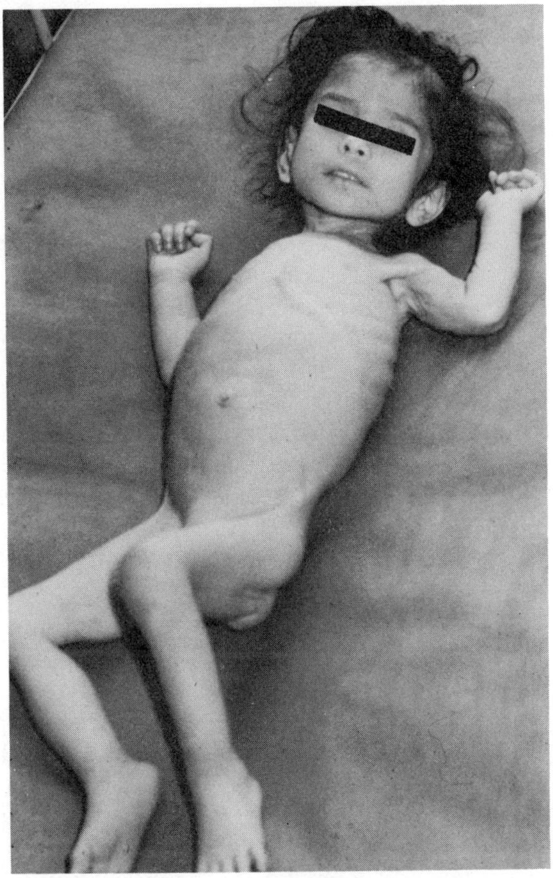

Figure 4–3. Marasmus in a child 2 years and 4 months old. (From S. L. Robbins and R. S. Cotran, *Pathologic Basis of Disease*, 2nd ed. W. B. Saunders Co., Philadelphia, 1979, p. 485.)

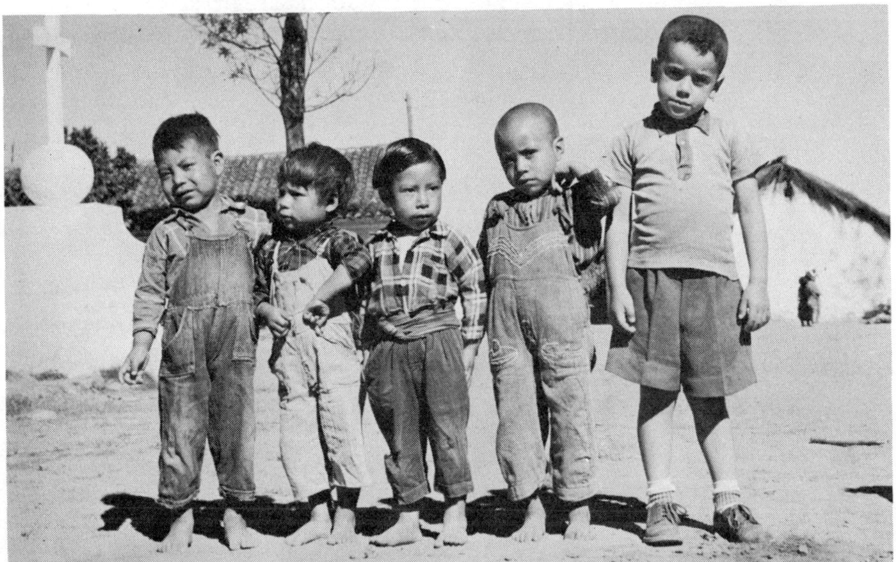

Figure 4–4. Growth failure in four Guatemalan boys 4 to 5 years old (*left*), caused by chronic malnutrition. The fifth boy (*right*), of the same age group, is from a family in which the diet is superior. His height and weight are normal for his age. (From G. M. Briggs and D. H. Calloway, *Bogert's Nutrition and Physical Fitness*, 10th ed. Copyright 1979 by W. B. Saunders Company. Reprinted with permission of W. B. Saunders Company, CBS College Publishing.)

In the United States, three of the extensive surveys of nutritional status conducted in recent years have reached similar conclusions — marasmus and kwashiorkor are quite rare, but chronic undernutrition and iron deficiency are surprisingly common. A child's growth record is a more accurate criterion of whether a child is receiving sufficient nutrients than are Recommended Dietary Allowances—the gross estimates of nutritional needs are not designed to assess an individual's nutritional status. Except for iron, the national surveys found little dietary or clinical evidence of vitamin or mineral deficiencies among the children in this country.

Malnutrition impairs the body's defense against disease. Therefore, infection, rampant in undeveloped regions of the world owing to poor sanitary conditions, occurs more frequently in malnourished children. Very severe malnutrition in infancy, if of long duration and followed by childhood undernutrition, produces irreversible effects in behavior, which in turn impair a child's ability to learn. Certain studies have shown that chronically undernourished children tend to lag behind their well-nourished counterparts in behavioral development.[8]

WHAT ARE THE IMPORTANT CONSIDERATIONS IN FEEDING THE PRESCHOOL CHILD (1 TO 5 YEARS OLD)?

As children grow, their eating habits change. These changes are reflective of their stage in development (Fig. 4–5). For the preschool child, in comparison to the infant, there is a slowing in the rate of growth and development. A decrease in the consumption of food parallels this decrease in metabolic rate. A parent should not become alarmed if the following changes in eating behavior exist; rather, they are considered "normal" for the preschool child:[3]

1. A pattern of strong food preferences and aversions (see Tables 4–10 and 4–11).
2. General disinterest in food.
3. Erratic desires for foods (food jags)—settling on a few foods only to discard them for another pattern of food choices shortly thereafter.

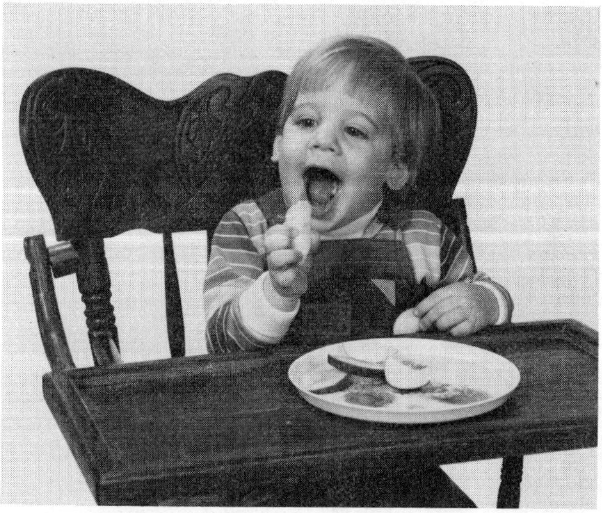

Figure 4–5. Finger foods are popular among preschool children.

TABLE 4–10. Favorite Foods by Category (Per Cent)*

Food	Preschool	Elementary
Meats	38.8%	52.3%
Snack items	16.7	4.5
Dairy foods	11.1	4.5
Mixed dishes	11.1	20.4
Breads, cereals	5.5	4.5
Fruits	5.5	—
Vegetables	5.5	4.5

*From L. S. Peavy and A. L. Pagenkopf, *Grow Healthy Kids: A Parent's Guide to Sound Nutrition from Birth through Teens.* Grosset and Dunlap, New York, 1980, p. 128. Adapted from N. R. Beyer and P. M. Morris, "Food Attitudes and Snacking Patterns of Young Children," *Journal of Nutrition Education,* Vol. 6, 1974, p. 131.

If a parent is becoming increasingly concerned about the food intake of the child, keeping a food diary may help. "The purpose of this food record is to determine *which* major categories of foods are, or are not, being eaten and *when* the child does most of his eating."[9] The child's diet can then be modified by offering previously omitted foods at the times when the child is most hungry.

The preschool child seems to prefer foods that are simply prepared. Mixed foods are unpopular with this age group. Finger foods are well accepted (see Table 4–12), and differences in food textures interest children. Each meal might include something soft and easy to chew (such as creamed potatoes), something crispy (such as carrot sticks), and something chewy (moist hamburger patty) to promote the use of newly learned chewing skills.[10]

TABLE 4–11. Disliked Foods by Categories (Per Cent)*

Food	Preschool	Elementary
Cooked vegetables	50.9%	47.7%
Mixed dishes, casseroles	14.1	10.7
Meat	8.8	7.7
Liver	7.0	12.4
Raw vegetables	5.3	6.2
Cottage cheese	3.5	1.5
Fish	3.5	6.2
Fruit	3.5	1.5
Eggs	1.7	4.6
Milk	1.7	1.5

*From L. S. Peavy and A. L. Pagenkopf, *Grow Healthy Kids: A Parent's Guide to Sound Nutrition from Birth through Teens.* Grosset and Dunlap, New York, 1980, p. 128. Adapted from N. R. Beyer and P. M. Morris, "Food Attitudes and Snacking Patterns of Young Children," *Journal of Nutrition Education,* Vol. 6, 1974, p. 131.

TABLE 4–12. Suggested Snacks and Finger Foods*

Fruits	Vegetables
Apple wedges	Cabbage wedges
Banana slices	Carrot sticks
Berries	Cauliflowerets
Dried apples	Celery sticks†
Dried apricots	Cherry tomatoes
Dried peaches	Cucumber slices
Dried pears	Green pepper sticks
Fresh peach wedges	Tomato wedges
Fresh pear wedges	Turnip sticks
Fresh pineapple sticks	Zucchini or summer squash strips
Grapefruit sections (seeded)	
Grapes	*Meats*
Melon cubes or balls	Cheese cubes
Orange sections (seeded)	Cooked meat cubes
Pitted plums	Hard-cooked eggs
Pitted prunes	Small sandwiches (quartered)
Raisins	Toast fingers
Tangerine sections	Whole-grain crackers

*From *A Planning Guide for Food Service in Child Care Centers,* USDA, FNS-64, Food and Nutrition Service, Washington, D.C., revised 1976.

†May be stuffed with cheese or peanut butter.

Mealtime should be a pleasant experience for the child. The atmosphere should be relaxed and conducive to pleasant conversation. The child should be equipped with eating utensils and dishes that are easy to handle.

The child should be offered only small amounts of food at a time. By the age of 4 or 5 the child may be able to dish food onto a plate in accordance with appetite. A child should never be forced to eat. This encourages a habit of overeating.

Snacks should be planned to enhance the nutritional value of the diet. They should be served at least one hour prior to the meals to allow for sufficient intake of food at mealtime.

For a guide to foods included and amounts for the preschool child, see Table 4–13. Good food habits developed at this time will help ensure an adequate diet throughout the life cycle.

WHAT ARE THE IMPORTANT CONSIDERATIONS IN FEEDING SCHOOL CHILDREN (6 TO 12 YEARS OLD)?

Meeting the nutritional requirements of the 6 to 12 year old requires larger amounts of the same foods needed by the preschool child (see Table 4–14).

Growth during prepuberty is slow and steady, with gradual increases in height and weight.

With the introduction of school into the daily routine of the child, the meal pattern of the child is likely to change. Breakfast may have to be eaten earlier to allow sufficient time to get to school. Children who skip breakfast are less well fed, since it is difficult to make up missed nutrients at other

TABLE 4–13. Pattern of Feeding*

Meal	Children 1 to 3 years	Children 3 to 6 years
Breakfast		
Milk, fluid[a]	1/2 cup	3/4 cup
Juice or fruit	1/4 cup	1/2 cup
Cereal or bread, enriched or whole grain[b]		
cereal, or	1/4 cup[c]	1/3 cup[d]
bread	1/2 slice	1/2 slice
Midmorning or midafternoon supplement		
Milk, fluid[a]; or juice; or fruit; or vegetable	1/2 cup	1/2 cup
Bread or cereal, enriched or whole-grain[b]		
bread, or	1/2 slice	1/2 slice
cereal	1/4 cup[c]	1/3 cup[d]
Lunch or supper		
Milk, fluid[a]	1/2 cup	3/4 cup
Meat and/or meat alternate[e]		
Meat, poultry, or fish, cooked[f]	1 ounce	1 1/2 ounces
Cheese	1 ounce	1 1/2 ounces
Egg	1	1
Cooked dry beans and peas	1/8 cup	1/4 cup
Peanut butter	1 tablespoon	2 tablespoons
Vegetables and fruits[g]	1/4 cup	1/2 cup
Bread, enriched or whole-grain[b]	1/2 slice	1/2 slice

*From *A Planning Guide for Food Service in Child Care Centers.* USDA FNS-64, Food and Nutrition Service, Washington, D.C., revised 1976, p. 5.

[a]Includes whole milk, low-fat milk, skim milk, cultured buttermilk, or flavored milk made from these types of fluid milk which meet state and local standards.

[b]Or an equivalent serving of an acceptable bread product made of enriched or whole-grain meal or flour.

[c]1/4 cup (volume) or 1/3 ounce (weight), whichever is less.

[d]1/3 cup (volume) or 1/2 ounce (weight), whichever is less.

[e]Or an equivalent quantity of any combination of foods listed under Meat and Meat Alternates.

[f]Cooked lean meat without bone.

[g]Must include at least *two* kinds.

meals. They may be less able to perform well at school work than children who eat breakfast. If the family develops good breakfast habits, the child will likely continue this practice. The child may be taught to prepare a simple breakfast.

At school, the child is introduced to group feeding. Peers and teachers may influence eating behavior, and the child may be more or less willing to try an unfamiliar food, depending upon the eating behavior of others in the group.

Whether the child brings a lunch prepared from home or buys lunch from the National School Lunch Program, it should supply approximately one-third of the RDA for all nutrients. Nutrition education begun in the home and continued at school will help the child select nutritionally balanced meals.

TABLE 4–14. Foods Included in a Good Daily Diet (Average Amounts for Each Age)*

Food	Preschool *3–5 Years Old*	Early Elementary *6–9 Years Old*	Later Elementary *10–12 Years Old*	Early Adolescence *13–15 Years Old*
Milk	2 cups	2–3 cups	3 cups or more	3–4 cups or more
Eggs	1 whole egg	1 whole egg	1 whole egg	1 or more whole eggs
Meat, poultry, fish	2 ounces (1/4 cup) (1 small serving)	2–3 ounces (1 small serving)	3–4 ounces (1 serving)	4 ounces or more (1 serving)
Dried beans, peas (also an occasional replacement for meat, poultry or fish)	3–4 tablespoons	4–5 tablespoons	5–6 tablespoons	1/2 cup or more
Potatoes (may occasionally be replaced by equal amount enriched macaroni, spaghetti or rice)	3–4 tablespoons	4–5 tablespoons	1/2 cup or more	3/4 cup or more
Other cooked vegetables (often a green leafy or deep yellow vegetable)	3–4 tablespoons at one or more meals	4–5 tablespoons at one or more meals	1/3 cup or more at one or more meals	1/2 cup or more at one or more meals
Raw vegetables (lettuce, carrots, celery, etc.)	2 or more small pieces	1/4 cup	1/3 cup	1/2 cup or more
Vitamin C source (citrus fruits, tomatoes, etc.)	1 medium-sized orange or equivalent	1 medium-sized orange or equivalent	1 medium-sized orange or equivalent	1 large orange or equivalent
Other fruits	1/3 cup at one or more meals	1/2 cup or more at one or more meals	1/2 cup or more at one or more meals	2 servings
Cereal, whole-grain restored or enriched	1/2 cup or more	3/4 cup or more	1 cup or more	1 cup or more
Bread, whole-grain or enriched	2 or more slices	2 or more slices	2 or more slices	2 or more slices
Butter or fortified margarine	1 tablespoon	1 tablespoon	1 tablespoon or more	1 tablespoon or more
Sweets	1/3 cup simple dessert at 1 or 2 meals	1/2 cup simple dessert at 1 or 2 meals	1/2 cup or more simple dessert at 1 or 2 meals	1/2 cup or more at 1 or 2 meals
Vitamin D source		Enough to provide 400 I.U. (10 mcg) of vitamin D daily		

*From *Foods for Growing Boys and Girls.* Courtesy of Kellogg Company, Department of Home Economics Services, Battle Creek, Mich., 1964.

WHAT ARE THE NUTRITIONAL REQUIREMENTS OF THE ADOLESCENT (11 TO 18 YEARS OLD)?

Adolescence is a period of rapid growth and development. Females tend to grow more rapidly between 12 and 14 years of age, while males experience this rapid growth between 14 and 16 years of age. However, there are many individual variations to the growth pattern.

Sexual maturation occurs during adolescence. Females develop breasts, grow pubic hair, and start menses. Males have testicular and penis enlargement, grow facial and pubic hair, and experience voice changes. Both males and females increase in height, weight, muscle mass, and fat tissue. Females have greater increases in fat tissue and less in muscle mass than males.

During this rapid growth period, calorie and nutrient needs are higher to provide for increases in bone density, muscle mass, and blood volume and the developing endocrine system. There is an increased need for calories, calcium, iron, and iodine (see Table 4–15).

Nutrient needs can easily be met by increasing the serving size of the Basic Four Food Groups (see Table 4–14).

During adolescence, certain environmental and psychological changes may adversely affect food habits. They include:

1. Society's emphasis on slimness. This may cause the adolescent, especially females, to skip meals or drastically reduce calorie and nutrient intake to maintain a low body weight. This could result in marginal or low intakes of some vitamins and minerals.

2. Need for acceptance among peer groups. Individuals may forego sound eating practices in order to conform to peer standards.

3. Access to job and spending money. This allows the adolescent greater freedom in purchasing food. Fast-food outlets are a common lure to this population.

TABLE 4–15. RDA for the Adolescent Ages 11 to 18*

Nutrient	Age 11–14 Males	Age 11–14 Females	Age 15–18 Males	Age 15–18 Females
Kilocalories	2700	2200	2800	2100
Protein (gm)	45	46	56	46
Vitamin A (mcg R.E.)	1000	800	1000	800
Vitamin D (mcg)	10	10	10	10
Vitamin E (mg T.E.)	8	8	10	8
Ascorbic Acid (mg)	50	50	60	60
Folacin (mcg)	400	400	400	400
Niacin (mg)	18	15	18	14
Riboflavin (mg)	1.6	1.3	1.7	1.3
Thiamine (mg)	1.4	1.1	1.4	1.1
Vitamin B_6 (mg)	1.8	1.8	2.0	2.0
Vitamin B_{12} (mcg)	3.0	3.0	3.0	3.0
Calcium (mg)	1200	1200	1200	1200
Phosphorus (mg)	1200	1200	1200	1200
Iodine (mcg)	150	150	150	150
Iron (mg)	18	18	18	18
Magnesium (mg)	350	300	400	300
Zinc (mg)	15	15	15	15

*From *Recommended Dietary Allowances*, 9th ed. National Academy of Sciences–National Research Council, Washington, D.C., 1980.

4. After-school activities. Less time is spent having meals with the family, and meals may be skipped.

5. Snacking becomes a part of the adolescent's diet. Snacks can either enhance the nutrient value of the diet or provide empty calories. Excess snacking leads to obesity.

Nutrition Counseling

Nutrition counseling is especially important for the teenager who has failed to develop good food habits up to this point and for the teenager who has strayed from previously good habits.

Information should be presented in an interesting and motivating manner. Since teenagers are very interested in their physical appearance, it should be emphasized that adequate nutrients allow for optimal growth and development of their body.

It is important that the counselor respect the independence of the teenager. Flexible eating styles instead of a rigid eating pattern presented to the adolescent will increase the effectiveness of the counseling.

Special problems of teenagers such as obesity, alcoholism, anorexia nervosa, and pregnancy should be an important focus of nutrition counseling, as well as prevention of heart disease, cancer, diabetes, and other diseases that may occur later in life.

Study Questions and Activities

1. What do the terms "growth" and "development" mean to you?
2. List all the reasons why a good breakfast is important from early childhood throughout life.
3. Why is an adequate lunch important for everyone?
4. What suggestions can you give a mother who finds it difficult to get her young child to eat new and different foods? Who finds it difficult to get her children to eat adequate breakfasts?
5. Plan three different adequate lunches for a child to carry to school.
6. What effects later in life might be expected from foods inadequate in quantity and quality during the growing period?

Geriatric Nutrition

WHAT IS MEANT BY AGING?

Aging is a process in which there is a reduced capacity to replace worn-out cells. It is a continuous process that occurs throughout the life cycle, resulting in progressive body changes. It occurs at different rates in different individuals. Why aging occurs is unknown.

Susceptibility to disease increases with age, since there is a reduced capacity to handle physical stresses. *Gerontology* is the study of the problems of aging in all its aspects (physiological, economic, and social). *Geriatrics* is the branch of medicine concerned with the treatment and prevention of diseases affecting the elderly.

The population of "aged" persons (65 years of age and older) in the United States has dramatically increased since the 1900s. The elderly are the fastest growing segment of the population. It is estimated that by the year 2000 the elderly may comprise nearly 20 per cent of the population, as compared with 4 per cent in 1900. Factors contributing to the increase in longevity include improvements in health care services, better nutrition, and advances in medical technology.

HOW DOES AGING AFFECT NUTRITION?

The aged person experiences social, physiological, and economic changes that affect nutrition.

Physiological Changes

The aging process slows the basal metabolic rate (BMR) and reduces the amount of lean body mass (muscle tissue). These changes, combined with a decrease in physical activity, result in a decrease in energy requirements and an increase in fat tissue. The RDA guidelines (see Table 4–17) for energy needs will vary among individuals, but are lower for the elderly than for younger individuals.

Perceptual changes may affect eating behavior. Taste may be altered due to a decrease in the number of taste buds as part of the aging process, disease states, nutritional deficiencies, or medications. There is a reduced ability to detect odors. Hearing and sight impairments may reduce the enjoyment of the social aspects of eating. These perceptual changes may contribute to a lower food intake.

Loss of teeth is prevalent among this population. This may lead to altered food choices that may decrease the nutritive value of the diet. Avoidance of meats and fresh fruits and vegetables may occur.

With aging there is a decrease in the body's ability to move waste products through the gastrointestinal tract. This may lead to constipation if adequate fiber and fluids are not included in the diet.

Decreases in body secretions occur with aging. Protein digestion is less efficient because of decreased hydrochloric acid secretion. Swallowing may be difficult because of decreases in saliva. Table 4–16 lists physiological changes to consider in the care of the aged.

Economic Changes

For most individuals, advancing age eventually brings retirement from work. This usually results in a decrease in income, which may occur at a time when there is an increasing amount of money being spent for medical care. Consequently, less money may be available to buy food. Protein foods may be consumed in decreased amounts because they are expensive, require preparation, and may be difficult to chew and swallow. Excessive consumption of carbohydrate foods may occur because they are inexpensive, easily stored without refrigeration, and easy to prepare.

Social Changes

Losing a spouse, living alone or with a son or daughter's family, or entering a nursing home are only a few of the social changes to which an elderly person may have to adapt.

There is a loss of mobility if physical impairments make driving a car or using public transportation difficult. Isolation from others will result unless there are friends or family for the elderly person to rely on. The loss of inde-

TABLE 4–16. Physiological Changes to Consider in the Nutritional Care of the Aged

Component	Functional Change	Outcome
Body composition	↓ Muscle mass	↑ Fat tissue in muscle size and strength
	↓ BMR	↓ Caloric requirements
	↓ Bone density	↑ Risk of osteoporosis
Perceptual changes	↓ Hearing	Feeling of isolation Reluctance to eat in public places or at large social affairs
	Slowing of adaptation to darkness	Need of brighter light to perform tasks
	↓ Number of taste buds	↓ Ability to taste salt, sweet ↑ Ability to taste bitter and sour
	↓ Smell	↓ Threshold for odors
G.I. tract	↓ Motility	Constipation
	↓ HCL	↓ Efficiency protein digestion More prone to food poisoning
	↓ Saliva	Difficulty swallowing
Heart	↑ Blood pressure ↓ Ability to use oxygen	↓ Ability to handle physical work and stress
Lungs	Reduced capacity to oxygenate blood	↑ Fatigue ↓ Capacity for exercise
Endocrine	↓ Number of secretory cells	↓ In blood hormone levels
	↓ Insulin	↑ Blood sugar level
Kidney	↓ In renal blood flow	↓ Capacity for filtration and absorption

pendence that often accompanies these changes in social structure may reduce an elderly person's self-esteem. Such changes may cause an elderly person's food intake to suffer if he or she becomes depressed.

HOW WELL DO THE ELDERLY EAT?

The two factors with the greatest influence on the nutritional status of the elderly are disease and poverty.[11] How well an elderly person eats will depend on the ability to maintain a high-quality diet in the face of these and other social, economic, and physical changes previously discussed.

The nutrient intake of the elderly has been studied, but not as extensively as that of younger populations. In 1965, the USDA conducted a Nationwide Food Consumption Study. The study revealed that older persons had poorer diets than younger family members. Elderly women were low in calcium, riboflavin, iron, and vitamin A. Elderly males were low in vitamin C, calcium, riboflavin, and vitamin A. The Ten State Nutrition Survey (TSNS) in 1968 found iron and vitamin C consumption to be low in some older persons. The HANES study of 1971–1972 showed that the most frequent dietary deficiencies in the elderly were those of iron, vitamin A, vitamin C, and calcium.

The results of these nationwide studies, as well as studies of smaller populations of institutionalized and noninstitutionalized elderly persons, varied depending upon the standards used to evaluate the diets as well as the income level of the participants and the methods used to obtain dietary information (24-hour recall, 7-day food record, or 1-day food record).

Not all elderly persons have below standard nutrient intakes. However, what these studies do tell us is that the aged are clearly vulnerable to nutrient deficiencies.

Nutrition Programs for the Elderly

Federal, state, and local agencies have made efforts to improve the quality of nutrition among the elderly (Fig. 4–6).

The federal Older Americans Act provides the states with money to conduct nutrition programs for the elderly. Under this Title III legislation (formerly known as Title VII), a hot noon meal is served five days a week to elderly persons in senior centers. This funding also provides transportation for individuals who are otherwise unable to get to the center. Nutrition education, health services, and recreational activities are planned around meals. For the homebound elderly, meals are prepared at the center and delivered. These meals provide one-third of the RDA of nutrients.

"Meals-on-Wheels" is a community-sponsored program that provides hot noon meals and cold evening meals to homebound elderly persons. The elderly person is charged for the meals based on ability to pay.

The Food Stamp Program is available to the low-income elderly. In some states food stamps can be used to purchase "Meals-on-Wheels."

These nutrition programs have helped improve the nutritional status of the elderly population. Participation in these programs is enhanced by social work agencies that can direct the elderly to the appropriate programs.

WHAT ARE THE NUTRITIONAL NEEDS OF THE ELDERLY?

Energy. Because of the decrease in basal metabolic rate and physical activity, energy needs are reduced. This decrease in kilocalorie needs means that adequate nutrients must be consumed in less food, which requires more careful meal planning.

Protein. Requirements for protein are not decreased with age. The RDA remains at .8 gm per kilogram of body weight.

Vitamins. Although little is known about the vitamin requirements of the elderly, there is no evidence to indicate that requirements are reduced. See Table 4–17 for a complete listing of vitamin needs.

Minerals. The RDA for minerals is the same as for younger adults, with one exception. Because iron needs are decreased after menopause, women 51 years of age and older need 10 mg of iron, compared with 18 mg of iron for younger women. See Table 4–17 for a complete listing of mineral requirements.

PLANNING MEALS FOR ELDERLY PERSONS

An elderly person's nutritional needs, like those of other individuals, can be met by planning meals according to the Basic Four Food Groups.

Since calorie needs are lower while nutrient needs remain high, the use of skim milk and lean meats and the limited use of sauces, gravies, fats, alcohol, and high-calorie desserts will help. Lower calorie desserts can be substituted and enhance the nutritional value of the diet (e.g., canned fruits packed in their own juice, puddings, and custard).

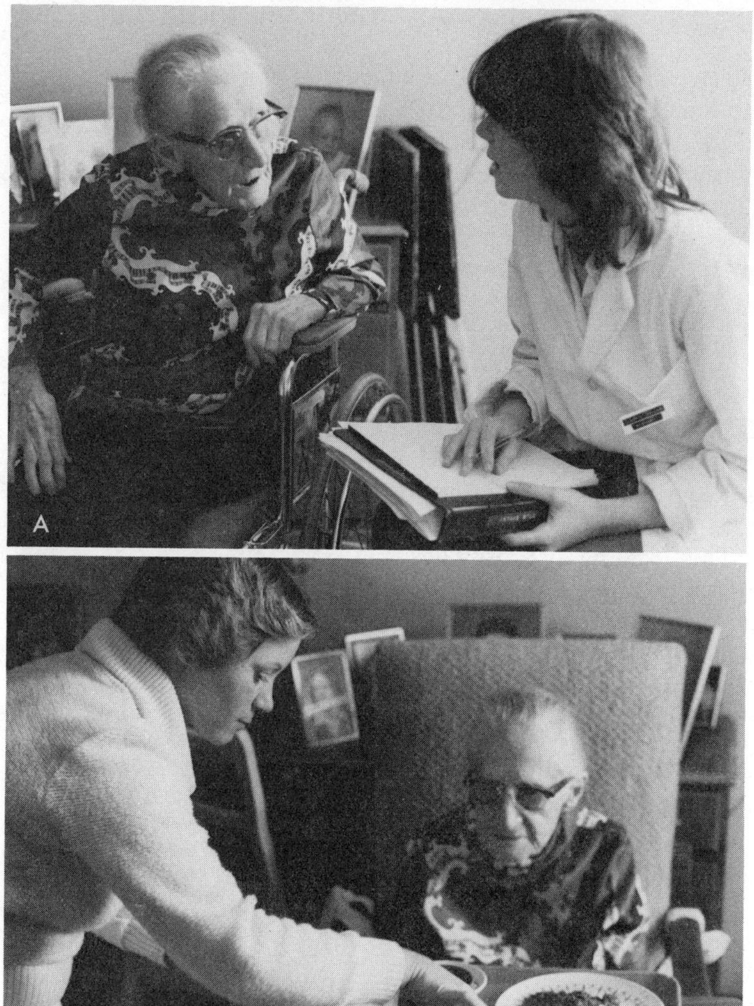

Figure 4–6. Improving nutrition among the elderly. *A*, Nutrition student taking a dietary history in a nursing home. *B*, A nurse's aide providing assistance at mealtime. *C*, Baking creates an interest in food in an institutional setting. (Courtesy of Lakeside Nursing Home, Ithaca, New York.)

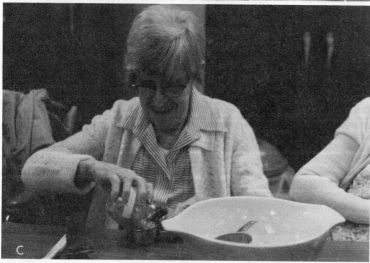

TABLE 4–17. RDA for Elderly*

	Males	Females
Energy (kcal) 51–75 years	2,400	1,800
76+ years	2,050	1,600
Protein (gm)	56	44
Thiamine (mg)	1.2	1.0
Niacin (mg)	16	13
Riboflavin (mg)	1.4	1.1
Vitamin B_6 (mg)	2.2	2.0
Folacin (mcg)	400	400
Vitamin B_{12} (mcg)	3.0	3.0
Ascorbic acid (mg)	60	60
Vitamin A (mcg R.E.)	1,000	800
Vitamin D (mcg)	5	5
Vitamin E (mg T.E.)	10	8
Calcium (mg)	800	800
Phosphorus (mg)	800	800
Magnesium (mg)	350	300
Iodine (mcg)	150	150
Iron (mg)	10	10
Zinc (mg)	15	15

*From *Recommended Dietary Allowances*, 9th ed. National Academy of Sciences–National Research Council, Washington, D.C., 1980.

If chewing is a problem, emphasizing tender, ground, or puréed meats, meat or fish loaves, and eggs may provide an acceptable solution. Adding additional meat to soups will also help enhance the protein value of the diet. Breakfast-type foods are generally well accepted because they are easy to chew and swallow. When necessary, these foods can also be used at lunch and dinner.

The fiber content of the diet can be increased by the use of whole-grain breads and cereals. Raw bran may be added to cereals for additional fiber, especially if the person is unable to chew fresh fruits and vegetables. Adequate fiber and fluid intake will prevent or alleviate constipation.

If special dietary modifications are needed, the dietitian can provide the necessary counseling.

Elderly persons are likely to eat better and enjoy their meals more when dining with others. Whenever possible, meals should be planned with other persons.

Any of the following three food plans (Table 4–18) can be used as a shopping guide. Any one of them will provide for regular meals, including breakfast, and allow for a variety of foods. Meals based on the thrifty and low-cost plans, compared to those based on the moderate-cost plan, usually include the less expensive kinds of foods from each of the food groups; smaller or fewer servings of meat, poultry, fish, vegetables, and fruit; larger or more servings of dry beans and peas, peanut butter, and breads and cereals; and more home-prepared foods and fewer ready-to-heat and ready-to-eat foods.[12]

Sample menus for a week are shown in Table 4–19. See Table 3–4 on page 111 for weekly cost of food plans for individuals 55 and older.

TABLE 4-18. Thrifty, Low-Cost, and Moderate-Cost Food Plans; Daily Quantities for a Couple 55 Years and Over*

Kind of Food	Thrifty Plan		Low-Cost Plan		Moderate-Cost Plan	
	Man	*Woman*	*Man*	*Woman*	*Man*	*Woman*
Milk (cups)†	1 1/2	1 1/2	1 1/2–2	1 1/2–2	2	2
Cooked lean meat or alternate‡ (ounces)	4	3	5	3–4	6–7	4–5
Vegetables and Fruits§ (1/2 cup)	3–4	3–4	4–5	4	5–6	5
Cereal and baked goods‖ (portions)	7 or more	5 or more	6 or more	5 or more	5 or more	4 or more

*From *Family Food Budgeting.* Home and Garden Bulletin No. 94, U.S. Department of Agriculture, Washington, D.C., 1976, p. 12. Amounts shown allow for some plate waste.

†As alternates: 3/4 ounce of hard cheese or 3/4 cup of cottage cheese, ice cream, or ice milk, or 1/2 cup of unflavored yogurt may replace 1/2 cup of fluid milk.

‡As alternates: 1 ounce of cooked poultry or fish, one egg, 1/2 cup cooked dry beans or peas, or 2 tablespoons of peanut butter may replace 1 ounce of cooked lean meat.

§One-half cup of vegetable or fruit or a portion — one medium apple, banana, or half a medium grapefruit or cantaloupe. Smaller portions may be served.

‖A portion is two slices of bread, one hamburger bun, one large muffin or cupcake, 1 ounce ready-to-eat cereal, or 3/4 cup cooked cereal, such as oatmeal, rice, spaghetti, macaroni, or noodles. Smaller servings may be given, but the total daily amounts on the average should add up to portions listed.

Study Questions and Activities

1. Why is it necessary to understand the physiological changes in aging?
2. Why are the elderly vulnerable to nutritional deficiencies?
3. How have the nutritional programs for the elderly helped to improve their nutritional status?
4. Observe meal service at a local nursing home. How have the meals been modified to meet individual needs?

Nutrition and the Athlete

Athletes need careful guidance as to which dietary regime will meet their nutritional requirements for the best possible performance in all kinds of sports. However, generalizations, misconceptions, and myths that cause confusion need to be analyzed wisely. Sound dietary practices can be developed by following the basic guidelines that will be discussed in this unit. Coaches, school nurses, dietitians, teachers, and physicians should all be able to advise an active teenager about specific nutritional concerns. This advice can be carried on into adulthood, as the athlete continues to be physically active and in a position to offer the same common sense guidelines to others. Several misconceptions about nutrition and the athlete will be discussed in this unit.

TABLE 4–19. Sample Menus for a Week*

Sunday	Monday	Tuesday	Wednesday	Thursday	Friday	Saturday
Cooked prunes Puffed rice with milk Toast — spread Coffee or tea	Tomato juice Poached egg Toast Coffee	Orange Wheat flakes with milk Toast — spread Coffee or tea	Prune juice French toast with powdered sugar Coffee	Orange juice Cheese omelet Toasted cornbread Coffee	Tangerine Scrambled eggs Toast — spread Coffee	Grapefruit sections Raisin toast — spread Coffee
						Shredded wheat with milk
Chicken a la king Parsley potato Asparagus Chocolate pudding	Lamb stew Cole slaw Bread — spread Caramel pudding Tea	Glazed ham logs Escalloped potato Peas Bread — spread Coconut cream pie	Meat loaf Au gratin potatoes Broccoli Cornbread — spread Instant butterscotch pudding Tea	Ham divan Roll Butterscotch pudding Tea	Macaroni and cheese Brussels sprouts Orange-grapefruit salad — French dressing Bread — spread Tapioca pudding	Barbecued pork chop Baked potato Spinach Bread — spread Fresh peach Iced tea
						Ice Cream
Cream of pea soup Tuna sandwich Celery sticks Crushed pineapple	Ham logs sandwich Sweet pickle Tomato-cucumber salad Banana with milk	Hard cooked eggs with cheese sauce Toast — spread Broiled tomato Carrot sticks Gingerbread	Salmon salad Tomato-green pepper salad Bread — spread Apricots Milk	Meat loaf sandwich Pickle Tossed salad Apricots with custard sauce Tea	Fish chowder Carrot and raisin salad Bread — spread Apple crisp Milk	Creamed dried beef on toast Waldorf salad Hot tea
Oatmeal-raisin cookie Milk	Molasses or ginger cookie Coffee or tea		Toast Tea	Hot tea	Toast Tea	Cheese and crackers
	Cinnamon toast Milk					

*Modified from *Food Guide for Older Folks.* Home and Garden Bulletin No. 17, Food Guide, Washington, D.C., U.S. Department of Agriculture, 1974, pp. 4–7.

WHAT ARE THE BASIC NUTRITIONAL GUIDELINES FOR THE ATHLETE?

Planning the Diet

The best advice one can give an athlete is to eat a wide variety of foods from the Four Food Groups, which will supply all the Recommended Dietary Allowances if eaten in appropriate amounts. An athlete's nutritional needs do not differ from those of the average individual except for energy, thiamine, niacin, and riboflavin requirements. Because these vitamins participate in energy metabolism, when energy needs are increased—as with the athlete—these vitamins also need to be increased. A sample meal pattern for a 3,000-kilocalorie diet can be found in Table 4–20. Four or five smaller meals instead of three larger ones are usually recommended. Snacks play an important role in meeting the RDA.

TABLE 4–20. An Athlete's Diet*

Food from The Basic Four to Supply 3,000 Kcalories/day

4 cups 2% milk
7 ounces meat, fish, poultry, cheese, or eggs
1/2 cup citrus fruit
1 1/2 cups other fruits and vegetables
18 servings enriched or whole-grain breads, cereal, or potatoes
10 teaspoons fats (butter, margarine, or other fat spread)
2 small servings plain desserts or jelly, snacks, carbonated beverages, fruit juice ades, etc.

Note: Extra calories may be obtained from complex carbohydrates, fats, and sweets, which increase the palatability of the diet as well.

Menu Sample for 3,000 Kcalories

Breakfast	1/2 cup orange juice 1 cup oatmeal 2 slices toast, buttered 1 Tbsp jelly or sugar 1 cup low-fat milk
Lunch	Sandwich with 3 oz sliced ham, 1 oz cheese Hamburger bun 2 oz corn chips Carrot sticks 1 cup 2% milk Sherbet
Snack	Apple Ginger cookies—2 large
Dinner	3 oz chicken 1/2 cup mashed potatoes 1/2 cup peas Tossed salad with 2 tsp dressing 2 dinner rolls 4 tsp butter or margarine Fresh pear 1 cup 2% milk Pound cake
Evening Snack	1 cup 2% milk 1/2 cup ice cream 1 tbsp chocolate sauce

*Modified from *Nutrition for Athletes: A Handbook for Coaches*, 9th ed., 1980. American Alliance for Health, Physical Education, Recreation, and Dance, 1900 Association Drive, Reston, Va., 22091.

ENERGY

The kilocalorie needs of the athlete are those that will (1) maintain an efficient body weight for best performance, and (2) meet the increased energy demands of training. For the average event, the kilocalorie needs vary from 500 to 1,500, depending on the sport (see Table 4–21).[13] Under normal conditions, appetite and satiety help to adjust energy intake to meet increased caloric needs.

The most efficient source of energy is complex carbohydrate (CHO). CHO is stored in the liver and the muscles in the form of glycogen, and in the body fluid as glucose. Muscular efficiency and athletic performance will improve if glycogen is readily available before exercise begins. Sweets such as candy, pastries, and cake eaten just before short-term events will only be used by the body to supply quick energy during the contest. However, their consumption may result in gastrointestinal distress and impaired performance or earlier exhaustion, even though they help to keep body reserves filled.

It is suggested that 50 per cent or more of food calories should come from carbohydrate sources; the usual is about 40 per cent carbohydrate.[15]

BREADS AND CEREALS

The heightened demand for nutrients and energy can be met by increased servings from the bread and cereal group. As many as 12 to 18 servings are needed to help supply 3,000 kcalories a day for an athlete. One serving contains 2 grams of protein, 15 grams of carbohydrate, and 68 kcalories. Fortified or enriched products in the bread and cereal group are especially good sources of vitamins and minerals.

Glycogen loading[16] (carbohydrate loading) is often beneficial for endurance-type activities lasting one hour or longer, such as long-distance running, cycling, and cross-country skiing, and also for high-altitude performance. This is a dietary regime also known as "muscle glycogen supercompensation," which means that muscle glycogen stores are increased beyond normal levels. The procedure involves the following steps:

1. Exercise to the point of exhaustion one week prior to the competition to significantly decrease glycogen levels.

TABLE 4–21. Caloric Cost of Exercise Per Minute*

Sport	Kcal/Min*	Sport	Kcal/Min*
Long-distance running	19.4	Gymnastics	6.5
Wrestling	14.2	Gymnastics	5.0
Swimming	11.2	Walking at 3.5 mph	5.2
Basketball	8.6	Baseball	4.7
Bicycle	8.2	Volleyball	3.5
Tennis	7.1	Reclining	1.3

*From S. Vitousek, "Is more better?" *Nutrition Today*, Vol. 14, No. 6, 1979.

There will be obvious variability in these numbers depending on the intensity of exercise and skill of the athlete. The relative order is more significant than the actual numbers.

2. During the next three days, a high-protein, high-fat, low-carbohydrate diet is consumed.

3. For the remaining four days of the week a diet of 95 to 90 per cent carbohydrate should be consumed. Exercise should be decreased so that the glycogen stores are spared. Complex carbohydrates seem to produce a longer-lasting effect in raising blood glucose and stimulate insulin usage.

Carbohydrate loading must be used with caution. It is not recommended for adolescent or preadolescent athletes.[19] An increase in body water is associated with increased glycogen stores, and may cause muscle stiffness, sluggishness, or reduced maximum oxygen utilization during competition. Eight glasses of water daily will guard against certain complications, including kidney damage.[17]

MILK

Consumption of low-fat and skim milk should be encouraged to help reduce the risk of developing obesity and coronary heart disease in later life. High-quality protein, B-complex vitamins, vitamin A, and minerals are obtained from the milk group.

It is a misconception that milk causes "cotton mouth" (dryness and discomfort in the mouth). Also, milk does not cause a sour stomach, as some athletes are led to believe.

Coaches and trainers have been known to discourage milk consumption. This is unfortunate, because milk supplies valuable nutrients and is a good source of extra energy between meals.

MEAT AND HIGH-PROTEIN FOODS

Another way of reducing the amount of saturated fat in the diet is to encourage the athlete to eat lean meat. High-protein foods included in this group also supply B vitamins and iron. Good quality protein is not used as a primary source of energy for the healthy athlete but is necessary for building muscle tissue. About 1 gram of protein per kilogram of body weight is recommended,[15] but if there is increased need for calories, 2 gm of protein/kg body weight is not harmful.

According to a recent survey, it was found that protein was thought to be the most important factor in increasing muscle mass. However, this is a common misconception. Muscle mass can only be increased by appropriate exercise. Protein is only important in the diet for the purpose of building and repairing tissues.[15]

Liver, oysters, raisins, dried fruit, or dried peas and beans should be eaten once weekly as a good source of iron. Some female athletes may have difficulty meeting their daily requirement of iron. Highly trained athletes process the oxygen they have more efficiently, thus decreasing the need for serum hemoglobin.[16]

Vegetarian diets that do not supply animal protein can also be adequate if planned carefully so that all the essential amino acids are supplied[17] (see p. 121 on vegetarianism). The diet should contain 12 to 15 per cent protein.

VEGETABLES AND FRUITS

These foods, which are a good source of essential vitamins and minerals, should also be used as snacks to provide good nutrition. At least ½ cup of a citrus fruit and ½ cup of a dark-green leafy vegetable are "musts" in the athlete's daily dietary regime. Two other servings of fruits and vegetables should be eaten as well. Fruits contain 10 grams of carbohydrate and 40 calories. Greens and lettuce have very little carbohydrate content. Other vegetables contain 2 grams of protein, 7 grams of carbohydrate, and 35 kcalories in each serving.

Body Weight

Appropriate weight must be attained if an athlete is to perform effectively in various sports. At the same time, the athlete must be well nourished and well hydrated, and have a healthy minimum fat reserve. Some sports require an increase in lean body mass; others, a decrease. In determining efficient body weight, levels of body fat are a more helpful method than using height-weight tables. Height-weight tables may indicate that an athlete who is very muscular is overweight. Acceptable levels of fat range from 7 to 15 per cent for men and from 12 to 25 per cent for women.[14] Taking skinfold measurements using calipers is an easy method for determining percentages of body fat (see Fig. 5–1).

If a lower percentage of body fat is desired in order to perform a sport more efficiently, a slow weight loss program at the rate of 1 to 2 pounds per week and a well-balanced diet is recommended. This will insure that actual body fat is being lost gradually, and not lean muscle mass lost in quick weight loss regimes.

Starvation, semistarvation, and dehydration are to be avoided because such practices may endanger health and impair performance.

WHAT IS AN APPROPRIATE PRE-GAME MEAL?

Any food that might cause discomfort and limit the potential of the athlete should be avoided. A light carbohydrate meal low in protein and fat and of approximately 500 calories is recommended for endurance events. The consumption of concentrated sugars may result in gastrointestinal distress and impaired performance.[16] The meal should be eaten at least three hours before the event to give the food enough time to be digested. Blood glucose and insulin levels will have time to stabilize, and the athlete will not feel hungry during competition. High-cellulose foods and carbonated beverages are not recommended in the pre-game meal, since they may cause gastrointestinal distress.

The emotional as well as the physical needs of the athlete should be considered in planning the pre-game meal. The individual should be allowed to eat foods that are personally appealing and not be forced to eat foods that may be distasteful.

Liquid pre-game meals are often useful for the athlete who experiences nausea after eating a regular meal. See Table 4–22 for a convenient homemade liquid meal. Natural foods rather than synthetic or predigested substances are recommended for liquid meals, since they are less likely to cause discomfort.

TABLE 4–22. Homemade Liquid Meal*

MIX:
- 1/2 cup water
- 1/2 cup nonfat dry milk
- 1/4 cup sugar
- 3 cups skim milk
- 1 tsp flavoring

2 cups supplies 400 calories

*From *Nutrition for Athletes: A Handbook for Coaches,* 9th ed., 1980. Reprinted by permission of the American Alliance for Health, Physical Education, Recreation, and Dance, 1900 Association Drive, Reston, Va., 22091.

Beverages should include milk. Tea and coffee should be used in moderation, since they contain caffeine, a stimulant that does not relieve fatigue. Alcohol affects coordination and should not be consumed. Some beverages that may be included in the pre-event meal, if well tolerated by the athlete, include:[15]

Skim milk	Limeade
Apple juice	*Clear beef or chicken broth
Orange juice (perhaps diluted)	*Bouillon
Pineapple juice (perhaps diluted)	*Consommé
Lemonade	

Guidelines for choosing the pre-event meal are listed in Table 4–23.

WHAT IS AN APPROPRIATE POST-EVENT MEAL?

Since athletic competition results in a feeling of exhaustion, it is important to relax and let the appetite return to normal before offering food. Until then, fruit juice may be taken. When the appetite returns to normal, sandwiches, fruit, and milk may be appealing to the hungry athlete. Later on, a larger meal is often welcome.

WHAT IS THE FLUID REQUIREMENT OF THE ATHLETE?

A loss of even as little as 1 to 2 per cent of body fluid can be detrimental to athletic performance. The body contains 55 to 60 per cent water and it cannot function properly without it. Heat exhaustion occurs after 5 per cent loss of water, and heat stroke and death if 10 per cent is lost. A good recommendation is to drink 2 cups of water (480 ml) for each pound of weight lost during exercise. Fluid should be replaced every 15 minutes with a beverage containing not more than 1 to 2 gm of sugar per 100 ml. This concentration will help maintain appropriate blood sugar levels as well as body strength.

Fruit juices quench the thirst and are quick energy sources. However, they should be diluted with equal amounts of cool water. An athlete should drink more fluid than needed to just satisfy thirst.

---

*A source of sodium (salt); no calories.

TABLE 4-23. Guidelines for Choosing the Pre-event Meal

1. Eat 3–4 hours before the competition.
2. Include a serving of roasted or broiled meat or poultry.
3. Include a serving of mashed or baked potato or 1/2 cup macaroni, noodles, or the like.
4. Include one serving of vegetables.
5. 1 cup skim milk.
6. 1 tsp fat spread and 2 tsp jelly or other sweet.
7. 1/2 cup or serving of fruit.
8. Sugar cookie or plain cake (angel food, sponge, or white cake).
9. 1–2 cups extra beverages.
10. Salt food well.

*From *Nutrition for Athletes: A Handbook for Coaches*, 9th ed., 1980. Reprinted by permission of the American Alliance for Health, Physical Education, Recreation, and Dance, 1900 Association Drive, Reston, Va., 22091.

Two pounds of weight loss represents 1 quart of sweat loss. The need for water can be determined by having the athlete weigh in before and after an event. If the weight loss is more than 6 pounds, the body needs extra salts as well as fluids. Food can be salted liberally or electrolyte replacement drinks can be used (Table 4–24). Bouillon and broth are liquids that supply needed sodium as well as water.[17]

ARE DIETARY SUPPLEMENTS DESIRABLE?

An overdose of fat-soluble vitamins can be harmful, and an excess of water-soluble vitamins is excreted in the urine. A well-balanced diet supplies all the necessary vitamins and minerals. However, the levels of sodium, potassium, and iron are most often affected by heavy exercise or insufficient intake. Liberal salting of food and the inclusion of potassium and iron-rich foods will meet needs.

Protein supplements are expensive and wasteful and can cause cramping, diarrhea, and loss of appetite. There is no need to emphasize protein-rich foods. One gm protein/kilogram of body weight is easily obtained from a varied diet.

There is no evidence that certain "wonder foods," such as wheat germ oil, bee pollen, or royal jelly, have any beneficial effect on athletic performance.[15,16]

TABLE 4–24. Electrolyte Drink*

1 gallon orange juice
4 gallons water
4 Tbsp salt

*From J. E. Falkel, "Basic Nutritional Guidelines for Athletes," in James H. McMaster, *The ABC's of Sports Medicine*. Robert Krieger Publishing Co., Huntington, N.Y., 1982.

Makes 5 gallons.

Study Questions and Activities

1. How do the nutritional needs of the athlete in training vary from when he or she is not in training? What food group supplies these nutrient needs?
2. Why is water so important to the athlete's activity?
3. How can electrolytes be replaced in the athlete's diet?
4. High-protein diets alone will not increase muscle mass. Why?
5. Why should carbohydrate loading only be used for endurance activities?

REFERENCES

1. R. M. Petkin, "Assessment of Nutritional Status of Mother, Fetus, and New Born," *American Journal of Clinical Nutrition*, Vol. 34, No. 4, 1981, pp. 658–668.
2. M. V. Krause and L. K. Mahan, *Food, Nutrition and Diet Therapy*, 6th ed. W. B. Saunders Co., Philadelphia, 1979, p. 276.
3. P. S. Howe, *Basic Nutrition in Health and Disease*, 7th ed. W. B. Saunders Co., Philadelphia, 1982, p. 174.
4. L. Anderson, et al., *Nutrition in Health and Disease*, 17th ed. J. B. Lippincott Co., Philadelphia, 1982, p. 308.
5. B. Alford and M. Bogle, *Nutrition During the Life Cycle*, Prentice-Hall, Inc., Englewood Cliffs, N.J., 1982.
6. *Food from Birth to Birthday*. National Diary Council, Rosemont, Ill., 1978.
7. M. V. Krause and L. K. Mahan, *Food, Nutrition and Diet Therapy*, 6th ed. W. B. Saunders Co., Philadelphia, 1979, p. 323.
8. M. S. Read, *Malnutrition, Learning and Behavior*. National Institute of Child Health and Human Development, U.S. Department of Health, Education, and Welfare, Washington, D.C., 1976.
9. J. J. Wurtman, "What Do Children Eat? Eating Styles of the Preschool, Elementary School, and Adolescent Child," in R. M. Suskind, ed., *Textbook of Pediatric Nutrition*. Raven Press, New York, 1981, pp. 597–607.
10. L. S. Peavy and A. L. Pagenkopf, *Grow Healthy Kids: A Parent's Guide to Sound Nutrition from Birth through Teens*. Grosset and Dunlap, New York, 1980, p. 126.
11. B. M. Posner, *Nutrition and the Elderly*. D. C. Heath Co., Lexington, Mass., 1979, p. 18.
12. *Family Food Budgeting*, Home and Garden Bulletin No. 94. U.S. Department of Agriculture, Washington, D.C., 1976, p. 12.
13. S. Vitousek, "Is More Better?" *Nutrition Today*, Vol. 14, No. 6, 1979, p. 10.
14. E. L. Fox, *Sports Physiology*. W. B. Saunders Co., Philadelphia, 1979.
15. American Alliance for Health, Physical Education, Recreation, and Dance, *Nutrition for Athletes: A Handbook for Coaches*. Reston, Va., 1980.
16. "Nutrition and Human Performance," *Dairy Council Digest*, Vol. 51, No. 2, May-June 1980, pp. 13–16.
17. J. E. Falkel, "Basic Nutritional Guidelines for Athletes," in James H. McMaster, *The ABC's of Sports Medicine*. Robert Krieger Publishing Co., Huntington, N.Y., 1982, pp. 59–70.
18. *Nutrition and Physical Fitness—A Review*. The State Education Department, Nutrition Education and Training Program, University of the State of New York, 1980, p. 7.
19. G. Mirkin, "Carbohydrate Loading: A Dangerous Practice," Journal of the American Medical Association, Vol. 223, 1973, p. 1511.

ADDITIONAL REFERENCES

NUTRITION IN PREGNANCY AND LACTATION

B. Alford and M. Bogle, *Nutrition During the Life Cycle*. Prentice-Hall, Inc., Englewood Cliffs, N.J., 1982.

NUTRITION OF INFANTS

L. Anderson, et al., *Nutrition in Health and Disease*, 17th ed. J. B. Lippincott Co., Philadelphia, 1982, Chapter 18.

P. S. Howe, *Basic Nutrition in Health and Disease*, 7th ed. W. B. Saunders Co., Philadelphia, 1981, Chapter 15.

M. V. Krause and L. K. Mahan, *Food, Nutrition and Diet Therapy*, 6th ed. W. B. Saunders Co., Philadelphia, 1979, Chapter 14.

L. S. Peavy and A. L. Pagenkopf, *Grow Healthy Kids: A Parent's Guide to Sound Nutrition from Birth through Teens.* Grosset and Dunlap, New York, 1980.

C. H. Robinson, *Basic Nutrition and Diet Therapy*, 4th ed. Macmillan Publishing Co., Inc., New York, 1980, Chapter 14.

R. M. Suskind, ed., *Textbook of Pediatric Nutrition.* Raven Press, New York, 1981.

NUTRITION IN CHILDHOOD AND ADOLESCENCE

National Dairy Council, "Nutrition Concerns During Adolescence," *Dairy Council Digest*, Vol. 52, No. 2, 1981, pp. 7–11.

E. Wasserman and L. J. Newman, "Nutrition in the Adolescent," in *Sourcebook on Food and Nutrition*, 2nd ed. Marquis Academic Media, Chicago, 1980, pp. 174–177.

GERIATRIC NUTRITION

B. Alford and M. Bogle, *Nutrition During the Life Cycle.* Prentice-Hall, Inc., Englewood Cliffs, N.J., 1982.

L. Anderson, et al., *Nutrition in Health and Disease*, 17th ed. J. B. Lippincott Co., Philadelphia, 1982.

E. W. Bussee, "Eating in Late Life: Physiologic and Psychologic Factors," *Contemporary Nutrition*, Vol. 4, No. 11, Nov. 1979.

A. E. Harper, "Dietary Guidelines for the Elderly," *Geriatrics*, Vol. 36, 1981, pp. 34–42.

E. Luros, "A Rational Approach to Geriatric Nutrition," *Dietetic Currents*, Vol. 8, No. 6, Nov.-Dec. 1981.

NUTRITION AND THE ATHLETE

L. J. Bogert, G. M. Briggs, and D. H. Calloway, *Nutrition and Physical Fitness*, 9th ed., W. B. Saunders Co., Philadelphia, 1973.

E. M. Hamilton and E. N. Whitney, *Nutrition: Concepts and Controversies*, West Publishing Co., St. Paul, 1979.

M. V. Krause and L. K. Mahan, *Food, Nutrition and Diet Therapy*, 6th ed. W. B. Saunders Co., Philadelphia, 1979.

Nutrition for Sports: A Coach's Guide to a Winning Diet. Florida Department of Citrus, Lakeland, Fla., 1981.

C. H. Robinson and M. R. Lawler, *Normal and Therapeutic Nutrition*, 16th ed. Macmillan Publishing Co., New York, 1982, p. 376.

R. E. Serfass, "Nutrition for the Athlete," *New York State Journal of Medicine*, Sept. 1976. Reprinted in *Contemporary Nutrition*, Vol. 2, No. 5, May 1977, pp. 1–2.

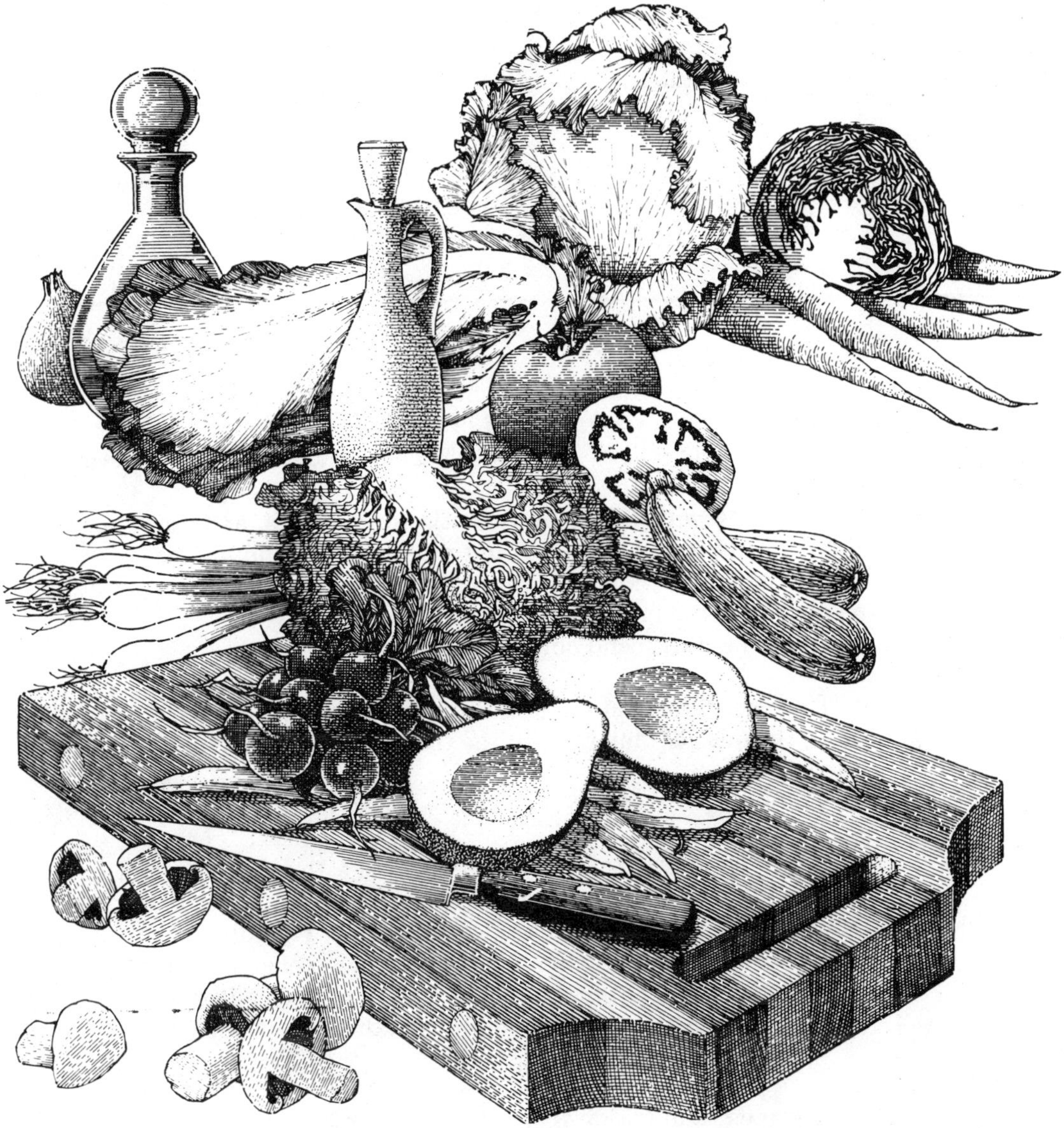

Section Two
THERAPEUTIC NUTRITION

OBJECTIVES

- ☐ To define terms
- ☐ To discuss topics for consideration in planning nutritional care for an ill or injured person
- ☐ To discuss important considerations in feeding patients

In the previous section on normal nutrition, the relationship of good nutrition to health was discussed in terms of:

1. Nutrients—their functions, recommended dietary allowances, food sources, and use by the body.
2. Foods—nutritional contributions, selection and care, daily requirements, family food budgeting, and principles of food buying.
3. The application of basic nutrition principles to family feeding and to the various stages in the life cycle.
4. Public health and community nutrition.

The nutritional care process continues as the reader learns to apply the basic principles of nutrition to the treatment of disease and other conditions of stress.

HOW ARE DIET PRINCIPLES RELATED TO TREATMENT OF DISEASE?

Evidence showing the value of food as a therapeutic agent has accumulated rapidly over the years. Corresponding changes and developments have occurred in medical practice. More is known regarding the maintenance of good nutrition during acute illness, convalescence, and rehabilitation. Also better understood is the manner in which certain illnesses and drugs affect requirements for the usual recommended dietary allowances.

WHAT IS THERAPEUTIC NUTRITION?

Therapeutic nutrition is simply the role of food and nutrition in the treatment of various diseases and disorders. Also referred to as diet therapy, nutritive therapy, or diet in disease, it involves the modification or adaptation of the normal diet in one or more ways to meet the physiological needs of an ill or injured person.

The normal diet may be modified by any one or a combination of the following:

Consistency. The diet may be changed to make it low fiber, high fiber, soft, or fluid.

Flavor. Strong flavors may be omitted, e.g., spices, sweetness, etc., especially if not tolerated.

Types of foods. Fried foods, citrus fruits, raw vegetables, etc., may be eliminated from the diet if not tolerated.

Preparation methods. Food may need to be ground, chopped, or pureéd.

Feeding techniques. Oral or tube feedings may be necessary.

Amounts of specific foods. An overall increase or decrease may be necessary as in reduction and diabetic diets.

Amounts of specific nutrients. These may be increased or decreased, as in sodium-restricted or high-protein diets.

All therapeutic diets start with a basic normal adequate diet, which is then modified in the manner required by the individual patient. (See also the nutrition evaluation of the foundation diet on page 26.)

HOW IS NUTRITIONAL CARE A PART OF TOTAL PATIENT CARE?

Meals served to a patient in the hospital make an important contribution to recovery from illness and are a fundamental aspect of total care. Good nutritional condition needs to be maintained, or poor nutritional condition improved, while the patient is treated for an illness or injury. The diet is no less important than other special therapies and medications. While the correct diet is important for all patients, it carries special importance in diseases of long duration and for anyone in a stressful condition.

5 The Nutritional Care Process

CHAPTER OUTLINE

THE NUTRITION CARE PLAN
- Assessment
- Implementation
- Evaluation
- Discharge Planning
- Malnutrition — Signs and Types

PATIENT MEAL SERVICE
- Important Considerations in Feeding
- General Considerations in Meal Service

OBJECTIVES

- ☐ To learn what is involved in the nutritional care planning process.
- ☐ To learn how to make the patient meal service attractive and appealing to promote recovery from an illness.

TERMS TO UNDERSTAND

Amylase	Hemorrhage	Marasmus
Anthropometry	Immune	Papillae
Antigen	Kwashiorkor	Transferrin
Edema	Lipase	Trypsin

The Nutrition Care Plan

WHAT IS THE MEANING OF NUTRITIONAL CARE PLANNING?

The nutritional care process is the way a person's changing nutritional needs are met. This process varies with specific circumstances; for example, educating someone about eating habits is usually sufficient to insure that the special demands of each state of the life cycle can be properly met. However, when the individual becomes ill and/or placed in a hospital or nursing home, it is necessary to start a more complex form of nutritional care called *nutritional care planning.* This requires the cooperation of the entire health team in order to be effective.[1]

WHAT ARE THE STEPS IN NUTRITIONAL CARE PLANNING?

Nutritional care planning involves several steps, the first of which is *assessment.* This step makes possible the identification of nutritional needs or problems. A *plan* for meeting these needs is then formulated, and *implemented*, keeping in mind the changing condition of the patient. The effectiveness of the plan in terms of the patient's progress must then be documented and *evaluated.* The nutritional care plan should always be incorporated into the total patient care plan, which is formulated by various members of the health care team as soon as possible in order to establish patient-centered goals to be met before *discharge.* The physician will then review the plan. The nutritional care planning process, therefore, includes:

1. Nutritional assessment
2. Identification of nutritional needs
3. Planning how to meet nutritional needs
4. Carrying out the plan of care
5. Evaluating nutritional care
6. Nutritional discharge planning

How is Nutritional Status Assessed?

As soon as the patient arrives at the health care center, members of the health team proceed to gather pertinent and accurate information. Professionally standardized techniques are used in assessing three main areas: (1) dietary history, (2) anthropometry, and (3) biochemical and clinical data. The patient is weighed and several body measurements including height are taken. The nurse inquires about food intolerances and allergies. If family members are present, they may also contribute to the assessment in regard to the individual's past eating and health habits. The social worker writes the social history, which the dietitian uses in gathering dietary information. The physician's report of the physical examination; results of blood, urine and skin tests; anthropometric measurements; and the diet history are equally important in assessing nutritional status, the first step in nutritional care planning. The data obtained is recorded and analyzed so that the professional can identify those individuals who may need prompt nutritional support and those who may need only a modified diet and counseling. Very often a person looks well nourished but, through proper assessment, is found to be in a high-risk state. See Table 5–1 for signs suggesting malnutrition.

DIET HISTORY

There are many factors that influence a person's nutritional status that should be taken into account in a diet history. Asking what types of foods the individual eats and how often—over a 24-hour period or for an average of three to seven days—will help the dietitian determine if the patient is in the habit of consuming the Basic Four Food Groups regularly. Appetite and weight changes may be significant and should be analyzed. It is important to note if the patient has lost more than 10 pounds within the last six months. Chewing and swallowing difficulty can hamper the individual's intake of food and thus be detrimental to nutritional status. A sore mouth and ill-fitting dentures are therefore potential problems to be noted in the diet history. Medications and illnesses, especially those involving the gastrointestinal tract, are noted because these may affect the appetite or nutrient utilization or both. (See page 100 for more information on drugs in relation to nutritional

TABLE 5-1. Physical Indicators of Malnutrition*

Hair	Lack of natural shine; hair dull and dry, thin and sparse, fine, silky, and straight; color changes; can be easily plucked.
Face	Skin color loss; skin dark over cheeks and under eyes; lumpiness or flakiness of skin of nose and mouth; swollen face; enlarged parotid glands; scaling of skin around nostrils.
Eyes	Eye membranes are pale; redness and fissuring of eyelid corners; dryness of membranes; cornea has dull appearance; scar on cornea; ring of fine blood vessels around cornea.
Lips	Redness and swelling of mouth or lips.
Tongue	Swelling; scarlet and raw tongue; magenta color of tongue; smooth tongue; swollen sores.
Teeth	May be missing or erupting abnormally; gray or black spots; cavities.
Gums	"Spongy" and bleed easily; recession of gums.
Glands	Thyroid enlargement (front of neck); parotid enlargement (cheeks become swollen).
Skin	Dryness of skin; sandpaper feel of skin; flakiness of skin; skin swollen and dark; excessive lightness or darkness of skin; black and blue marks due to skin bleeding; lack of fat under skin.
Nails	Nails are spoon-shaped; brittle, ridged nails.
Muscles and Skeleton	Muscles have "wasted" appearance; baby's skull bones are thin and soft; round swelling in front and side of head; swelling of ends of bones; small bumps on both sides of chest wall; knock-knees or bow legs; bleeding into muscle; person cannot get up or walk properly.
Internal Systems	Rapid heart rate (above 100 tachycardia); enlarged heart; abnormal rhythm; elevated blood pressure; liver enlargement; enlargement of spleen; mental irritability and confusion; burning and tingling of hands and feet; weakness and tenderness of muscles; decrease and loss of ankle and knee reflexes.

*Modified from Christakis, G. "Nutritional Assessment in Health Programs," *American Journal of Public Health*, Vol. 63, Suppl. 1, 1973.

status.) Elimination practices may indicate the need for additional roughage and liquids.

Cultural habits influence eating patterns and may be significant in determining appropriate nutritional therapy, and therefore must not be overlooked.[2] Also, food tastes and habits cannot be changed overnight. There must be some understanding of the psychological significance food may hold for the individual patient.

No nutrition care plan, including the therapeutic diet, will be effective if the meals are not eaten. The patient's own acceptance of the plan is as important a factor in recovery (or more important in some cases) as medication or physical treatment. Some attention to food preferences, as far as possible with the necessary diet restrictions and limited hospital and personnel facilities, as well as attention to the appearance and service of the food and the attitude of the one who serves it, all contribute to the acceptance of the diet and the success of therapeutic treatment.

ANTHROPOMETRY

Anthropometric assessments are based on measurements such as height, weight, wrist circumference, mid-upper arm circumference, arm muscle circumference, and skinfold thickness.[2] If these measurements vary to any great extent from the standards, over- or undernutrition may be suspected, since the extent of the body's fat stores and degree of muscle mass can be determined. For example, a low skinfold thickness measurement may indicate malnutrition. A decreased arm muscle circumference indicates malnutrition and that the body is using muscle protein to meet energy needs. Figure 5–1 shows how measurements of mid-upper arm circumference and triceps skinfold are made. Body build or frame type may be assessed fairly accurately by measuring the wrist (Fig. 5–2). Height-weight tables then become meaningful when used in conjunction with wrist measurements. See Tables 5–2 to 5–4 for standards of some of these anthropometric measurements.

Body weight is often expressed as relative weight, desirable weight, or as a percentage of usual weight. It is probably more appropriate to express the weight of sick, hospitalized patients in terms of relative body weight than lower ideal body weight. Relative body weight (RBW) is calculated as follows:

$$\text{RBW} = \frac{\text{observed body weight}}{\text{standard reference weight}} \times 100$$

Any assessment of body weight can be misleading if the patient is retaining fluid or is dehydrated.

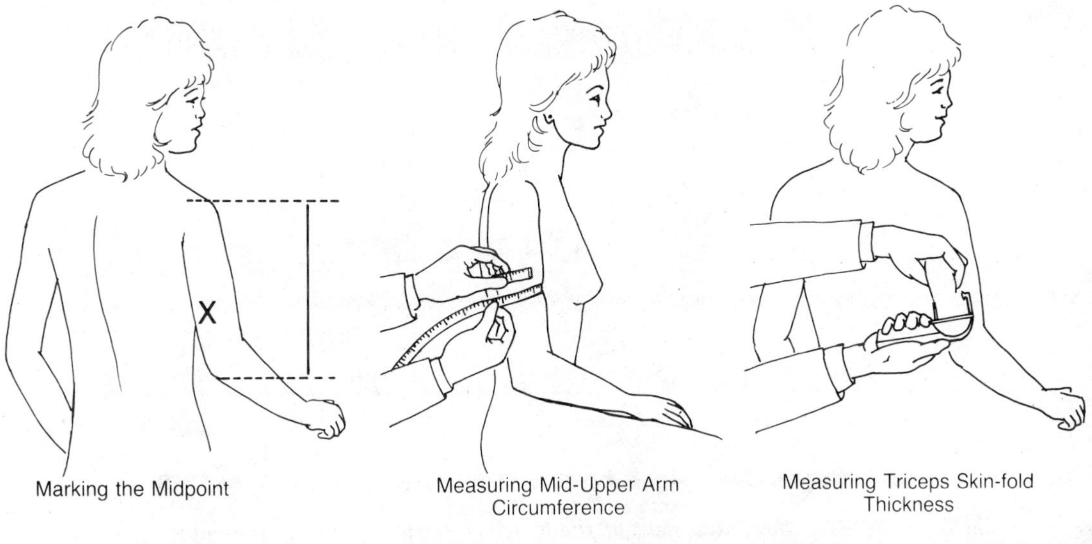

Figure 5–1. Measuring mid-upper arm circumference and triceps skinfold thickness.

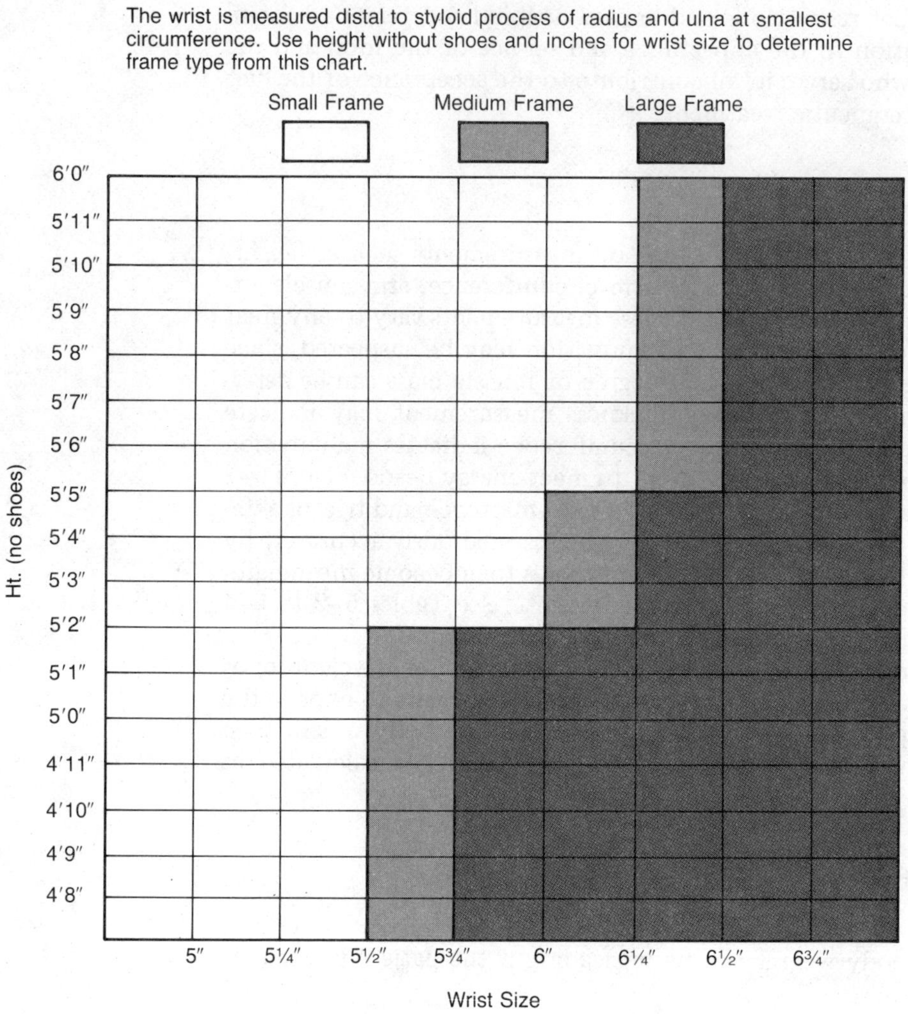

Figure 5–2. Assessing body frame type. (From Peter G. Lindner, M.D. Copyright 1973. Reproduced with permission.)

TABLE 5–2. Triceps Skinfold (mm), Adults*

Sex	Standard	90% Standard	90–60% Standard	60% Standard
Male	12.5	11.3	11.3–7.5	7.5
Female	16.5	14.9	14.9–9.9	9.9

*From D. B. Jelliffe, *The Assessment of the Nutritional Status of the Community*. WHO Monograph No. 53. World Health Organization, Geneva, 1966. Courtesy of Ross Laboratories, Columbus, Ohio.

TABLE 5-3. Mid-Arm Circumference (cm), Adults*

Sex	Standard	90% Standard	90–60% Standard	60% Standard
Male	29.3	26.3	26.3–17.6	17.6
Female	28.5	25.7	25.7–17.1	17.1

*From D. B. Jelliffe, *The Assessment of the Nutritional Status of the Community.* WHO Monograph No. 53. World Health Organization, Geneva, 1966. Courtesy of Ross Laboratories, Columbus, Ohio.

BIOCHEMICAL AND CLINICAL DATA

The results of a number of routine laboratory tests can have nutritional implications.[3] For example, a malnourished person produces less creatinine in 24 hours than someone of the same height and weight who is well nourished (see Table 5–5 for ideal urinary creatinine values). Protein requirements can be determined through urine studies. Certain proteins (albumin and transferrin) may be less concentrated in malnourished individuals. A complete blood count (CBC) is also a useful tool in nutritional assessment. For example, a malnourished patient cannot fight infection as well, and this is shown by a low lymphocyte count. Also, skin tests show how a person responds to certain antigens, and may indicate that he or she is not immune to certain diseases.

A person may be considered to be moderately malnourished if three of the following measurements are abnormal, and severely malnourished if all four measurements are abnormal[3]:

1. A loss of more than 10 pounds within the last six months.
2. A total lymphocyte count of less than 1,500/cubic mm.
3. A serum albumin of less than 3.5 gm.
4. Anthropometric measurements, including triceps skinfold and mid-arm circumference less than 70 per cent of the standard.

Figure 5–3 shows a sample initial nutritional assessment and care plan form that incorporates the information just discussed.

TABLE 5-4. Mid-Arm Muscle Circumference (cm), Adults*

Sex	Standard	90% Standard	90–60% Standard	60% Standard
Male	25.3	22.8	22.8–15.2	15.2
Female	23.2	20.9	20.9–13.9	13.9

*From D. B. Jelliffe, *The Assessment of the Nutritional Status of the Community.* WHO Monograph No. 53. World Health Organization, Geneva, 1966. Courtesy of Ross Laboratories, Columbus, Ohio.

TABLE 5-5. Ideal Urinary Creatinine Values (mg), Adults*

Male†		Female‡	
Height (cm)	*Ideal Creatinine (mg)*	*Height (cm)*	*Ideal Creatinine (mg)*
157.5	1288	147.3	830
160.0	1325	149.9	851
162.6	1359	152.4	875
165.1	1386	154.9	900
167.6	1426	157.5	925
170.2	1467	160.0	949
172.7	1513	162.6	977
175.3	1555	165.1	1006
177.8	1596	167.6	1044
180.3	1642	170.2	1076
182.9	1691	172.7	1109
185.4	1739	175.3	1141
188.0	1785	177.8	1174
190.5	1831	180.3	1206
193.0	1891	182.9	1240

*From B. R. Bistrian, G. L. Blackburn, M. Sherman, and N. S. Scrimshaw, "Therapeutic Index of Nutritional Depletion in Hospitalized Patients." *Surgery, Gynecology and Obstetrics*, Vol. 141, No. 4, Oct. 1975, p. 512. Courtesy of Ross Laboratories, Columbus, Ohio.

†Creatinine coefficient (males) = 23 mg/kg of ideal body weight.

‡Creatinine coefficient (females) = 18 mg/kg of ideal body weight.

Implementation

Various activities or interventions are needed to carry out plans to meet patient-centered nutritional goals. These activities include the diet prescription, any necessary modification of food consistency, nutritional supplements, assistance and encouragement at mealtime, counseling, and advice about meeting the individual's nutritional needs after discharge. Implementation includes ongoing monitoring of laboratory data, weight records, and food and fluid intake.

Each member on the health care team has an opportunity to aid in implementing the nutritional care plan, whether it be in the form of encouragement to eat at mealtime, the provision of adaptive eating equipment, or the encouragement of exercise and socializing.

Evaluation

All of the methods used to achieve a nutritional goal must be evaluated for effectiveness so that changes can be made as necessary. Evaluation is achieved through observation of the individual's condition and his or her acceptance of a dietary regimen, and by understanding laboratory data. Weight status must also be evaluated. Progress should be written in the medical record so that the entire health team will understand the rationale for the nutritional care given. Reasons for the effectiveness or ineffectiveness of a plan should be noted and new methods for achieving a nutritional goal can then be tried and evaluated.

Name____________________ Age______ Sex______ Diet__________

Diagnosis:	*Pertinent Medications:*

Mental Status: ____________________

Activity Level: Low_____ Moderate_____ High_____

Height: ________ Weight: ________ Amount of Wt. Change Last 6 Months: ______

Body Frame: S_____ M_____ L_____ Usual Weight: ________

Bowel Function: ________ Bladder Function: ________

Skin Integrity: ________ Allergies: ________

Eyesight: ________ Hearing: ________

Meal Pattern: ________________

Cultural/Religious Food Habits: ________________

Observed Food and Fluid Intake: ________________

Assistance Needed at Mealtime: ________________

Chewing and Swallowing Ability: ________________

Communication Ability: ________________

Lab Findings: Hgb______ HCT______ FBS______
Na______ K______ Cl______ BUN______

Lymphocytes: ________ Albumin: ________

Anthropometric Measurements: ________________
(% of standard)

Skin Antigen Test______ TSF______ MAC______ AC______

PLAN FOR NUTRITIONAL CARE

Problem/Need	Goal	Method

By: Date:

Figure 5–3. Initial Nutritional Assessment and Care Plan.

Discharge Planning

The last step in the nutrition care planning process, called discharge planning, begins as soon as the patient is admitted to the health care facility. By the time the patient is ready to leave, needs have already been assessed and nutritional status evaluated, and changes have been made in the nutrition care plan in response to the patient's progress. Recommendations can then be given to the family or to the person responsible for the continuing care, whether it be at home or at another facility. Diet instruction should include counseling on weight control, diet in relation to the patient's medications and physical condition, and a review of the foods allowed and avoided on a modified dietary regime.

The illness itself and the different conditions imposed on eating when a patient goes from home to hospital or nursing home, diet restrictions, and changes imposed by a therapeutic diet (possibly with different foods and different forms of foods), all accompanied by a patient's fears, must be considered in discharge planning. Part of nutritional care is educating the patient in new food habits that he or she will take home and that will require some adjustment in the home environment and family group. See Figure 5–4 for a sample discharge summary form.

WHAT ARE THE TYPES OF PROTEIN-CALORIE MALNUTRITION?

Malnutrition can be classified into two types, marasmus and kwashiorkor (see also Chapter 4).

Kwashiorkor (protein malnutrition) is generally the result of an inadequate intake of protein in relation to calories. It typically affects children who, after a period of breast-feeding, are weaned onto starchy staples low in protein—such as the tropical roots and tubers—or sugary foods. It is most common in those parts of tropical Africa where roots, tubers, and bananas are the dominant starchy staples; kwashiorkor means "disease that occurs when displaced from the breast by another child."[4] It is assessed by proper biochemical analysis in the laboratory. The following are characteristics of kwashiorkor (see also Figure 4–2):

Name: ______________________ Age: ________ Birthdate: ________

Weight: ________ Height: ________

Diagnosis: ______________________

____

Diet: ______________________

Meal Pattern: ______________________

Appetite: ______________________

Approximate Caloric Intake: ________

Food Preferences

Beverage: ______________________

Meat & Meat Sub: ______________________

Vegetables: ______________________

Fruit: ______________________

Other: ______________________

Allergies: ______________ Dislikes: ______________

Recommendations (Include special needs in relation to weight, medications, present illness)

____

____

Signature ______________

Date ______________

Figure 5–4. Nutritional Discharge Summary

1. Lack of growth due to poor protein intake.
2. Profound apathy, general misery.
3. Changes in skin and hair texture and color (dry, flaky skin, especially in the pelvic region and thighs; hair is thin and easily plucked out and takes on a reddish color).
4. Diarrhea.
5. Fatty liver.
6. Fluid retention in tissues (shown by pot belly, swollen legs and face).
7. Normal or even above normal weight, triceps skinfold, creatinine-height index, and mid-arm circumference.
8. Markedly reduced levels of serum transferrin and albumin.
9. Reduced levels of serum triglycerides, phospholipids, and cholesterol.
10. Low hemoglobin.
11. Decreased production of amylase, lipase, and trypsin.
12. Low serum vitamin A.

Marasmus (protein-calorie malnutrition), on the other hand, arises from an insufficiency of both energy intake and protein. The condition usually occurs in the first year of life and among the children of undernourished women. These infants are often of low birthweight and even in their first few months will show considerable low weight for age. The assessment of marasmus is based on physical evidence noted in the clinic, as opposed to laboratory data as with kwashiorkor.[5] The following are characteristics of marasmus (see also Figure 4–3):

1. Severe growth failure in children.
2. Emaciation — wasting of muscles and lack of body fat due to inadequate intake of calories.
3. Reduced weight, skinfold thickness, creatinine-height index, and mid-arm circumference.
4. Serum transferrin and albumin levels are usually normal.
5. Fatty liver and edema are not present.

Most severely malnourished children will show signs and symptoms of both kwashiorkor and marasmus, and may alternate between the two. The main danger to these children is lowered resistance to disease. Even if they survive, they may permanently be impaired both mentally and physically.[4] The period of recovery from marasmus is much longer than with kwashiorkor. See page 147 regarding the effect this disease has upon children's learning and behavior.

Now it is also generally acknowledged that the incidence of protein-calorie malnutrition in hospitalized patients is higher than previously recognized.[2] Adult kwashiorkor occurs when the patient is unable to eat and is under stress of an acute illness or major surgery. The condition may develop within two weeks.[5] In the hospitalized patient who is under acute stress from surgery or illness, there is a high risk of infection and other complications.

Patient Meal Service

WHAT ARE IMPORTANT CONSIDERATIONS IN FEEDING PATIENTS?

Attractive food service plays an important role in stimulating the appetite and enjoyment of food. Mealtime is often the major event of the day for the patient, and every effort must be made to ready the room and the patient to receive the meal. The patient's attitude towards food may reflect a more general attitude towards illness.

WHAT ARE SOME SUGGESTIONS FOR FEEDING A PATIENT?

1. It is important for the person feeding a patient to be seated and relaxed.
2. Engage in pleasant conversation with the patient.
3. Explain the reasons for various foods offered, especially if the patient does not understand the diet well.
4. Alternate one food with another.
5. Offer liquids frequently or when requested.
6. If the patient is blind, describe the foods before feeding.
7. Avoid criticism of the meal and of the patient.

General Considerations in Meal Service

1. The table should be appropriately and properly set.
2. Clean linen or good quality paper products, and clean, lightweight, and attractive china, glassware, and silverware should be used.
3. Silverware should be placed in order of use (from outside in).
4. Food portions should be of appropriate size, attractively arranged on dishes, and garnished.
5. Hot foods should be served *hot;* cold foods, *cold.*
6. Mealtime conversation should be pleasant, without discussion of disagreeable subjects or "shop talk" and without disparaging remarks about the food or mention of likes and dislikes.
7. Trays, if used, should be lightweight and sufficiently large to hold all the necessary articles and foods and permit convenient and neat arrangement, without overcrowding (see Fig. 5–5).
8. The patient must receive assistance, if necessary, for assuring adequate intake, e.g., containers need to be opened, meat cut, and condiments applied to foods.
9. There should be no spilled foods or liquids.
10. The tray should be served on time with a smile and with only complimentary remarks about the food.
11. The tray or meals should be solidly placed in front of the patient and the foods within easy reach with the patient in a comfortable position.
12. Plenty of time should be allowed for eating.
13. The tray should be removed without any appearance of hurry.

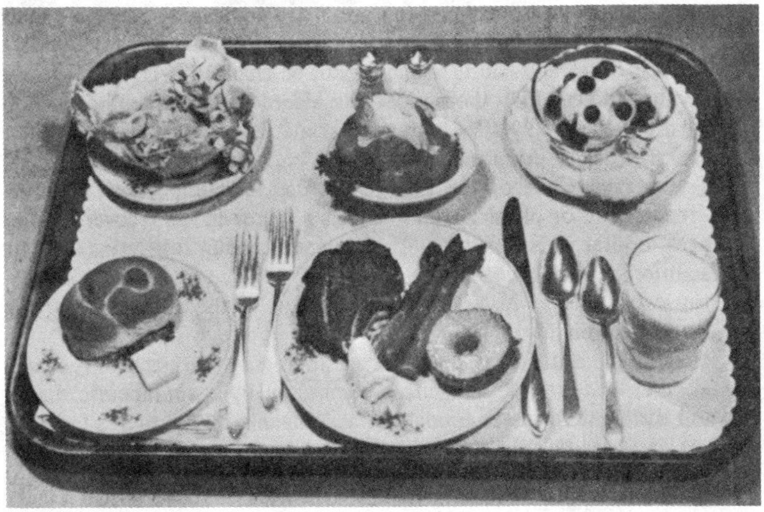

Figure 5–5. A tray adequate in size and correctly set for dinner for a patient. (From M. V. Krause, *Food, Nutrition and Diet Therapy*. W. B. Saunders Co., Philadelphia.)

Study Questions and Activities

1. For an overall picture of good food service, set up a table properly for breakfast, luncheon, and dinner.
2. Set up sample trays from the hospital dietary department for breakfast, noon, and night meals and for nourishment service. Discuss trays: size, cover, napkins, china, glassware, silver, etc. If trays are not available from the hospital, set up a series of tray service for hospital patients.
3. Comment on the dinner setting on a tray, Figure 5–5.
4. Observe a clinical conference on a patient receiving a therapeutic diet. What information from Figure 5–3 was discussed?
5. Write a short paper on the important considerations in feeding a patient.
6. List factors that might affect a patient's nutrition during illness.

REFERENCES

1. M. V. Krause and L. K. Mahan, *Food, Nutrition and Diet Therapy*, 6th ed. W. B. Saunders Co., Philadelphia, 1978, pp. 417–428.
2. J. Keithley, "Proper Nutritional Assessment Can Prevent Hospital Malnutrition," *Nursing*, Vol. 9, No. 2, Feb. 1979.
3. M. H. Seltzer, "Nutritional Assessment for the Practicing Physician." *Nutrition and the M.D.*, Vol. VII, No. 4, April 1981.
4. T. T. Poleman, "World Hunger: Extent, Causes, and Cures," Cornell/International Agricultural Economics Study, Cornell University, Ithaca, N.Y., May 1982.
5. R. S. Goodhart and M. E. Shils, *Modern Nutrition in Health and Disease*, 6th ed. Lea & Febiger, Philadelphia, 1980.

6 Basic Hospital Diets and Therapeutic Modifications

CHAPTER OUTLINE

BASIC PROGRESSIVE HOSPITAL DIETS
- Liquid Diet
- Soft Diet
- Regular Diet

THERAPEUTIC DIETS
- Indications for Use
- Modifications of Regular Diet

NUTRITIONAL NEEDS IN STRESS CONDITIONS
- Types of Stress
- Effect on Nutritional Status
- Nutritional Needs

NUTRITION IN CANCER
- Effect of Tumor Growth
- Nutritional Problems from Treatments

DIET IN MISCELLANEOUS DISEASES AND CONDITIONS
- Allergies
- Inborn Errors of Metabolism
- Miscellaneous Diets
- Test Diets

NUTRITIONAL SUPPORT
- Oral
- Tube Feeding
- Peripheral Parenteral Nutrition
- Total Parenteral Nutrition

OBJECTIVES

☐ To discuss basic routine hospital diets.
☐ To learn the ways the basic normal diet is modified for therapeutic purposes.
☐ To learn about nutrition in cancer and stress.
☐ To discuss diets in miscellaneous diseases and conditions.
☐ To understand the importance of nutritional support and the different methods by which it is administered.

TERMS TO UNDERSTAND

Adrenal medulla	Hemoglobin	Osmolality
Albumin	Hemorrhage	Osteoporosis
Allergen	Histidinemia	Parenteral
Anabolic	Hypochromic	Peripheral
Catabolic	Homocystinuria	Peripheral parenteral nutrition
Catheter	Hyperlipoproteinemia	Periodontal
Callus	Intravenous	Pernicious anemia
Chemotherapy	Jejunostomy	Phenylketonuria
Decubitus ulcer	Ketogenic diet	Physical stress
Dumping syndrome diet	Lymphocytes	Psychological stress
Edema	Metabolize	Radiation
Electrolyte	Metabolites	Steroids
Elemental diet	Muscosites	Total parenteral nutrition
Enteral	Macrocytic	Toxin
Epinephrine	Microcytic	Transferase
Gastrostomy	Nasogastric	Tyramine
Gustatory	Nasojejunal	Tumor
Hematocrit	Oropharyngeal	Uremia

Basic Progressive Hospital Diets

WHAT IS MEANT BY A BASIC HOSPITAL DIET?

A basic routine diet is a necessity in the many hospitals and other types of institutions that care for the sick, for reasons of economy, efficiency, convenience, and uniformity of service. Such a routine diet must be nutritionally adequate to maintain good nutrition or improve nutritive status. It is based on the same foundation diet pattern for normal nutrition stressed throughout this book: certain numbers of servings daily from each of the Four Food Groups which in total meet the Recommended Dietary Allowances for all the essential nutrients, combined into attractive and palatable meals (see pp. 24–25 and p. 27).

The basic routine diet, variously referred to from hospital to hospital as House, General, Regular, Standard, or Full Diet, is served to ambulatory patients and those patients who do not require a therapeutic diet. Many factors affect the choice of foods within each group to be served on this General or House Diet; type of hospital (private, state, etc.), budget, socioeconomic level of patients, adaptability to large quantity preparation, etc. It may contain any or all foods that any healthy person may eat, but possibly with fewer calories. There will be a minimum of rich foods and foods requiring a long time for digestion, because hospital patients are less active than average people. This basic normal nutritionally adequate diet is the foundation for planning any or all adaptations or modifications needed by any patient to meet his or her particular needs due to illness of one kind or another, accident or injury.

When the General Diet is modified in consistency to become a Soft Diet or a Liquid Diet, these three diets are known as Basic Hospital Diets and represent the progressive steps through which a regular hospital patient, requiring no therapeutic food prescription, is carried. In some hospitals, a Light Diet is included in the list as a transitional convalescent diet between a Soft Diet and a General Diet for minor illnesses or if the patient is not ready for a regular diet. Semisolid foods and liquid foods are allowed on the soft diet.

Table 6–1 lists information about each of the routine hospital diets. There are some differences from hospital to hospital in the foods allowed in each category, as well as in the number of kinds of diets. When a patient is admitted to the hospital, the type of diet will be selected by the physician. This may be changed if and when the patient's condition makes it desirable.

The method of feeding and the time for feeding may vary with patients. For example, tube or intravenous feedings may be desirable to meet an individual's needs. Sometimes hourly feedings or several small meals a day are preferred to three meals (see also Nutritional Support, p. 215).

Activities

1. The class makes a tour of the Dietary Department, with the dietitian explaining the various units and their relation to each other.

2. List your own hospital's routine Hospital Diets. A copy should be available to you. Compare the foods on your hospital's diets with those on Table 6–1.

3. Sketch tray settings used in your hospital for breakfast and dinner service.

Comments:

Linen	Silver	Extras
China	Glassware	Convenience
Attractiveness	Other points	Ways to improve

4. Class observes at every mealtime for one day the tray set-ups for the regular diet, soft diet, full liquid diet, and clear liquid diet, in their own or other hospital, and writes menus below. If hospital has printed menus, student may attach a copy to this page and use it for checking foods allowed on each type diet.

Typical Hospital Diets Served from One Menu *Date*

Menu	Regular Diet	Soft Diet	Full Liquid Diet	Clear Liquid
Breakfast				

Midmorning

Dinner

Midafternoon

Supper

Night

Therapeutic Diets

WHAT ARE THE OBJECTIVES AND INDICATIONS FOR THERAPEUTIC DIETS?

Therapeutic diets are necessary for one or more of the following reasons:

1. To maintain or improve nutritive status.
2. To improve nutritional deficiencies — clinical or subclinical.
3. To maintain, decrease, or increase body weight.
4. To rest certain organs or the whole body.
5. To eliminate particular food constituents to which patient may be allergic.
6. To adjust the composition of the diet to meet the ability of the body to adjust, metabolize, and excrete certain nutrients and other substances.

TABLE 6–1. Progressive Basic Hospital Diets

	Clear Liquid Diet	Full Liquid Diet	Soft Diet*	Regular, House, General, or Full Diet
Characteristics	Temporary diet of clear liquids without residue. Nonstimulating, non-gas-forming, nonirritating. 400–500 kilocalories.	Foods liquid at room temperature or liquefying at body temperature.	Normal diet modified in consistency to have limited fiber. Liquids and semisolid food; easily digested.	Practically all foods. Simple, easy-to-digest foods, simply prepared, palatably seasoned; to have a wide variety of foods and various methods of preparation. Individual intolerances, food habits, ethnic values, and food preferences considered.
Adequacy	Inadequate; deficient in protein, minerals, vitamins, and kilocalories.	Can be adequate with careful planning; adequacy depends on liquids used. If used longer than 48 hours, high-protein, high-calorie supplements to be considered.	Entirely adequate liberal diet.	Adequate and well balanced.
Use	Acute illness and infections. Postoperatively. Temporary food intolerance. To relieve thirst. Reduce colonic fecal matter. One- to two-hour feeding intervals. Prior to certain tests.	Transition between clear liquid and soft diets. Postoperatively. Acute gastritis and infections. Febrile conditions. Intolerance for solid food. Two- to four-hour feeding intervals.	Between full liquid and light or regular diet. Between acute illness and convalescence. Acute infections Chewing difficulties. Gastrointestinal disorders. Three meals with or without between-meal feedings.	For uniformity and convenience in serving hospital patients. Ambulatory patients. Bed patients not requiring therapeutic diets.

Foods	Water, tea, coffee, coffee substitutes. Fat-free broth. Carbonated beverages. Synthetic fruit juices. Ginger ale. Plain gelatin. Sugar. No milk or fats. Orange juice may cause distention. Salt, plain hard candy, fruit ices, all fruit juices without pulp.	All liquids on clear liquid diet plus: All forms of milk. Soups, strained. Fruit and vegetable juices. Eggnogs. Plain ice cream and sherbets. Junket and plain gelatin dishes. Soft custard. Cereal gruels. Puréed meat and meat substitutes only; for use in soups only. Butter, cream, margarine, sugar, honey, hard candy, syrup; salt, pepper, cinnamon, nutmeg, and flavorings; puréed vegetables for use in soups only.	All liquids. Fine and strained cereals. Cooked tender or puréed vegetables. Cooked fruits without skin and seeds. Ripe bananas. Ground or tender meat, fish, and poultry. Eggs and mild cheeses. Plain cake and puddings. Moderately seasoned foods. Enriched white, refined whole-wheat bread (no seeds).	All foods from the "Basic Four."
Modification	Liberal clear liquid diet includes fruit juices, egg white, whole egg, thin gruels.	Consistency for tube feedings: foods that will pass through tube easily.	Low residue—no fiber or tough connective tissue. Traditional bland—no chemical, thermal, physical stimulants. Cold soft—tonsillectomy. Mechanical or "dental" soft—requiring no mastication—diced, chopped, mashed foods in place of puréed. Light or convalescent diet—intermediate between soft and regular.	For a light or convalescent diet, fried foods, rich pastries, fat-rich foods, coarse vegetables, possibly raw fruits and vegetables, and gas-forming vegetables may be omitted.

*Because of trend toward more liberal interpretation of diets and foods, in some hospitals the soft diet may be combined with the light diet, with cooked low-fiber vegetables allowed in place of purées.

HOW ARE HOSPITAL DIETS MODIFIED FOR THERAPEUTIC PURPOSES?

In addition to the modifications to hospital diets listed on page 192, the foundation basic normal diet may be further modified as follows:

1. Energy value (kilocalories) may be increased or decreased.
2. Fiber (bulk, roughage) may be increased or decreased.
3. Specific nutrients (one or more) may be increased or decreased.
4. Specific foods or types of foods (such as allergens for persons with allergies, fried foods, or gas-forming foods) may be increased or decreased.
5. Any of these modified diets may be further altered to become a soft or liquid diet.
6. Spices, condiments, and foods with extractives or strong flavors may be eliminated from the diet.

HOW ARE THERAPEUTIC DIETS NAMED AND PRESCRIBED?

Therapeutic diets (no longer called "special diets") are named in terms of the diet modification without reference to the name of the disease (except in the case of the diabetic diet) or its symptoms or to the name of the person(s) who may have originated or modified the diet. This makes possible a universal understanding of terms and also reduces the number of therapeutic diets. Adaptations are sometimes classified as *qualitative* when the adaptations are in types of foods or consistency and *quantitative* when the modifications are increases or decreases of certain nutrients or calories. It is desirable that every therapeutic diet be planned for the particular patient for whom such a diet is ordered.

The diet prescription is written in terms of caloric requirements based on the individual's weight and activity, and requirements for protein, fat, carbohydrate, minerals, vitamins, and fiber, with due regard for increased or decreased needs for each because of the patient's illness. This prescription is translated into foods and meals by the dietitian, who, in turn, instructs the patient regarding the diet, its importance as a single therapeutic measure or as a supplement to medication, and how to prepare and serve it at home.

WHAT ARE EXAMPLES OF THERAPEUTIC DIETS AND INDICATIONS FOR USE?

Modifications in Consistency

Other than liquid, soft, or regular diets, the following additional modified diets are used: mechanical (edentulous), tube feeding, bland diet, restricted residue diet, and high-residue or high-fiber diet.

Mechanical Diet (Edentulous). This type of diet is used for the individual who has difficulty in chewing because of lack of dentures or teeth, or because of inflammation of the oral cavity.

Tube Feeding. Tube feedings are used for patients who have an esophageal obstruction, severe burns, gastric surgery, or additional inability to chew or swallow. They are also sometimes necessary for patients with anorexia nervosa.

Bland Diet. This diet is used for patients with ulcerative colitis, gastritis, or diarrhea. A progressive regime, it has been found to be successful in treating gastric and duodenal ulcers.

Restricted Residue Diet. This may be used for patients with severe diarrhea, ulcerative colitis, diverticulitis, typhoid fever, or partial intestinal obstruction, and after G.I. surgery.

High-Residue or High-Fiber Diet. This type of diet may be prescribed for atonic constipation (intestinal stasis) or for diverticulosis.

Modifications in Carbohydrate, Protein, and Fat

The diabetic diet; the low-calorie diet; the high-protein, high-fat, low-carbohydrate diet; and the ketogenic diet are all examples of controlled carbohydrates, proteins, and fats.

Diabetic Diet. The diabetic diet is carefully calculated for each patient to minimize the occurrence of hyperglycemia and glycosuria and to attain or maintain ideal body weight.

Low-Calorie Diet. This diet is used to achieve weight loss among those with cardiovascular and renal diseases, hypertension, gallbladder disease, gout, or hyperthyroidism, and for severely ill patients with low food tolerances.

High-Protein, High-Fat, Low-Carbohydrate Diet. This diet is used for patients with hypoglycemia.

Ketogenic Diet. In some cases, a ketogenic diet is used to control epilepsy.

Modifications in Fat

Fat-modified diets include the restricted fat diet, the fat-controlled low-cholesterol diet, and the dietary management of hyperlipoproteinemia.

Restricted Fat Diet. Fat is restricted for patients with diseases of the liver, gallbladder, or pancreas in which disturbances of digestion and absorption of fat may occur.

Fat-Controlled Low-Cholesterol Diet. This diet is used in individuals with elevated blood cholesterol levels and for those with atherosclerosis.

Dietary Management of Hyperlipoproteinemia. This diet is necessary for individuals with the five types of hyperlipoproteinemia.

Modifications in Protein

Protein modified diets include the restricted protein, gluten-free, restricted phenylalanine, restricted purine, and high-protein diets.

Restricted Protein Diet. This diet is used for patients in hepatic coma or with chronic uremia, renal disease, or liver disease.

Gluten-Free Diet. Individuals with celiac disease or nontropical sprue have gluten intolerance and must be on a gluten-free diet.

Restricted Phenylalanine Diet. This diet is used in confirmed cases of phenylketonuria (PKU), in which phenylalanines cannot be processed by the body.

Restricted Purine Diet. A decrease in purines is useful in lowering the blood uric acid level in gout.

High-Protein Diet. A high-protein diet is used to correct a protein inadequacy from any source — pre- and postoperative, high fever, burns, injuries, increased metabolism, nephrosis (children), chronic nephritis (unless there is nitrogen retention), pernicious anemia, ulcerative colitis, hepatitis, celiac and cystic fibrosis, tuberculosis and other wasting diseases, wounds, or anemia (nutritional).

Modifications in Carbohydrate

Both the lactose-free diet and the dumping syndrome diet have modifications to carbohydrate intake.

Lactose-Free Diet. Patients who have the total or partial inability to metabolize this milk sugar must avoid lactose in their diet.

Dumping Syndrome Diet. Patients who have had a gastrectomy or gastric bypass surgery may require this special diet.

Modifications in Electrolytes and Minerals

In these diets sodium may be increased or restricted, potassium and copper may be restricted, and calcium and phosphorus may be increased, as may iron and general vitamin consumption.

Increased Sodium Diets. These may be useful in Addison's disease.

Restricted Sodium Diets. These are far more common and are prescribed for patients with congestive heart failure, hypertension, renal disease with edema, cirrhosis of the liver with ascites, pre-eclampsia and eclampsia (toxemia), and ACTH therapy.

Restricted Potassium Diet. If potassium is not excreted from the body properly, a restricted diet may be necessary.

Restricted Copper Diet. Wilson's disease, oliguria, or anuria all call for a restriction of copper intake.

High-Calcium and Phosphorus Diet. An increase in calcium and phosphorus intake is desirable in rickets, osteomalacia, tetany, dental caries, and acute lead poisoning.

High-Iron Diet. Nutritional or hemorrhagic anemia calls for a high intake of dietary iron.

High-Vitamin Diet. An increase in vitamin A is necessary to combat night blindness and xerophthalmia; increased intake of vitamin D is recommended for rickets and osteomalacia; increased vitamin K is needed in liver and gallbladder disease, in which the vitamin is not stored; increased thiamine is necessary to avoid beriberi and polyneuritis; increased niacin is needed to combat pellagra; and increased ascorbic acid (vitamin C) will improve wound healing and fight scurvy.

Acid-Ash or Alkaline-Ash Diet. This diet is used for certain types of kidney stones, depending on solubility in either one.

Suggested Activity

The instructor will provide a list of therapeutic diets currently being prepared and served in the hospital with name of disorder or disease for which each has been prescribed. Any pertinent details regarding the patient and care might be discussed incidentally. The student will list these therapeutic diets below. Student should become acquainted with any diet manual prepared by the hospital's dietary department. A personal copy would be desirable, if possible.

Nutritional Needs in Stress Conditions

The focus of this part will be on the effect of excessive physical stress upon health and will emphasize ways to cope with the nutritional demands of a patient who is either critically ill, undergoing surgery, or suffering from major burns, fevers and infections, or multiple fractures. For a discussion of the physical stress produced by exercise, see Chapter Four, "Nutrition and the Athlete," p. 162.

WHAT IS STRESS?

Stress may be either physical or psychological or both; it consists of a number of nonspecific biological responses brought about by the influence of adverse external conditions. Although the body and mind are normally able to adapt to the stresses of such situations, this ability has definite limits, which vary among individuals. Beyond this point, continued stress may result in a mental or physical breakdown.

WHAT ARE THE TYPES OF STRESS?

Physical Stress. A situation such as a near accident or injury, which is sudden and poses an immediate threat to the individual, elicits what is called "emergency stress." Physical stress may also be of a more continuing type, due to long-term conditions such as pregnancy, acute and chronic disease, surgery, fractures, exposure to extremes of temperature, trauma, or continued exposure to noise, vibration, fumes, or chemicals. Although the body's stress reaction is different in the emergency and long-term cases, in general it is mediated by the adrenal glands. The hormone epinephrine from the adrenal medulla increases heart rate and blood pressure, and the sugar content of the blood rises to supply needed energy.

Psychological Stress. The source of stress may sometimes be psychological rather than physical. When a person foresees or imagines danger, the body may respond with an increase in muscle tenseness and heart rate and, if under this type of stress for a long period of time, may even develop a peptic ulcer. Another familiar example of a reaction to psychological stress is "stage fright." A healthy person can usually learn to cope with such stressful situations through repeated exposure to them.[1]

HOW DOES NUTRITIONAL STATUS AFFECT A PERSON'S RECOVERY FROM STRESS?

Good nutritional status before, during, and after a stressful situation is a health asset to any patient. Its importance is especially visible in such situations as surgery: The patient's nutritional status can determine the success of an operation as well as the degree of postoperative progress in withstanding the particular stresses imposed by surgery and convalescence. A well-nourished patient can expect fewer complications, quicker and better wound healing, and a shorter convalescence. In contrast, an individual in a poor nutritional state is vulnerable to many problems and complications. Gastrointestinal discomfort, decubitus ulcers, dehydration and edema, and poor wound healing are likely in such patients, due in part to a low level of certain nutrients and possibly low hemoglobin, serum protein, and electrolyte levels.

IN WHAT WAYS DOES STRESS AFFECT NUTRITIONAL NEEDS?

The need for substances such as calories, protein, fluids, electrolytes, vitamins, and minerals is heightened during stress (Table 6–2). The increase in calories is necessitated by certain hormonal actions. Upon initiation of stress, hormones from the adrenal glands pour into the bloodstream, with effects on heart rate, blood pressure, and dilation of blood vessels. They also give cells an enhanced capacity to absorb glucose; the glucose is then broken down to provide energy needed to meet the challenge of the stressful situation. An individual's caloric requirement is therefore raised in proportion to the degree of stress experienced. The emotional response of a very ill person will increase caloric requirement if fear, anxiety, and tension are present. Fat digestion may also be affected for this reason.[1a]

TABLE 6–2. Summary of Nutritional Needs for Specific Stress Conditions

Type of Stress	Possible Effects of Condition	Nutritional Therapy
Surgery	Blood loss, shock, hemorrhaging	Increase protein and calories (35 calories per kg body weight (BW)
	Depletion of protein, or increase in protein metabolism	1–1.5 gm protein per kg BW
	Negative nitrogen balance	Therapeutic doses of vitamins if poor nutritional status before surgery and for patient fasting more than 4 days: vitamin A for normal tissue formation; B-complex vitamins for CHO, protein and fat metabolism; vitamin K and calcium for clotting of blood; vitamin C for formation of collagen; zinc if levels are low
	Dehydration	
	Edema	
	Nausea, vomiting, diarrhea	
	Need to build antibodies to prevent infection	Reduce sugar and fat in meals if nauseated
	Insulin shock in diabetic patient	Supply glucose to prevent insulin shock in diabetic
		Parenteral feeding for first few hours after surgery
		Fluids to prevent electrolyte imbalance and maintain circulatory volume
Fractures of long bones and other trauma	Increase in protein metabolism	Increase protein to 150 gm
	Loss of phosphorus, potassium, sulfur	Increase calories to 2,000–4,000
	Development of osteoporosis due to immobilization and loss of calcium	Increase all other nutrients
	Electrolyte imbalance	Intravenous administration of fluids (400–600 calories)
	Loss of fluids	3% amino acid solution
	Renal failure and uremia	High-protein, high-calorie beverages if patient cannot tolerate enough at mealtime
		Tube feedings

TABLE 6-2. Summary of Nutritional Needs for Specific Stress Conditions *(Continued)*

Type of Stress	Possible Effects of Condition	Nutritional Therapy
Dumping syndrome (following gastric surgery)	Foods eaten are not held in the new pouch formed by the remaining stomach tissue. Foods pass quickly into the jejunum before any digestion takes place in the stomach. Pain and other symptoms result.	High protein, high-fat, low-carbohydrate foods. Give 6–8 small meals/day. Eat regularly. No fluids at meals. Whole milk may not be tolerated
Burns	High loss of nitrogen Neurohormonal catabolic changes Increased water loss Anorexia Fluid loss Weight loss Electrolyte imbalance Mineral losses	50–90 kcal per kg BW before burn 2–3 gm protein per kg BW before burn Vitamin-mineral supplement Antacids and frequent feedings to prevent ulcers Supplements, tube feedings, parenteral nutrition, or combination Service of attractive, appetizing food in warm environment
Infection	Increased metabolism Dehydration Fever Body tissue breakdown Need for production of antibodies and lymphocytes Anorexia Nausea and vomiting Antibiotics interfere with intestinal synthesis of B-complex vitamins Loss of sodium and potassium if fever is present	High-protein, high-calorie, high-vitamin diet: .8–1.0 gm protein per kg BW After 3–4 days, .5–2 gm Progress consistency from liquid to soft to regular Increase calories 35–45 calories per kg BW to restore nitrogen losses 3–4 liters of fluids Protein containing liquids that are not too sweet. Parenteral feeding if necessary. Increase vitamins B_1 and B_2 and niacin as calories are increased Vitamin supplements Potassium- and sodium-rich foods Frequent small feedings Tube feedings if necessary
Fevers, including those of *short duration*, such as tonsillitis, colds, influenza, measles, chickenpox, and scarlet fever, and those of *long duration*, such as tuberculosis and recurrent malaria.	Protein metabolism increased Stored fat and body protein utilized for energy if food intake is inadequate — also loss of body protein Stored carbohydrate (glycogen) is depleted Sodium chloride and potassium levels are lowered	*Typhoid fever* — Large quantity of milk is the basis Low fiber 3–6 eggs daily if tolerated Frequent, small feedings High-calorie, high-protein diet

Table continued on following page.

TABLE 6-2. Summary of Nutritional Needs for Specific Stress Conditions (*Continued*)

Type of Stress	Possible Effects of Condition	Nutritional Therapy
	Disturbances of appetite, digestion and absorption may occur	*Poliomyelitis* — Liquid to soft diet during acute state. Then high-calorie, high-protein, high-vitamin
		Protein supplements may be better tolerated than milk
		Vitamin supplements may be indicated
		Tube feeding may be necessary in early stages
		Rheumatic fever — High-calorie, high-protein liquid in early stages
		Diet gradually increased to one high in iron, vitamin A, protein, and calories
		Restricted sweets to avoid reduction in appetite
		Possible sodium restriction with ACTH therapy
		Tuberculosis — 2500–5000 calories; 100–150 grams protein. Optimum minerals and vitamins with special attention to calcium and ascorbic acid
		Easily digested, simple food, attractively served. Forced feeding undesirable

During fever, which often accompanies infection, the caloric need is increased by 7 per cent for every 1°F above normal (or 13 per cent for every 1°C), by 10 per cent for counteracting sepsis, and by an additional 10 to 13 per cent for restlessness.[2] In general, it has been found that a 50 per cent increase in calories above basal metabolic needs will prevent breakdown of body tissues and promote anabolism. Recovery from stress involves two phases: (1) the catabolic stage, involving breakdown of body protein, followed by (2) the anabolic phase, during which the body tissues are rebuilt. The first few days after surgery, during the catabolic phase, a patient requires between 2,500 and 4,000 calories per day. If not supplied through feedings, the body will use its glycogen stores first, its fat stores second, and then its own body protein. The patient will lose weight and become weak. The breakdown of body protein during the catabolic phase leads to the loss of nitrogen through the urine, along with a loss of potassium, phosphorus, and sulfur. A diet high in protein is necessary to replace these mineral losses. Therefore, adequate calorie and protein intake should be the first consideration in helping a patient reach the anabolic phase of healing and convalescence. Protein needs are also increased when the body is trying to produce antibodies and lymphocytes to fight infection.

Liberal protein for the fracture patient favors deposition of calcium in the bones and the formation of good callus. Whenever there is complete immobilization and no weight bearing, as in the case of fractures and long-term bed rest, there is excessive loss of calcium.[3] It is beneficial to increase the protein content of the diet right away. Calcium therapy should begin after there is some mobilization.

It is easier to meet the body's needs for electrolytes, fluids, vitamins, and minerals, but the lack of these nutrients has a less serious consequence than the lack of protein and calories. Nutritional requirements may be met through a variety of nutritional support methods, as discussed on page 215.

Vomiting, diarrhea, fever, and rapid blood loss are conditions which require that the patient receive as much as 3 to 4 liters of fluid daily to guard against dehydration. This large quantity of fluid intake also helps the body eliminate toxins, which are carried out by the circulatory system and excreted by the kidneys.

When there is excessive loss of blood, as in surgery, the electrolyte balance is likely to be upset as sodium and potassium levels are lowered (see p. 198 for a discussion of electrolytes). It is important that the patient's intake and output of fluids be recorded, which will indicate whether or not a potential problem exists.

In addition to protein, salts, and fluids, the person in stress particularly needs specific vitamins, depending on the condition and previous nutritional status of the patient. For example, vitamins A and C aid in wound healing (Table 6–3), while the B-complex vitamins are most important during periods of increased metabolism and high caloric intake. The National Research Council, in its pamphlet *Therapeutic Nutrition*, advises the following for the postsurgical patient:

1. A healthy person with no previous history of malnutrition who is ambulatory and eating well has no need to take vitamin supplements.
2. The patient who does not meet the above qualifications needs only 1 to 2 times the normal RDA.
3. The patient who is receiving an intravenous diet should receive from 1 to 2 times the minimum requirement for parenteral injection, with additional amounts of vitamin C.
4. The patient with a severe burn, serious illness, or severe trauma should be given 5 to 10 times the usual RDA the first few days; thereafter, only 2 to 3 times the basic allowance until recovery is complete.[2]

Even well-nourished individuals under stress conditions experience a catabolic phase before the anabolic phase of healing occurs. When new tissue is formed to repair damage, a positive nitrogen and potassium balance is reached, and bodily functions such as digestion, urination, and hydration return to normal. This anabolic phase should be reached as quickly as possible by supplying sufficient nutrients and fluids to counteract the depletion caused by stressful situations.

Therefore, in order to prepare a patient for a stressful situation such as surgery, preoperative dietary treatment may be required for a time, dependent upon the condition of the patient and the type of operation, whether major or minor. Special attention is given to high protein, high-carbohydrate meals, with mineral and possibly vitamin supplementation (particularly ascorbic acid) and fluids. Table 6–4 gives a sample high-protein, high-kcalorie diet. Obese patients, anemic patients, and diabetics may need special diet

TABLE 6–3. Nutrients Affecting Wound Healing*

Nutrient	Specific Component	Contribution to Wound Healing
Proteins	Amino acids	Needed for neovascularization, lymphocyte formation, fibroblast proliferation, collagen synthesis, and wound remodeling. Required for certain cell-mediated responses including phagocytosis and intracellular killing of bacteria.
	Albumin	Prevents wound edema secondary to low serum oncotic pressure.
Carbohydrates	Glucose	Needed for energy requirement of leukocytes and fibroblasts to function in inhibiting activities of wound infection.
Fats	Essential unsaturated fatty acids a. Linoleic b. Linolenic c. Arachidonic	Serve as building blocks for prostaglandins that regulate cellular metabolism, inflammation, and circulation. Are constituents of triglycerides and fatty acids contained in cellular and subcellular membranes.
Vitamins	Ascorbic acid	Hydroxylates proline and lysine in collagen synthesis. Enhances capillary formation and decreases capillary fragility. Is a necessary component of complement that functions in immune reactions and increases defenses to infection.
	B Complex	Serve as cofactors of enzyme systems.
	Pyridoxine, pantothenic and folic acid	Required for antibody formation and white blood cell function.
	A	Enhances epithelialization of cell membranes. Enhances rate of collagen synthesis and cross-linking of newly formed collagen. Antagonizes the inhibitory effects of glucocorticoids on cell membranes.
	D	Necessary for absorption, transport, and metabolism of calcium. Indirectly affects phosphorus metabolism.
	E	No special role known; may be important if there is a fatty acid deficiency.
	K	Needed for synthesis of prothrombin and clotting factors VII, IX, and X. Required for synthesis of calcium-binding protein.
Minerals	Zinc	Stabilizes cell membranes. Needed for cell mitosis and cell proliferation in wound repair.
	Iron	Needed for hydroxylation of proline and lysine in collagen synthesis. Enhances bactericidal activity of leukocytes. Secondarily, deficiency may cause decrease in oxygen transport to wound.
	Copper	Is an integral part of the enzyme, lysyloxidase, that catalyzes formation of stable collagen crosslinks.

*From L. Avakian, C. Ball, and E. Weiss, "Wound Care and the High-Risk Patient," *Life Support Nursing*, Oct. 1982, p. 41. Developed from S. Levenson and E. Seifter, "Dysnutrition, Wound Healing, and Resistance to Infection," *Clinics in Plastic Surgery*, Vol. 4, No. 3, July 1977, pp. 375–388.

TABLE 6-4. High-Protein, High-Calorie Diet*

Breakfast	Lunch	Dinner	Evening Snack
Fruit, 1/2 cup citrus	Chicken breast, 3 oz	Roast beef, 4 oz	Milkshake, 1 glass
Eggs, 2 scrambled	Potato salad, 1/2 cup	Mashed potato, 1/2 cup	Cheese sandwich
Cereal, 1/2 cup cooked	Hard roll	Gravy	
Bread, 1 slice whole-grain or enriched	Butter or margarine	Peas, 1/2 cup	
Butter or margarine	Sliced tomato salad	Bread, 1 slice whole wheat	
Milk, 1 cup	Peaches, 1/2 cup fresh	Butter or margarine	
Coffee or tea	Milk, 1 cup	Baked custard	

*Approximately 125 gm protein, 2,500 kilocalories.

adjustments. The preoperative diet is equally important for the patient in good nutritive condition, to meet the shock of surgery and the following days when food is curtailed and nutritive balance impaired.

WHAT IS USUAL PREOPERATIVE DIET PROCEDURE?

1. No food is allowed immediately before the operation, the time dependent on the type of operation and anesthesia.
2. Minor surgery: No food is allowed the day of the operation, unless surgery is scheduled for the P.M.
3. G.I. tract surgery: A fluid diet is required for several days preceding the operation. No fluid or food is allowed after midnight of the day previous to the operation.

Study Questions

1. What types of stress have you experienced and how has your body reacted?
2. Describe the nutritional needs of (1) a fracture patient and (2) a burn patient.
3. What types of snacks would you provide a person with rheumatic fever?

Nutrition in Cancer

WHAT IS THE RELATIONSHIP BETWEEN NUTRITION AND CANCER?

Discussion of the relationship between nutrition and cancer falls into one of the following categories:

1. Dietary factors influencing tumor growth
2. Tumor growth influences on the nutritional status of the host
3. Nutritional problems resulting from cancer treatment

This section will discuss the nutritional problems arising from both the disease and its treatments.

HOW DOES CANCER EFFECT THE NUTRITIONAL STATUS OF THE HOST?

Anorexia

In cancer patients, as the disease progresses, dietary intake is likely to decline. Anorexia, lack of desire to eat, is very common. Factors contributing to anorexia include anxiety, depression, and pain. Its etiology is not clearly understood at the present time, but research has given us some insight into the cause.

Metabolites, chemical substances produced by the tumor, may exhibit an anorexic effect on the hypothalamus, the portion of the brain believed to regulate hunger and satiety.

Taste changes are experienced by some cancer patients and may influence appetite. Among the most common changes are a lowered threshold for bitter flavors and an elevated threshold for sweetness. This may account for the common aversion to meat and the difficulty in tasting sweet foods. These gustatory changes may be the result of nutritional deficiencies as well as a decrease in the normal cell mass of taste buds.[4] Tumor competition may make it increasingly difficult for foods to taste "normal," since there are not enough taste buds being produced.

Tumor-Host Competition

Tumor tissue competes with host tissue for available nutrients, with the tumor prevailing. This competition is not well understood; however, alterations in the metabolism of proteins, carbohydrates, lipids, vitamins, electrolytes, and trace elements as well as energy metabolism have been noted among cancer patients.[5] The extent of nutritional problems imposed by these altered states of metabolism is the subject of much research. With this understanding, an improved nutrient prescription for nutritional support in cancer will follow.

Cachexia

Cachexia, the severe tissue wasting and malnutrition seen in cancer patients, is aggravated by anorexia, tumor-host competition, and altered states of metabolism. Figure 6–1 depicts these factors, as well as others that contribute to cancer cachexia.[5]

WHAT ARE THE NUTRITIONAL PROBLEMS RESULTING FROM CANCER TREATMENT?

Cancer is treated by (1) radiation, (2) chemotherapy, and (3) surgery, used alone or in combination. Each form of therapy imposes nutritional risks on the patient. The following are nutritional goals during cancer treatment:

1. Prevent weight loss (a short-term goal)
2. Achieve and maintain normal weight (a long-term goal)
3. Replace nutritional losses from side effects of treatment (i.e., fluid and electrolyte losses from vomiting, diarrhea, malabsorption, etc.)
4. Provide adequate calories, protein, carbohydrates, fat, vitamins, and minerals

These goals cannot be achieved without an understanding of individual food tolerances and preferences.

In a survey of 89 major cancer hospitals in the United States, the Diet, Nutrition, and Cancer Program of the National Cancer Institute set out to find which dietetic practices are the most helpful in feeding cancer patients. This 160-page report is now available.[6]

Group dining of ambulatory patients, access to kitchen facilities to prepare snacks and meals, cafeteria-style food service, food-related activities such as pizza parties and picnics are only a few of the report's suggestions on how to help increase the food intake of cancer patients.

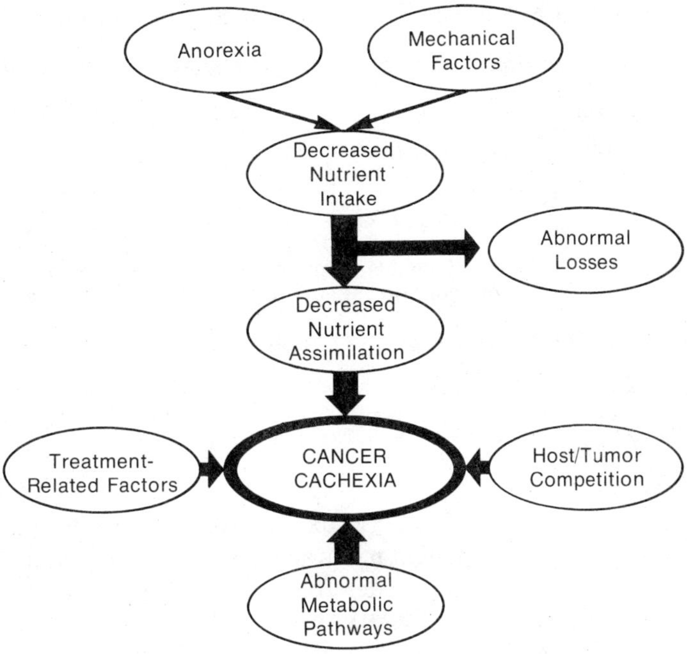

Figure 6–1. The pathways contributing to cancer cachexia. (From G. P. Buzby and J. J. Steinberg, Nutrition in cancer patients. *Surgical Clinics of North America*, Vol. 61, 1981, p. 694.)

Radiation

Exposure to radiation will help to decrease the size of the tumor. At the same time, damage to the surrounding healthy tissue may cause nutritional problems. Radiation to the oropharyngeal region can destroy the sense of taste, thus leading to "mouth blindness" as well as dental caries, mucositis, decreased salivation, and progressive periodontal disease.[7] These side effects make it increasingly difficult to taste, chew, and swallow food.

The abdomen and pelvic area are very sensitive to radiation. Diarrhea, malabsorption, and obstruction are potential hazards during therapy. Nausea, vomiting, anorexia, and weight loss are associated with extensive radiation therapy.[8]

Dietary Recommendations. If signs of malnutrition are present, these should be corrected before treatments are initiated (see Nutritional Assessment, p. 177). Good nutritional status will increase the likelihood of a positive response to therapy. Treatments of higher doses of radiation are better tolerated in well-nourished patients and more effective against cancer cells.

For patients receiving head and neck radiation, food should be moist and easy to chew and swallow. Very hot, cold, or spicy foods and citrus foods should be avoided.

For those receiving abdomen or pelvic radiation, fiber-restricted foods help prevent or alleviate diarrhea. Lactose intolerance may develop and should be watched for.

Chemotherapy

Chemotherapeutic drugs kill cancer cells by inhibiting one or more of the key steps in the metabolism of the cancer cells; unavoidably, normal cells are also affected. Nausea, vomiting, and anorexia are the most common side

TABLE 6–5. Foods Well Accepted when Experiencing Chemotherapy Side Effects*

Side Effect	Well-Accepted Foods
Stomatitis	Popsicles, custards and puddings, milk shakes, ice cream, nectars and other bland juices, soups, jello, eggnogs
Nausea	Carbonated beverages, jello, crackers, broth, popsicles, fruit juice
Diarrhea	Low-residue diet, applesauce, cheese, cottage cheese, jello For pediatric patients: bananas, applesauce, toast, carbonated beverages

*Data obtained from A. Gormican, "A Survey of Dietetic Practices and Procedures used in Feeding Cancer Patients," National Technical Information Service (NTIS No. 22161), Springfield, Va., Vol. 5, No. 1, 1977, pp. 31–35.

effects. If toxic dosages of the drug are given, sores may develop along the alimentary tract, accompanied by malaise, abdominal pain, and diarrhea.[8] These side effects may be lessened by dose alterations.

Dietary Recommendations. As mentioned with radiation therapy, the goal is to provide optimal nutrition before, during, and after treatment.

Steroids used in chemotherapy may require the use of dietary sodium and carbohydrate restrictions due to fluid retention and high blood glucose levels. The side effects experienced during chemotherapy treatments may make it difficult to consume optimum nutrients. Some foods well accepted when experiencing side effects are shown in Table 6–5.

Surgery

Surgery is used in the treatment of cancer in an attempt to remove tumors or alleviate symptoms (e.g., obstruction). The nutritional problems that may develop are dependent on the type of surgical procedure performed.

Dietary Recommendations. Providing optimal nutrition may require dietary modifications based on the patient's ability or inability to consume, digest, and absorb nutrients. Table 6–6 is a list of common dietary modifications needed after certain surgical procedures.

TABLE 6–6. Surgical Procedures Requiring Postoperative Dietary Modifications

Procedure	Nutritional Problems	Dietary Modifications
Radical neck resection	Inability to chew or swallow	Nasogastric tube feeding
Gastrectomy	"Dumping syndrome"	Restrict concentrated carbohydrate, small frequent meals, liquids between meals
Small bowel resection	Diarrhea, malabsorption	Elemental diet
Ileostomy Colostomy	Fluid and electrolyte imbalances	Replacement of fluids and electrolytes

Study Questions and Activities

1. Discuss some of the reasons why cancer patients experience anorexia.
2. Name some of the factors contributing to cancer cachexia.
3. What are some of the nutritional problems imposed by cancer therapies? What dietary modifications are necessary?
4. Why is it important to individualize the diet of the cancer patient?

Diet in Miscellaneous Diseases and Conditions

ALLERGIES

What is Food Allergy?

When a person is sensitive to a certain food or foods, an allergy develops and various symptoms are noted. These may involve the skin, nasal passages, respiratory system, or gastrointestinal tract. Occasionally, the entire circulatory system is affected and shock occurs.[9] Hypersensitivity is evidenced by the following:

1. Skin lesions
2. Gastrointestinal disturbances
3. Headaches
4. Asthma

A protein allergen that passes through the gastrointestinal tract is usually responsible for the reaction. The foods that most often cause allergic reactions include milk, eggs, wheat, oranges, tomatoes, grapefruit, chocolate, fish, nuts, spinach, oats, and corn.

How is Food Allergy Diagnosed?

A detailed allergic history is an important procedure used in diagnosing and managing food allergy.[9] Foods that are thought to be causing an allergy are eliminated for a week or two, then consumed in an excessive amount for several days to see if the symptoms reappear. If this procedure causes symptoms after repeated tests, food allergy may be indicated.

Skin tests, though not always reliable, are valuable for patients who have immediate reactions to foods.

Different test diets, called Rowe Elimination Diets, are used to determine the causative food allergen. The diets contain a few carefully chosen foods, with common allergens omitted from one or more of the diets. A nutritionally adequate diet is then planned to exclude the specific foods to which the individual is allergic. Tables 6–7 to 6–9 list common foods to be omitted on the wheat-free diet, egg-free, and milk-free diets. Table 6–10 lists foods allowed on the egg-, wheat-, and milk-free diet. A list of sources of allergy recipes may be found in the references at the end of this chapter. There are many commercial products for allergy diets available. Careful reading of the labels on such products is necessary to detect any specific allergen to be omitted in the diet.

Very often a person who is allergic to one food will be allergic to other foods in the same food family. For example, someone allergic to peanuts usually cannot eat peas or beans either, simply because they are members of the pea family. Lists of "food families" are available.

TABLE 6–7. Foods Excluded on the Wheat-Free Diet*

Beverages — Instant coffee unless 100% coffee, coffee substitutes, beer, gin, whiskey. Check flavored milk drinks (malted, chocolate, etc.).
Bread — Commercial breads, including rye (unless 100 per cent rye), soy, cracked wheat, graham, and whole wheat. Most corn bread contains wheat flour. Matzoh, pretzels, melba toast, and zwieback are also wheat products.
Cereals — Dry or cooked wheat cereals.
Crackers and Cookies — All commercial cookies (even arrowroot cookies contain some wheat).
Desserts — Cakes, doughnuts, pastries, ice cream cones, commercial ice cream, prepared mixes for cakes and cookies. Commercial pie fillings generally are thickened with wheat flour. Many custards and puddings use wheat flour for thickening.
Gravies, sauces or cream soups — Commercially canned soups are usually prepared with wheat flour.
Macaroni, noodles, spaghetti, and vermicelli.
Meats — Breaded or prepared with wheat flour. Cold cuts such as bologna, wieners, and some sausages. Canned meat dishes with sauce, such as chili.
Pancakes and Waffles — Unless made from special recipes. Commercial mixes, including buckwheat, may contain some wheat.
Miscellaneous — Cream cheese dips, seasoned potato chips, soy sauce, salad dressings, and baked beans, unless prepared at home.

*Modified from *Allergy Recipes.* American Dietetic Association, Chicago, 1979.

TABLE 6–8. Foods Excluded on the Egg-Free Diet*

Beverages — Eggnog, root beer, malted drinks, any prepared drinks made with eggs or egg powder.
Breads — Breads and rolls with glazed crust, sweet rolls, pancakes, waffles, doughnuts, pretzels, french toast, etc.
Broth or consommé.
Cookies and Cakes — Check labels on commercial mixes and products. Frostings must be egg-free.
Desserts — Cream pies, meringues, custards, ice cream, sherbet, candy (e.g., almond paste, cream, chocolate, fondant, marshmallow).
Noodles — Made with eggs.
Meats — Containing egg such as meat loaf, meat balls, croquettes, and breaded meats.
Salad dressings and mayonnaise (unless egg-free) — Egg sauces such as hollandaise.

*Modified from *Allergy Recipes.* American Dietetic Association, Chicago, 1979.

TABLE 6-9. Foods Excluded on the Milk-Free Diet*

Cow's milk in all forms — Fresh, buttermilk, dry, evaporated, condensed (although some persons are not sensitive to dry or evaporated milk), yogurt, whey.
Beverages — Chocolate milk, hot cocoa, or any beverage made with milk.
Breads — Commercial breads or rolls with milk added to ingredients. Check prepared mixes.
Butter.
Cheese — All kinds.
Cookies and cakes — Check labels on commercial mixes and products.
Cream — Including whipped cream and sour cream.
Cream sauces — Cream soups, creamed vegetables, milk gravy, milk chowder.
Desserts — Cream pies, custards, ice cream, sherbet, candy such as chocolate and caramel.
Mashed potatoes.
Meats — Meat loaf, cold cuts, frankfurters, etc.

*Modified from *Allergy Recipes.* American Dietetic Association, Chicago, 1979.

TABLE 6-10. Egg-, Wheat-, and Milk-Free Diet*

Milk substitutes	Soybean milks and other lactose-free supplements
Fruits and vegetables	All fruits and vegetables
Breads and cereals	Rye flour, Rye Krisp, rice flour, cornmeal, oatmeal, enriched rice, barley, rice and barley cereals, tapioca, cornstarch, all potatoes
Meats and substitutes	All meats, poultry, fish, and shellfish; dried peas and beans; nuts; peanut butter; soybeans
Fats	Butter and fortified margarine without added milk solids; vegetable fats and oils; olive oil; lard; bacon fat
Soups	Meat stock soups made with vegetables
Sweets and desserts	Sugar, syrup, jelly, jam, honey, gelatin desserts, fruits, water ices, pure sugar candies
Beverages	Coffee, tea, decaffeinated coffee, carbonated beverages
Miscellaneous	Iodized salt, pepper, herbs and spices, flavorings; foods with cornstarch such as gravies and fruit puddings (Danish dessert)

*Modified from *Allergy Recipes.* American Dietetic Association, Chicago.
Eggs and egg products, wheat and wheat products, and milk and milk products are omitted.

INBORN ERRORS OF METABOLISM

Inborn errors of metabolism refers to genetic defects in metabolism in children born without the ability to produce an enzyme needed for metabolic process.

Galactosemia

Characteristics. Features that characterize galactosemia include a lack of transferase, liver enzyme that converts galactose to glucose; toxic levels of galactose in the blood; diarrhea; drowsiness; edema; liver failure; hemorrhage; and mental retardation.

Dietary Modifications. The lack of the enzyme transferase requires the following dietary modifications. Any foods containing milk, lactose, nonfat dry milk solids, casein, whey, or whey solids must be avoided (see Table 6–9). Acceptable infant formulas are Isomil, Neo-Mull-Soy, ProSobee, Soylac, meat base formulas, Nutramigen, and Pregestimil. Additional nutrients are provided according to the RDA.

It is very important that all ingredient labels for processed and packaged foods be read carefully. As discussed, any foods containing milk, lactose, nonfat dry milk solids, casein, whey, or whey solids cannot be tolerated. Lactate, lactic acid, and lactalbumin are acceptable. The complete list of ingredients may not be found on some foods, such as bread and imitation milk. Therefore, frequent monitoring of red blood cell galactose and galactose-1-phosphate is recommended to assure adequacy of the diet.

Phenylketonuria

Characteristics. Phenylketonuria is characterized by a lack of the enzyme necessary to metabolize phenylalanine, one of the essential amino acids. Since phenylalanine is not metabolized, high levels accumulate and there is a characteristic excretion of phenylketones in the urine. Infants are usually blond, blue-eyed, and fair, and often have eczema. When untreated, the infants are hyperactive and irritable, with an unpleasant personality, and have a musty or gamy odor. Severe retardation results if treatment is delayed.

Dietary Modifications. Special infant formulas are necessary to prevent build-up of toxic levels of phenylalanine. Lofenalac, Phenyl-Free, and PKU-Aid are acceptable. A 10 to 30 per cent increase of protein over the RDA is necessary to assure adequate absorption of amino acids. Calories need to be adjusted to the age, appetite, and growth pattern of the child. Special tables showing the phenylalanine content of various foods are available. Only one fourth of the phenylalanine provided by the protein of the RDA should be consumed.

Homocystinuria

This disease is characterized by a lack of the enzyme necessary for sulfur amino acid metabolism. The purpose of the diet for homocystinuria is to lower blood methionine and homocystine levels. Adequate L-cystine must be supplied. It is used to prevent the build-up of methionine and homocystine in the plasma and homocystine in the urine. Typically, the untreated child is retarded, with a fair complexion and detached retinas. Death usually occurs from spontaneous thrombosis.

Tyrosinosis

This disorder is a result of an error in tyrosine metabolism. The purpose of the diet for tyrosinosis is to reduce plasma tyrosine and phenylalanine levels, and to prevent liver and kidney damage. It may prevent mental deterioration if started early in life.

Maple Syrup Urine Disease

In this disease there is an inability to utilize branched chained amino acids. The purpose of the diet for maple syrup urine disease (MSUD) is to reduce leucine, isoleucine, and valine plasma levels to normal. The diet is used to prevent neurological damage and rapid death by reducing these branched chain amino acids in the diet.

Histidinemia

This inborn error is caused by a lack of the enzyme for histidine metabolism. The purpose of the diet is to lower the plasma histidine level and to treat the symptoms of histidinemia, which results in speech disorders and mental retardation.

MISCELLANEOUS DISORDERS

Gout

Characteristics. Gout resembles arthritis and is characterized by pain in a single joint (often starting with the large toe), followed by complete remission. As the disease progresses, the attacks become more prolonged and more frequent. Eventually there are degenerative joint changes and deformity. Obesity is frequently associated with gout, which is thought to be related to excessive eating, drinking, and exercise. Food allergies may also precipitate an attack.

Diet Modifications. The most important dietary change is to avoid foods rich in purines (Table 6–11). This is accomplished by minimizing protein foods high in purine while maintaining adequate carbohydrate intake to prevent tissue metabolism. Alcohol is avoided, as are fatty foods, since they may inhibit excretion of urate and hinder weight control. Maintenance of sufficient fluid intake as well as ideal body weight is important. Rapid weight losses should be avoided, since ketonemia may trigger an acute gout attack. A sample menu for the gout patient can be found in Table 6–12.

It should be noted that drugs are usually more effective in lowering blood uric acid than dietary modifications.

Iron Deficiency Anemia

Characteristics. In iron deficiency anemia there is a decrease in the number of red blood cells or in the quantity of hemoglobin carried in those cells. The red cells may be small in size (microcytic) or low in hemoglobin (hypochromic). Iron deficiency anemia may be caused by a major loss of blood (hemorrhage), although slow, chronic blood loss, inadequate intake of iron, or inadequate absorption of dietary iron and protein may also result in anemia.

Dietary Modifications. In order to correct this form of anemia it is important to eat a high-protein, high-iron diet that is also liberal in ascorbic acid. The diet is often supplemented with iron salt (ferrous oxide) therapy.

The following foods should be included in a diet rich in protein, iron, and vitamin C: liver, lean meat, eggs, kidney, heart; green leafy vegetables; dried fruits and legumes; citrus fruits; whole-grain and enriched breads and cereals; potatoes; and molasses.

TABLE 6–11. Foods Grouped According to Purine Content*

Group 1: High Purine Content
(100 to 1,000 mg of purine nitrogen per 100 gm of food)

Anchovies	Mackerel
Bouillon	Meat extracts
Brains	Mincemeat
Broth	Mussels
Consomme	Partridge
Goose	Roe
Gravy	Sardines
Heart	Scallops
Herring	Sweetbreads
Kidney	Yeast, baker's and brewer's
Liver	

Foods in this preceding list should be omitted from the diet of patients who have gout (acute and remission stages).

Group 2: Moderate Purine Content
(9 to 100 mg of purine nitrogen per 100 gm of food)

Meat and fish (except those on Group 1):	*Vegetables:*
Fish	Asparagus
Fowl	Beans, shell
Meat	Lentils
Shellfish	Mushrooms
	Peas
	Spinach

One serving (2 to 3 ounces) of meat, fish or fowl or one serving (1/2 cup) vegetable from this group is allowed each day or five days a week (depending upon condition) during remissions.

Group 3: Negligible Purine Content

Bread, enriched white and crackers	Herbs
Butter or fortified margarine (in moderation)	Ice cream
Cake and cookies	Milk
Carbonated beverage	Nuts
Cereal beverage	Olives
Cereals and cereal products (refined and enriched)	Pickles
Cheese	Popcorn
Chocolate	Puddings
Coffee	Relishes
Condiments	Rennet desserts
Cornbread	Rich desserts (in moderation)
Cream (in moderation)	Salt
Custard	Spices
Eggs	Sugar and sweets
Fats (in moderation)	Tea
Fruit	Vegetables (except those in Group 2)
Gelatin desserts	Vinegar
	White sauce

Foods included in this group may be used daily.

*From M. V. Krause and L. K. Mahan, *Food, Nutrition and Diet Therapy*, 6th ed. W. B. Saunders Co., Philadelphia, 1978, p. 550.

TABLE 6-12. Sample Menu for the Gout Patient (Approximately 150 mg Purine)

Breakfast	Lunch	Dinner
1/2 cup orange juice	6 oz vegetarian vegetable soup	1/2 cup tomato juice
1/2 cup farina	2 oz beef patty on bun	2 oz broiled chicken
8 oz milk (whole or low fat)	Sliced tomato and lettuce	1/2 cup mashed potatoes
1 poached egg or egg substitute	French dressing	1/2 cup peas
1 slice toast	Catsup, mustard	1/2 cup fruited gelatin salad
1 tsp butter or margarine	3 apricot halves	1 slice bread
1 tbsp jelly	2 sugar cookies	1 tsp butter or margarine
1 cup coffee	8 oz milk (whole or low fat)	1 cup coffee
1 oz cream or nondairy creamer		1 oz cream or nondairy creamer
		2 tsp sugar

MACROCYTIC (LARGE CELL) ANEMIA

In this form of anemia the diet should meet or exceed dietary allowances for iron. In folic acid deficiency anemia, the diet should be supplemented with folic acid therapy, and in pernicious anemia, with vitamin B_{12} by injection. (Individuals with pernicious anemia lack intrinsic factor and therefore cannot absorb dietary B_{12}.)

Functional Hypoglycemia (Hyperinsulinism)

Characteristics. In functional hypoglycemia the serum glucose levels fall below 50 mg/dl. The symptoms include headache, tremor, sweating, rapid heart beat, emotional instability, extreme hunger, anxiety, weakness, and, eventually, loss of consciousness.

Dietary Modifications. Changes in diet that help moderate this disorder include a decreased level of carbohydrate (75 to 110 gm per day) and a protein content of 120 to 140 gm per day. Since the glucose from protein is released slowly, there is minimal stimulation of insulin secretion. The remainder of calories should be taken as fat. In individuals who are overweight, fat intake must be limited. Concentrated sweets and sugars are omitted altogether. Coffee, tea, cola beverages, and alcohol should be avoided. Often, six to eight small, frequent feedings help to alleviate symptoms. A sample menu for the individual with functional hypoglycemia can be found in Table 6-13.

Test Diets

A variety of diets have been established to aid in the assessment of certain disorders or as part of diagnostic tests. The following are among the most common.

Low-Tyramine Diet. This diet is designed to restrict foods containing tyramine and related compounds. It is used for patients who are taking monoamine oxidase (MAO) inhibitors for clinical depression. The diet helps to prevent such adverse reactions as palpitation, severe headache, and hypertension. Table 6-14 lists foods excluded in a low-tyramine diet.

TABLE 6–13. Sample Menu for the Hypoglycemic Patient

Breakfast	Lunch	Dinner
2 slices bacon or bacon substitute 2 eggs or egg substitute 1/2 slice toast 2 tsp butter or margarine 1/2 cup milk (whole or low fat) Artificial sweetener 1 cup decaffeinated coffee	6 oz beef broth 3 oz beef patty Lettuce salad 2 Tbsp French dressing 1/2 hamburger bun 2 tsp butter or margarine 3 halves canned unsweetened apricots Artificial sweetener 1 cup decaffeinated coffee	3 oz baked ham 1/2 cup mashed potato 1/2 cup spinach Lettuce salad 1 Tbsp mayonnaise 2 halves unsweetened pears in dietetic gelatin dessert 1 tsp butter or margarine Artificial sweetener 1 cup decaffeinated coffee
Midmorning snack	*Midafternoon snack*	*Evening snack*
3 oz sliced cheese 3 squares saltines 1/2 cup milk (whole or low fat)	2 oz cold sliced beef 1/2 slice bread 1/2 cup milk (whole or low fat)	1/2 cup cottage cheese 1 square graham cracker 1 tsp butter or margarine 1/2 cup milk (whole or low fat)

Fat-Free Test Diet. Patients scheduled for x-ray visualization of the gallbladder are put on a fat-free test diet.

Fecal Fat Determination Diet. It is necessary to measure fecal fat for the diagnosis of cystic fibrosis or malabsorption syndromes. The test diet includes a minimum of 100 gm of fat per day for two to three days prior to the test.

Glucose Tolerance Test Diet. Unless contraindicated, the patient scheduled for a glucose tolerance test (used to aid in the diagnosis of diabetes mellitus) will have a high-carbohydrate diet (300 gm for three days) prior to the test.

Meat-Free Test Diet. Meat, poultry, and fish contain hemoglobin, myoglobin, and enzymes that may give a false-positive result in tests for gastrointestinal bleeding. Therefore, patients scheduled for these tests may be on a meat-free diet for as many as four days before the tests.

TABLE 6–14. Foods Excluded on a Low-Tyramine Diet

Aged cheese — All cheeses except cottage, cream, and other unripened cheeses
Fermented sausage — Bologna, salami, pepperoni, and liver sausage
Pickled herring and salted dried fish
Broad beans and pods — Lima and Italian beans, lentils, snow peas, dried beans and peas, and soybeans
Fruits — Bananas, avocados, canned figs, and raisins
Cultured dairy products — Buttermilk, yogurt, and sour cream
Chocolate and products made with chocolate
Caffeine — Coffee, tea, and cola drinks
Beer and ale
Wines (especially Chianti)
Yeast extracts
Licorice
Soy sauce and any food product that is made with soy sauce

Study Questions and Activities

1. Why is tyrosinosis considered to be an inborn error of metabolism?
2. Name some foods that would be excluded on a wheat- and egg-free diet.
3. What are some of the symptoms of an allergy?
4. Plan a day's menu for an egg-free diet for a child.
5. Plan a day's menu for a person allergic to eggs and milk.

Nutritional Support

WHAT ARE THE METHODS OF DELIVERING NUTRITIONAL SUPPORT TO THE PATIENT?

Techniques for providing the patient with optimal caloric and nutrient requirements range from very simple to complex (see Fig. 6–2).

This section will cover the following methods by which a patient receives nutritional support:

1. Oral nutritional support
2. Tube feedings
3. Peripheral parenteral nutrition (PPN)
4. Total parenteral nutrition (TPN)

WHAT IS MEANT BY ORAL NUTRITIONAL SUPPORT?

Whenever possible, the patient should be encouraged to ingest a normal diet by an oral route. This is the preferred and most natural method of nutritional support. It also has the psychological advantage of giving the patients control over at least one aspect of their treatment.

Individualization

Each person enters the hospital with eating habits developed since the introduction of solid foods as an infant. Cultural, social, religious, and economic influences play a major role in food selection.

Each patient should receive individual attention in planning out meals according to the prescribed diet. Some hospital selections may be unfamiliar to the patient. Alternative food selections may be necessary in order to satisfy the patient's food preferences and tolerances. Every attempt should be made to provide the patient with adequate nutrients in familiar, well-tolerated foods.

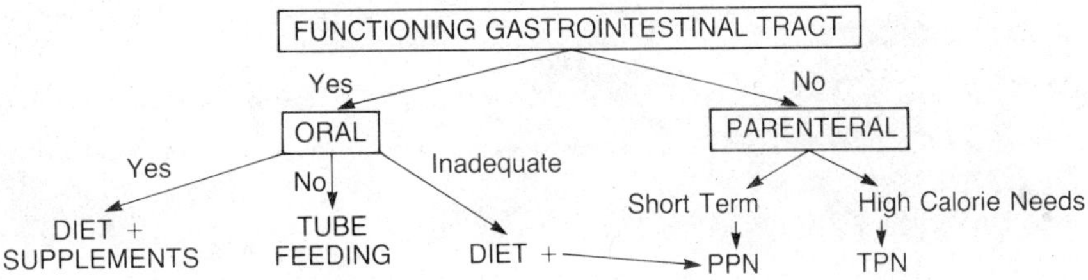

Figure 6–2. Determining the type of nutritional support for the patient.

Recording a patient's food intake will give a fairly accurate estimate of calories and nutrients consumed. From this information an assessment can be made as to whether the patient's nutritional needs are being met orally or if alternative methods of nutritional support should be considered.

Supplements

Ingestion of three meals a day may not be adequate to meet the increased nutrient and caloric requirements of some disease states. Additional foods between meals may help to satisfy this increased demand.

Supplemental foods must also adhere to the diet order prescribed for the patient. When selecting these foods it is important that the patient sample various supplements and choose those preferred for between meals (see Fig. 6–3). This has three advantages: (1) it gives the patient control over an aspect of treatment, (2) it increases the likelihood of the supplement being consumed, and (3) it avoids intolerances of foods due to taste perception changes.

Commercial formulas as well as eggnogs and milk shakes are among the most popular supplements. High-calorie and high-protein puddings, gelatins, and soups have also been developed. Table 6–15 lists the nutritional content of some of these commercial products; other more specialized formulations are listed in Appendix 7.

WHAT IS TUBE FEEDING?

A tube feeding consists of blenderized foods or a commercial formula administered by a tube into the patient's stomach or small intestine. It is sometimes referred to as enteral (by way of the small intestine) feeding.

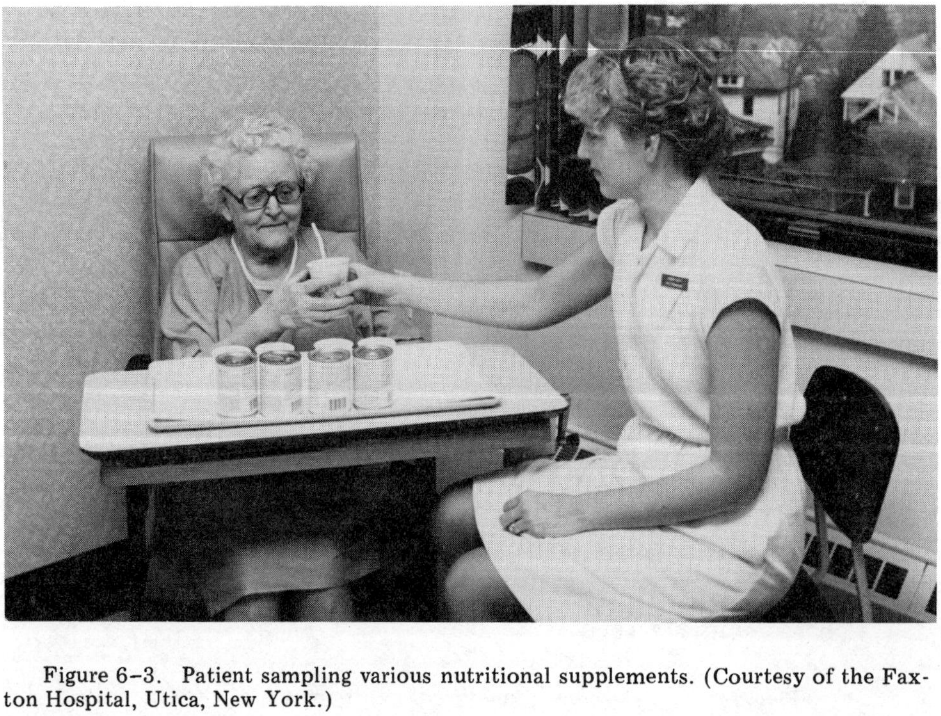

Figure 6–3. Patient sampling various nutritional supplements. (Courtesy of the Faxton Hospital, Utica, New York.)

TABLE 6–15. Enteral Hyperalimentation Chart*

	Blenderized				Milk Based	
	Vitaneed	*Formula 2*	*Compleat-B*	*Compleat-Modified*	*Meritene*	*Carnation Instant Breakfast*
Calories/ml	1	1	1	1	1	1
Carbohydrate Source	Maltodextrin, purėed fruit and vegetables	Wheat flour, sucrose	Hydrolyzed cereal solids, purėed foods, nonfat dry milk, maltodextrin	Hydrolyzed cereal solids, fruit and vegetable purėe	Lactose, corn syrup, sucrose	Sucrose, corn syrup, lactose
Protein Source	Beef, sodium and calcium caseinates, vegetables	Wheat, beef, egg, milk	Beef purėe, nonfat dry milk	Beef, calcium caseinate, vegetables	Skim milk	Milk, sodium caseinate, soy protein isolate
Fat Source	Soy oil, beef	Egg yolk, corn oil, beef fat	Corn oil	Corn oil	Corn oil	Whole milk
Protein gram/liter	35	38	40	43	58	58
Fat gram/liter	40	40	40	37	32	31
Carbohydrate gram/liter	125	123	120	141	110	135
Nonprotein Calories: g N	154:1	142:1	131:1	131:1	79:1	88:1
mOsm/kg Water	375	435–510	390	300	505–570[b]	—
Na/K mEq/Liter	22/32	26/45	52/34	29/36	38/41	41/70
Vitamins, ml to meet 100% U.S. RDA	2000	2000	1600	1500	1252	1400
Producer	Organon	Cutter	Doyle	Doyle	Doyle	Carnation
Flavors[b]	Natural flavor	Orange	Natural flavor	Unflavored	Varied	Varied
Form	Ready to use	Ready to use	Ready to use	Ready to use	Ready to use	Powder
Uses/Features	Blenderized tube feeding, low Na, lactose free, requires digestion.	Blenderized tube feeding, low Na, requires digestion.	Blenderized tube feeding, requires digestion.	Blenderized tube feeding, high protein, lactose free, requires digestion.	Supplement or tube feeding, high protein, requires digestion.	Supplement, high protein, requires digestion.

[a]Unflavored.
[b]Flavors may change values.
[c]Water-soluble vitamins only.

Table continued on following page.

TABLE 6–15. Enteral Hyperalimentation Chart* (*Continued*)

	Lactose Free					
	Citrotein	*Renu*	*Isocal*	*Osmolite*	*Precision Isotonic Diet*	*Precision L.R. Diet*
Calories/ml	1	1	1	1	1	1.1
Carbohydrate Source	Sucrose, maltodextrin	Maltodextrin, sucrose	Glucose oligosaccharides	Hydrolyzed corn starch	Glucose oligosaccharides, sucrose	Maltodextrin, sucrose
Protein Source	Egg albumin	Calcium and sodium caseinates	Calcium and sodium caseinates, soy protein isolate	Calcium and sodium caseinates, soy protein isolate	Egg albumin	Egg albumin
Fat Source	Soy oil	Soy oil	Soy oil, MCT oil	MCT oil, corn oil, soy oil	Soy oil	Soy oil
Protein gram/liter	43	35	34	37	29	26
Fat gram/liter	2	40	44	39	30	2
Carbohydrate gram/liter	129	125	132	145	144	248
Nonprotein Calories: g N	78:1	154:1	167:1	153:1	183:1	239:1
mOsm/kg Water	495–515[b]	300	300	300	300	480[a]
Na/K mEq/Liter	30/18	22/32	23/34	24/26	33/25	31/23
Vitamins, ml to meet 100% U.S. RDA	1152	2000	2000	1887	1560	1710
Producer	Doyle	Organon	Mead Johnson	Ross	Doyle	Doyle
Flavors[b]	Orange, grape	Vanilla	Unflavored	Unflavored	Vanilla, orange	Varied
Form	Powder	Ready to use	Ready to use	Ready to use	Powder	Powder
Uses/Features	Supplement, high protein, requires digestion.	Supplement or tube feeding, low Na, isotonic, requires digestion.	Supplement or tube feeding, low Na, isotonic, requires absorption.	Supplement or tube feeding, low Na, isotonic, requires digestion.	Supplement or tube feeding, isotonic, requires digestion.	Supplement or tube feeding, requires digestion.

[a]Unflavored.
[b]Flavors may change values.
[c]Water-soluble vitamins only.

Table 6–15. Enteral Hyperalimentation Chart* (*Continued*)

	Lactose Free				
	Precision HN Diet	*Ensure*	*Sustacal*	*Travasorb Whole Protein Liq. Nutrition*	*Travasorb MCT*
Calories/ml	1	1	1	1	1
Carbohydrate Source	Maltodextrin, sucrose	Hydrolyzed corn starch, sucrose	Sucrose, corn syrup	Sucrose, corn syrup solids	Corn syrup solids
Protein Source	Egg albumin	Sodium and calcium caseinates, soy protein isolate	Calcium and sodium caseinates, soy protein isolate	Sodium and calcium caseinates, soy protein isolate	Lactalbumin, potassium caseinate
Fat Source	Soy oil	Corn oil	Soy oil	Corn oil, soy oil	MCT oil, sunflower oil
Protein gram/liter	44	37	61	37	43.3
Fat gram/liter	1.3	37	23	37	29
Carbohydrate gram/liter	216	145	140	145	108
Nonprotein Calories: g N	125:1	153:1	79:1	154:1	100:1
mOsm/kg Water	525	450[a]	625	450	312
Na/K mEq/Liter	43/23	37/40	40/53	32/32	15/45
Vitamins, ml to meet 100% U.S. RDA	2850	1887	1080	2000	2000
Producer	Doyle	Ross	Mead Johnson	Travenol	Travenol
Flavors[b]	Citrus, vanilla	Varied	Vanilla, chocolate, eggnog	Varied	Unflavored
Form	Powder	Ready to use	Ready to use	Ready to use	Powder
Uses/Features	Supplement or tube feeding, high protein, requires digestion.	Supplement or tube feeding, requires digestion.	Supplement or tube feeding, high protein, requires digestion.	Supplement or tube feeding, requires digestion.	Supplement or tube feeding, low Na, high protein, requires digestion.

[a] Unflavored.
[b] Flavors may change values.
[c] Water-soluble vitamins only.

Table continued on following page.

TABLE 6–15. Enteral Hyperalimentation Chart* (*Continued*)

	Lactose Free			
	Ensure Plus	*Sustacal HC*	*Isocal HCN*	*Magnacal*
Calories/ml	1.5	1.5	2	2
Carbohydrate Source	Hydrolyzed corn starch, sucrose	Corn syrup solids, sugar	Corn syrup	Maltodextrin, sucrose
Protein Source	Sodium and calcium caseinates, soy protein isolate	Calcium and sodium caseinates	Calcium and sodium caseinates	Calcium and sodium caseinates
Fat Source	Corn oil	Soy oil	Soy oil, MCT oil	Soy oil
Protein gram/liter	55	61	75	70
Fat gram/liter	53	58	91	80
Carbohydrate gram/liter	200	190	225	250
Nonprotein Calories: g N	146:1	134:1	145:1	154:1
mOsm/kg Water	600[a]	650	690	590
Na/K mEq/Liter	50/60	36/38	35/36	44/32
Vitamins, ml to meet 100% U.S. RDA	2000	1200	1500	1000
Producer	Ross	Mead Johnson	Mead Johnson	Organon
Flavors[b]	Varied	Vanilla, eggnog	Unflavored	Vanilla
Form	Ready to use	Ready to use	Ready to use	Ready to use
Uses/Features	Supplement or tube feeding, requires digestion.	Supplement or tube feeding, low Na, requires digestion.	Tube feeding, low Na, high calorie, requires digestion.	Supplement or tube feeding, low Na, high calorie, requires digestion.

*Copyright 1980, Clinical Unit, University Hospital, Boston, Massachusetts.
[a]Unflavored.
[b]Flavors may change values.
[c]Water-soluble vitamins only.

Indications for Use

This type of nutritional support is used when the patient cannot consume adequate nutrients and calories orally but still has a functioning gastrointestinal tract.

A tube feeding is commonly used for psychiatric patients who refuse to eat, anorexic cancer patients, patients who have had head or neck surgery, comatose patients, and patients with obstructions of the esophagus or fractured jaws, or in any situation in which the patient is unable to chew or swallow.

Common Sites

The following are common routes for tube feedings (see Fig. 6–4):

1. Nasogastric — Tube passed from the nose to the stomach
2. Nasojejunal — Tube passed from the nose to the small intestine
3. Gastrostomy — Tube surgically inserted into the stomach
4. Jejunostomy — Tube surgically inserted into the small intestine

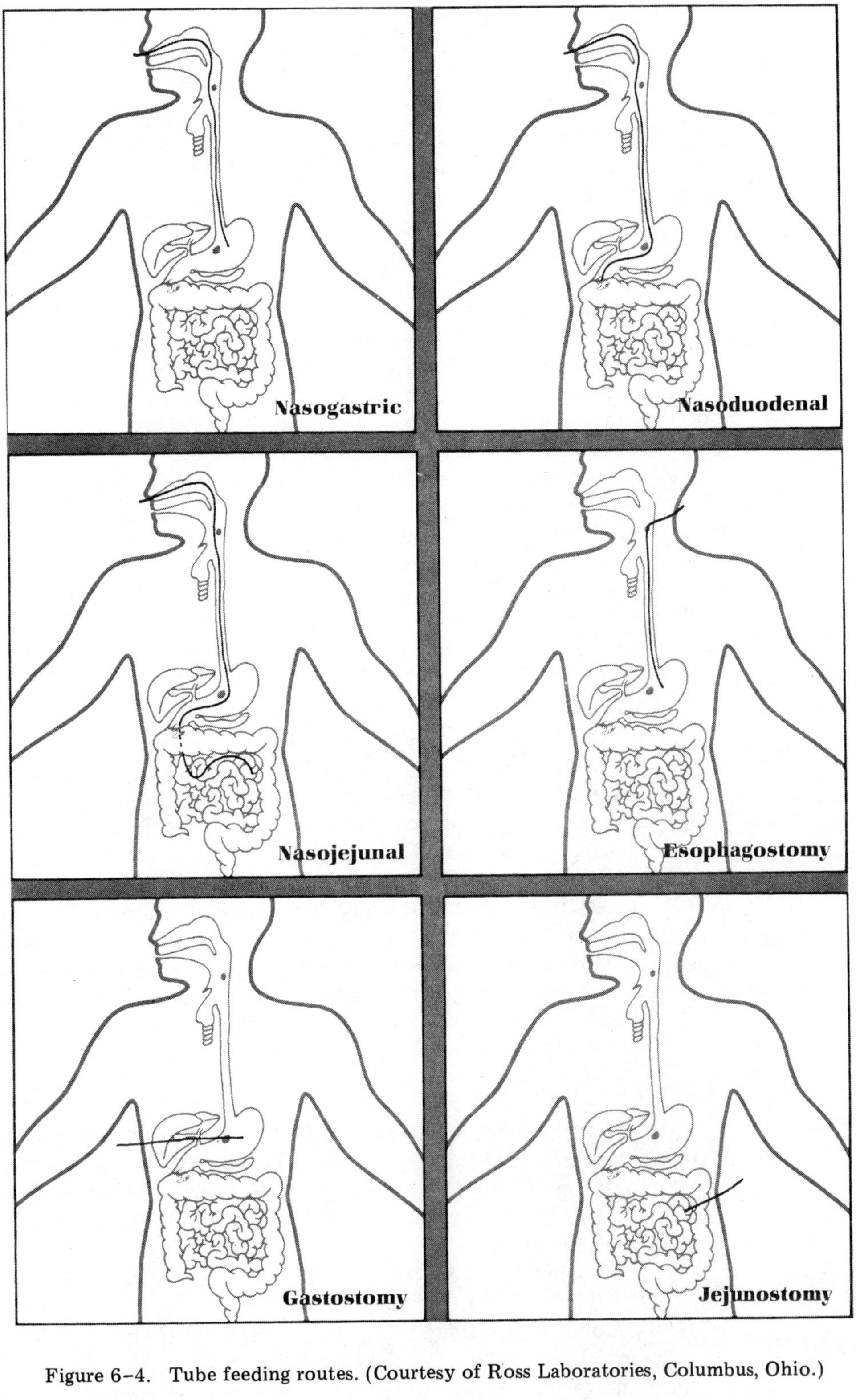

Figure 6–4. Tube feeding routes. (Courtesy of Ross Laboratories, Columbus, Ohio.)

Formulas

A tube feeding may consist of blenderized foods or a commerically prepared formula. The present trend is toward the increased use of commercially prepared formulas, since they are more convenient, decrease the risk of bacterial contamination, offer a wide variety of formulas to meet the needs of different clinical situations, and allow the use of a smaller tube to administer the feeding.

Commercial formulas vary in their composition of carbohydrates, proteins, fats, osmolality, and residue (see Table 6–15). The formula selected will depend on the clinical state of the patient. The dietitian is responsible for knowing when various formulas can and cannot be used.

If the patient's gastrointestinal tract is fully functioning, a formula requiring digestion of all its components can be used (e.g., Ensure, Ensure Plus, Magnacal, Compleat B, Blenderized Diet). If the patient's gastrointestinal tract is not fully functioning, a formula containing digested nutrients can be administered. These formulas are referred to as elemental or defined formula diets (e.g., Vivonex, Vivonex HN, Criticare, Vital). They are commonly used in short bowel syndrome, intestinal malabsorption, and pancreatitis. These formulas are absorbed in the upper part of the small intestine.

Lactose intolerance and fluid and electrolyte restrictions must also be considered when choosing a formula.

All formulas should be refrigerated once they are mixed or opened to prevent bacterial contamination. After 24 hours any unused portion of the formula should be discarded.

Administration

The preferred method of administration for tube feedings is continuous infusion with or without a pump (Fig. 6–5).

The recommended rate is usually between 30 and 50 ml/hr, beginning with a half-strength formula. It is increased at increments of 25 ml/hour until the ideal volume has been reached. The rate at which the feeding is increased will depend on the patient's tolerance, but it is usually increased at 25 ml intervals every 8 to 24 hours.

Once the desired volume has been reached, the formula should be increased in strength gradually from half strength to three quarters strength to full strength.

This gradual increase in the volume and strength of the formula gives the patient's gastrointestinal tract a chance to adjust to the formula. It helps to prevent diarrhea, gas, and cramping. (See Table 6–16 for a sample tube feeding progression.)

Monitoring

Serum albumin levels should be monitored. If this level is low (below 3.5 mg/per cent), it may hinder the patient's ability to absorb the formula. Albumin may then be administered parenterally (intravenously), and the strength of the formula should be at one quarter until the desired albumin level is reached.

Patients receiving tube feedings should be weighed daily. This will indicate if the patient is receiving adequate calories to promote weight gain. Adequate fluid intake is especially important with formulas containing high amounts of protein, so that the kidneys can efficiently excrete nitrogenous waste products. Encouraging the patient to drink fluids as well as rinsing the tube with water between feedings will help increase fluid intake.

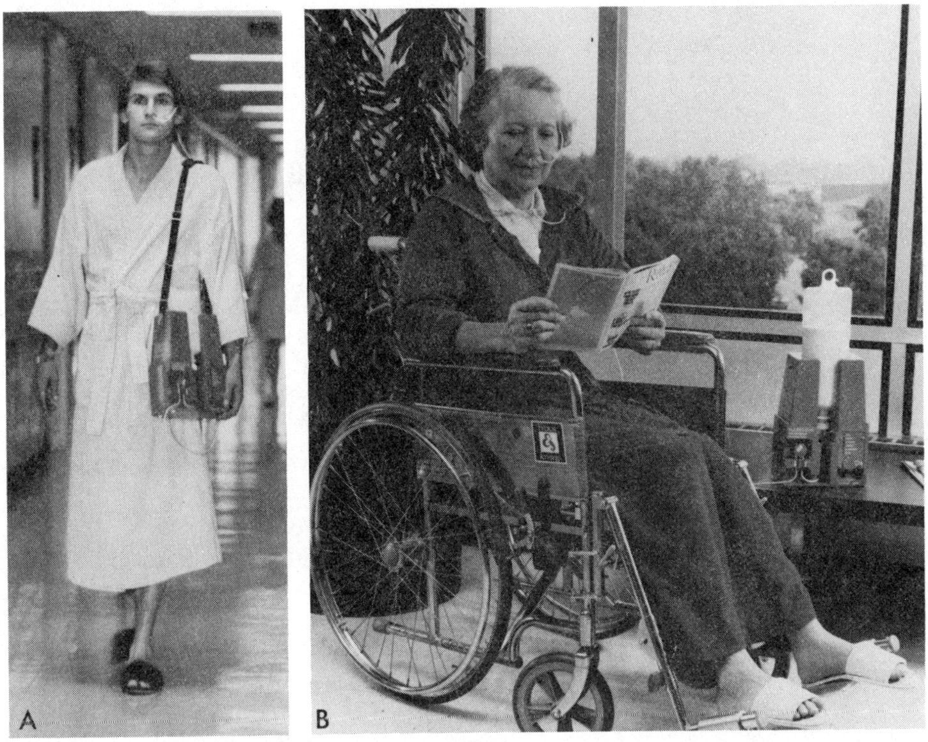

Figure 6–5. Tube feeding systems have been developed so that patients are not confined to a hospital bed. Some may even be used in the home. (Courtesy of Ross Laboratories, Columbus, Ohio.)

TABLE 6–16. Sample Tube Feeding Progression*

	Hour	Rate (ml/hr)	Strength		Calories
Day 1	7–3	50	1/2		200
	3–11	75	1/2		300
	11–7	100	1/2		400
				Total	900
Day 2	7–3	100	1/2		400
	3–11	125	1/2		480
	11–7	125	3/4		750
				Total	1630
Day 3	7–3	125	Full		1000
	3–11	125	Full		1000
	11–7	125	Full		1000
				Total	3000

*Goal = 3,000 calories per day; formula = 1 calorie/ml.

Electrolytes and appropriate nutritional assessment tests should be monitored weekly.

WHAT IS PERIPHERAL PARENTERAL NUTRITION?

Peripheral parenteral nutrition (PPN) is the administration of protein, carbohydrate, and fat substrates via the peripheral veins.

Indications for Use

PPN should be used when a patient is unable to take an adequate oral or enteral feeding for no more than five to seven days.[12] Those patients who cannot consume an adequate intake for several days due to diagnostic tests or surgery should be considered. It is a short-term method of nutritional support.

Candidates for PPN should have[10]:

1. Adequate peripheral veins
2. Albumin levels 3.0 mg/per cent or greater
3. Ability to tolerate fluid loads up to 3,000 ml/24 hours
4. Weight loss not greater than 10 per cent of pre-illness weight

Formulas

Dextrose is the carbohydrate substrate used in PPN. Amino acid solutions provide protein. Fat is provided in solutions of soybean or safflower oil (10 to 20 per cent solutions). The solutions are mixed by the pharmacist (Fig. 6–6).

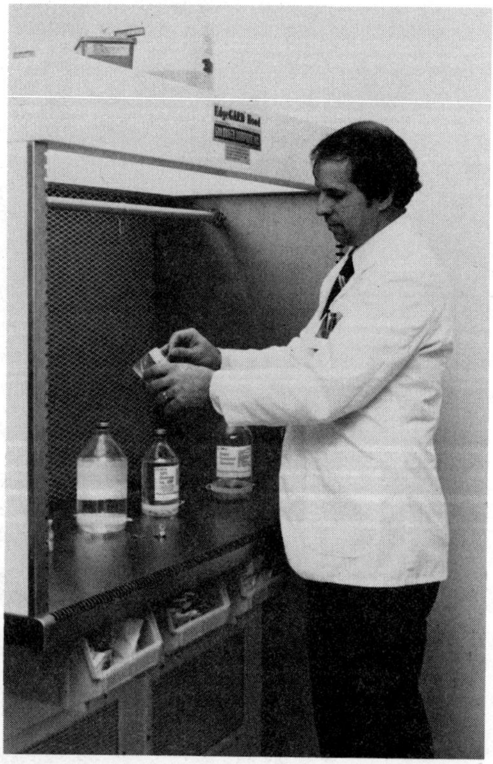

Figure 6–6. The pharmacist mixes TPN and PPN solutions under the laminar flow hood. (Courtesy of the Faxton Hospital, Utica, New York.)

The dextrose and amino acid solutions are mixed in one bottle. The fat solution is in another bottle. Both these bottles are connected at the site of infusion into the patient's peripheral vein (Fig. 6–7).

Monitoring

Phlebitis is a potential complication, so the infusion site should be closely observed.

Daily weights, as well as weekly nutritional assessment tests, are also monitored.

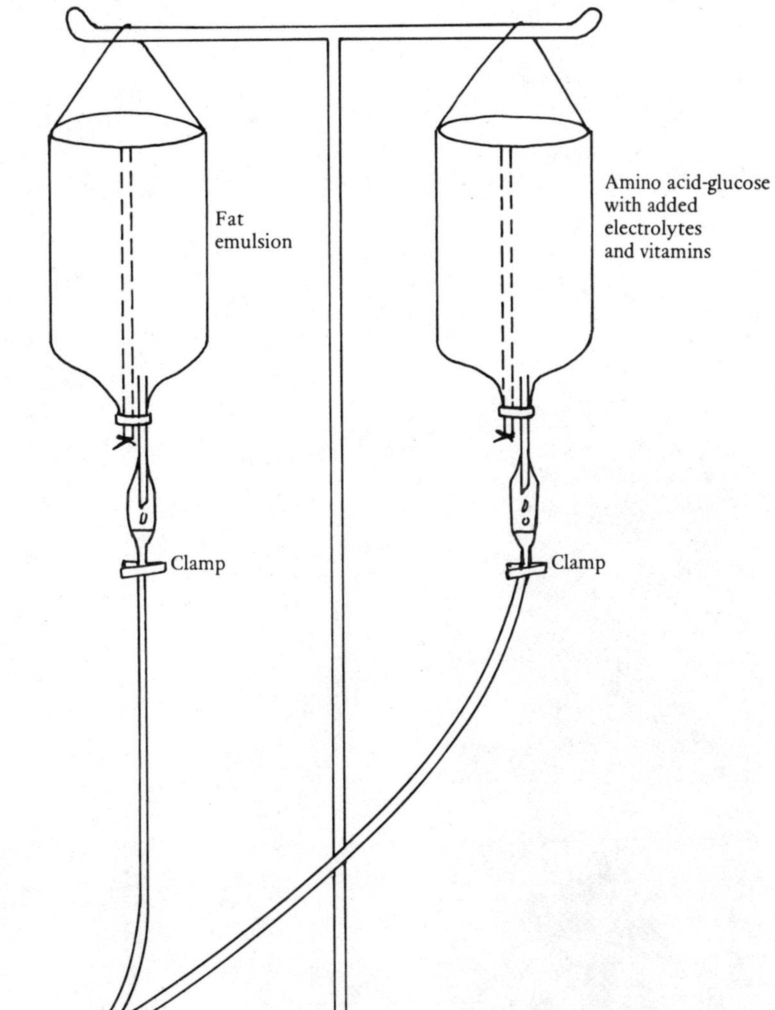

Figure 6–7. Y-tube connecting infusion sets from amino acid-glucose solution and fat emulsion bottles with the central venous catheter or peripheral vein. (From H. A. Schneider, et al., *Nutritional Support of Medical Practice.* Harper and Row Publishers, Inc., Hagerstown, Md., 1977.)

WHAT IS TOTAL PARENTERAL NUTRITION?

Total parenteral nutrition (TPN) is a method of nutritional support that introduces nutrients via a central venous catheter usually inserted into the superior vena cava.

Indications for Use

TPN is used when a patient's gastrointestinal tract is not functioning or when caloric needs are extremely high. It is used in patients with inflammatory bowel disease, partial or total obstruction of the gastrointestinal tract, massive burns, and severe malnutrition.

Formulas

Dextrose, amino acids, fat solutions, minerals, and vitamins can be administered in higher concentrations than PPN solutions. This is made possible because these solutions are introduced in a vein with a high rate of blood flow, which brings about rapid dilution of the solution.[11]

Monitoring

Daily weights and repeating nutritional assessment tests as needed will indicate if the patient is benefiting from the formula given. Electrolytes and trace minerals are monitored as the physician orders.

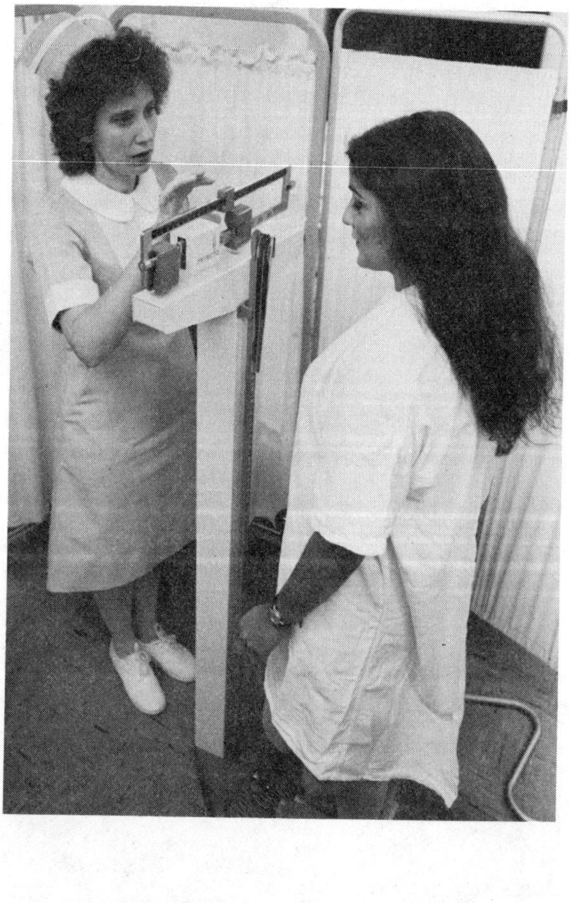

Figure 6–8. Daily weights indicate the effectiveness of the nutritional support received. (Courtesy of the Mohawk Valley Community College Nursing Department, Utica, New York.)

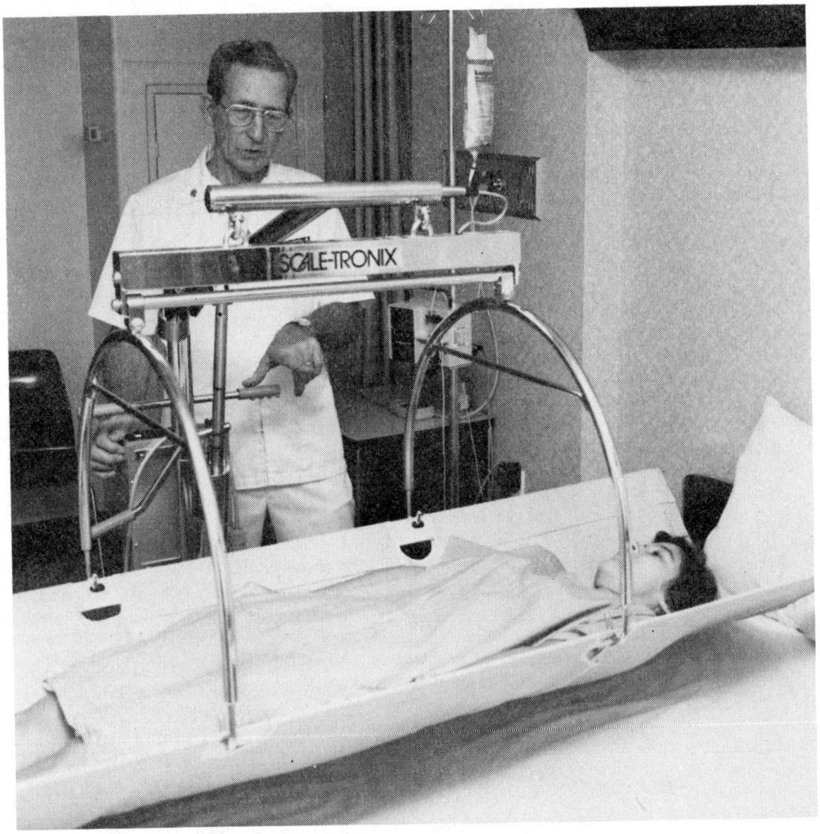

Figure 6–9. Bed scales will provide accurate weight for the patient unable to stand or get out of bed. (Courtesy of The Faxton Hospital, Utica, New York.)

WHEN IS NUTRITIONAL SUPPORT DISCONTINUED?

As the oral intake of the patient improves, the enteral, peripheral, or parenteral nourishment of the patient can gradually be decreased.

Tube feedings may be stopped one hour before and after meals to allow the patient an empty stomach before mealtime. As oral intake improves, the feeding may be infused at shorter intervals (e.g., overnight).

Parenteral solutions are gradually decreased at 1,000 ml per day increments to prevent hypoglycemia. Tube feedings may also be used to wean patients from TPN if adaptation to an oral diet is prolonged.[12]

Initially, food should be introduced in small amounts at frequent intervals. Diarrhea is sometimes a problem in patients who have been on TPN, because the intestinal tract has been bypassed and the mucosal lining may atrophy.[13] If this occurs, a low-residue diet may be necessary.

Once adequate oral intake can be maintained, nutritional support can be discontinued. This will be reflected in calorie intake studies and daily weights (Figs. 6–8 and 6–9).

Study Questions and Activities

1. How is the type of nutritional support to be used determined?
2. How do tube feeding formulas differ? Why is it necessary to have many formulas available?
3. Why is PPN used only for short periods of time?
4. Under what conditions is TPN the only method of nutritional support that can be used?
5. Write a tube feeding progression that will give 2,000 calories for a 1 calorie per ml formula.

REFERENCES

1. B. F. Miller and C. B. Keane, *Encyclopedia and Dictionary of Medicine, Nursing and Allied Health*, 3rd ed. W. B. Saunders Co., Philadelphia, 1982.
1a. "Nutritional Demands Imposed by Stress," *Dairy Council Digest*, Vol. 51, No. 6, Nov.-Dec. 1980.
2. P. S. Howe, *Basic Nutrition in Health and Disease*, 7th ed. W. B. Saunders Co., Philadelphia, 1981, pp. 142–144, 244.
3. M. V. Krause and L. K. Mahan, *Food, Nutrition and Diet Therapy*, 6th ed. W. B. Saunders Co., Philadelphia, 1979, p. 689.
4. J. S. Carson and A. Gormican, "Disease-Medication Relationships in Altered Taste Sensitivity," *Journal of the American Diatetics Association*, Vol. 68, No. 6, 1976, p. 550.
5. G. P. Buzby and J. J. Steinberg, "Nutrition in Cancer Patients," *Surgical Clinics of North America*, Vol. 61, No. 3, June 1981, p. 694.
6. A. Gormican, "A Survey of Dietetic Practices and Procedures Used in Feeding Cancer Patients," National Technician Information Service (NTIS No. 22161), Springfield, Va., Vol. 5, No. 1, 1977, pp. 1–158.
7. M. V. Krause and L. K. Mahan, *Food, Nutrition and Diet Therapy*, 6th ed. W. B. Saunders Co., Philadelphia, 1979, p. 730.
8. J. H. Butler, "Nutrition and Cancer: A Review of the Literature," *Cancer Nursing*, Vol. 3, No. 2, April 1980, pp. 131–137.
9. *Food Allergy*. Asthma and Allergy Foundation of America, New York, 1981, pp. 1–12.
10. J. Walker, S. Myers, and K. Schanzenbach, "Use and Abuse of Peripheral Parenteral Nutrition," *Nutritional Support Services*, Vol. 1, No. 8, Aug. 1981, p. 38.
11. F. Shatsky, "Substrates Available for Intravenous Nutrition," *Nutritional Support Services*, Vol. 1, No. 11, Nov. 1981, p. 27.
12. J. P. Grant, *Handbook of Total Parenteral Nutrition*. W. B. Saunders Co., Philadelphia, 1980, p. 114.
13. Y. Koga, K. Ikeda, K. Inokuchi, et al., "The digestive tract in total parenteral nutrition," *Archives of Surgery*, Vol. 110, No. 6, 1975, pp. 742–745.

ADDITIONAL REFERENCES

NUTRITIONAL NEEDS IN STRESS CONDITIONS

"Nutritional Demands Imposed by Stress," *Dairy Council Digest*, Vol. 51, No. 5, Nov.-Dec. 1980.

B. B. Gallucci and C. E. Rebeis, "Infection, Nutrition and the Compromised Patient," *Topics in Clinical Nursing*, Vol. 2, July 1979, pp. 30–32.

Journal of Parenteral and Enteral Nutrition, Vol. 4, No. 5, Sept.-Oct. 1980, inside cover.

C. E. Ennis and R. Jandrassy, "Nutrition Management of the Surgical Patient," *AORN Journal*, Vol. 31, No. 7, June 1980.

S. W. Salmond, "How to Assess the Nutritional Status of Acutely Ill Patients," *American Journal of Nursing*, Vol. 80, No. 5, May 1980, pp. 922–924.

R. Chernoff, "Nutritional Support: Formulas and Delivery of Enteral Feeding," *Journal of the American Dietetic Association*, Vol. 79, No. 4, Oct. 1981.

C. H. Robinson and M. R. Lawler, "Comprehensive Nutritional Services for Patients," "Immunity, Infections and Fevers," and "Nutrition in Surgical Conditions," in *Normal and Therapeutic Nutrition*, 16th ed. Macmillan Publishing Company, Inc., New York, 1982.

C. H. Robinson, "Nutrition in Surgical Conditions," in *Basic Nutrition and Diet Therapy*, 4th ed. Macmillan Publishing Company, Inc., New York, 1980.

NUTRITION AND CANCER

W. D. DeWys, "Changes in Taste Sensation in Cancer Patients," in M. Kare (ed.), *Correlation with Caloric Intake in the Chemical Senses and Nutrition.* Academic Press, New York, 1977, pp. 381–391.

W. D. DeWys and S. H. Herbst, "Oral Feeding in the Nutritional Management of the Cancer Patient," *Cancer Research,* Vol. 37, No. 7, 1977, pp. 2429–2431.

Dietary Modifications in Disease: Cancer. Ross Laboratories, Columbus, Ohio, 1978.

A. Gormican, "Influencing Food Acceptance in Anorexic Cancer Patients," *Postgraduate Medicine,* Vol. 68, No. 2, 1980, p. 145.

DIET IN MISCELLANEOUS DISEASES AND CONDITIONS

Baking for People with Food Allergies. Home and Garden Bulletin No. 147, U.S. Department of Agriculture, Washington, D.C., 1968.

C. G. Emerling and E. O. Joncheis, *The Allergy Cook Book.* Doubleday Company, New York, 1968.

Chicago Dietetic Association, *Manual of Clinical Dietetics,* 2nd ed. W. B. Saunders Co., Philadelphia, 1981.

C. H. Robinson, *Basic Nutrition and Diet Therapy,* 4th ed. Macmillan Publishing Company, Inc., New York, 1980.

ALLERGY RECIPES:

Tasty Rice Recipes... For Those With Allergies. Rice Council for Market Development, P.O. Box 22802, Houston, Texas, 77027. (no charge)

Allergy Recipes. The American Dietetic Association, 430 North Michigan Avenue, Chicago, Illinois, 60611. Booklet contains wheat-, milk-, and egg-free recipes. $1.50

Delicious and Easy Rice Flour Recipes. Marion N. Wood, Charles C Thomas, Publisher, Bannerstone House, 301–327 East Lawrence Avenue, Springfield, Illinois, 62703. $5.50

Gourmet Food on a Wheat-Free Diet. Marion N. Wood, Charles C Thomas, Publisher, Bannerstone House, 301–327 East Lawrence Avenue, Springfield, Illinois, 62703. $7.50

Low-Gluten Diet with Tested Recipes. A. B. French, M.D., Clinical Research Unit, University Hospital, 1405 E. Ann Street, Ann Arbor, Michigan. Booklet contains wheat-, rye-, oat-, and barley-free recipes. A separate list of some packaged and prepared foods by brand names that may be used in a modified gluten diet is also available. $5.00

Wheat-Gluten-Egg- and Milk-Free Recipes for use at High Altitudes and at Sea Level. Bulletin No. 544-S. Colorado State University, Food Science and Nutrition, Fort Collins, Colorado, 80521. $.50

The Chicago Dietetic Supply House, Inc. 405 East Shawmut Avenue, La Grange, Illinois, 60525. They will provide on request an allergy circular listing products which can be ordered.

NUTRITIONAL SUPPORT

H. A. Schneider, C. E. Anderson, and D. B. Coursin, *Nutritional Support of Medical Practice.* Harper and Row Publishers, Inc., Hagerstown, Md., 1977.

Tube Feedings: Clinical Applications. Ross Laboratories, Columbus, Ohio, 1980.

7

Disorders Requiring Kilocalorie-Controlled Diets

CHAPTER OUTLINE

DIABETES MELLITUS
- Etiology
- Classification
- Treatment
- Meal Planning

WEIGHT CONTROL: OVERWEIGHT AND UNDERWEIGHT
- Energy Needs
- Low/High Kilocalorie Diets
- Behavior Modification
- Surgery

THYROID DISTURBANCES: HYPOTHYROIDISM AND HYPERTHYROIDISM
- Definition
- Etiology
- Low/High Kilocalorie Diets

OBJECTIVES

To understand:

☐ How and why the normal basic diet is modified for the treatment of diabetes mellitus, weight control, and thyroid disturbances.

To apply:

☐ Knowledge of dietary treatment for diabetes, weight control, and thyroid disturbances to meal planning at various kilocalorie levels.

TERMS TO UNDERSTAND

Basal energy expenditure (BEE)
Behavior modification
Chemical regulation
Clinical regulation
Diabetic coma
Fad diet
Food Exchange List
Gastric bypass
Glycosuria
Hyperglycemia
Hyperlipidemia
Hyperthyroidism
Hypoglycemia
Hypothyroidism
Insulin-dependent diabetes mellitus (IDDM)
Insulin shock
Jejunoileal bypass
Ketoacidosis
Ketones
Ketonuria
Non–insulin-dependent diabetes mellitus (NIDDM)
Polydipsia
Polyphagia
Polyuria
Postural hypotension
Renal threshold
Sulfonylureas

Diabetes Mellitus
(Modified Carbohydrate, Protein, and Fat Diets)

WHAT ARE THE BASIC FACTS ABOUT DIABETES MELLITUS?

DEFINITION

Diabetes mellitus is a metabolic disorder in which the body is unable to utilize carbohydrates. As a result, protein and fat metabolism are affected.

ETIOLOGY

Diabetes mellitus results from partial or complete lack of insulin, a hormone produced in the pancreas (islets of Langerhans). It is also thought to be caused by a deficiency of receptor sites for insulin.[1] Viruses, obesity, and heredity have been cited as predisposing factors in the development of diabetes.

CLASSIFICATIONS

The National Diabetes Data Group has proposed the following classifications for diabetes[2]:

Non–Insulin-Dependent Diabetes Mellitus (NIDDM). This classification of diabetes was previously referred to as maturity-onset or adult diabetes mellitus because it occurs in persons 40 years of age or over. This group comprises the majority of diabetics, most of which are overweight.

In NIDDM, insulin may be produced in too short a supply for body needs, or it may be produced in normal amounts but meet insulin resistance at receptor sites.[2] This type of diabetes is slow and gradual in onset. Hyperglycemia is usually evident, but ketoacidosis is usually not a problem at the time of diagnosis. It is more stable, and can usually be controlled with diet alone or diet plus oral hypoglycemic drug therapy. Weight reduction in the obese is essential to successful treatment.

Insulin-Dependent Diabetes Mellitus (IDDM). This classification for diabetes was previously referred to as juvenile diabetes because it commonly occurs in children and young adults. It accounts for approximately 10 to 15 per cent of all diabetics.

Because insulin production is minimal or completely lacking in IDDM, insulin must be given in daily injections. The onset of this type of diabetes is usually sudden and severe. The person has most if not all of the clinical signs and symptoms that will be discussed next. Control is usually accomplished through diet and insulin regulation.

SYMPTOMS AND CLINICAL FINDINGS

Hyperglycemia. An elevation of the blood glucose level, or hyperglycemia, occurs because there is not enough insulin to allow glucose to be taken up by the cells for energy. Because insulin is unable to perform this vital body function, glucose remains in the blood, thus raising the blood glucose levels beyond normal limits.

Glycosuria. Glucose is excreted in the urine (glycosuria) when the kidneys exceed their capacity for reabsorption (renal threshold).

Ketonuria. Without insulin, carbohydrates are unavailable for energy utilization. Instead, the body calls upon fat as an energy source. Under normal conditions the liver breaks down small amounts of fatty acids to form ketones (acetone, beta-hydroxybutyric acid, acetoacetic acid). These ketones are further metabolized for energy. In uncontrolled diabetes, ketone production exceeds utilization. The excess is excreted in the urine. This is known as ketonuria.

Dehydration. The excretion of excess glucose and ketones by the kidneys requires more water. Water is taken from body tissues. This can result in dehydration if excessive amounts of glucose and ketones are excreted and water is not replaced.

Polydipsia and Polyuria. Increased thirst, known as polydipsia, is experienced as the body senses the need to replace excess fluids lost from frequent urination (polyuria) to rid the body of excess ketones and glucose.

Polyphagia. Increased appetite, known as polyphagia, is the body's response to the need for energy. However, this need is not being satisfied, since carbohydrates are unavailable for energy without insulin.

Weight Loss. Because glucose is unavailable, it is excreted in the urine along with excess ketones. Both represent wasted energy sources. Weight loss results because energy demand exceeds available sources.

HOW IS DIABETES TREATED?

Oral Compounds and Insulin

Although some non–insulin-dependent diabetics can be controlled by diet alone, others require additional oral hypoglycemic agents. These oral compounds, called sulfonylureas, are not insulin but stimulate insulin secretion. Table 7–1 gives a list of some commonly used sulfonylureas.

For the insulin-dependent diabetic, insulin must be taken by injection. If it were to be ingested, it would be digested because it is a protein. Different types of insulin may be given; the type and amount is determined by the physician. There are slow-acting, intermediate-acting, and rapid-acting insulins. Intermediate-acting insulin is the most frequently used. See Table 7–2 for a list of these insulins and their duration of action.

TABLE 7–1. Oral Hypoglycemic Agents

Hypoglycemic Agent	Duration of Action
Tolbutamide (Orinase)	6–12 hours
Chlorpropamide (Diabinese)	up to 60 hours
Tolazamide (Tolinase)	10–12 hours
Acetohexamide (Dymelor)	12–24 hours

TABLE 7–2. Types of Insulin

Type of Insulin	Peak Action (hours)	Duration of Action (hours)
Rapid acting (regular, semilente)	3–4	6–8
Intermediate (lente, NPH, globin)	9	24
Slow acting (PZI, ultralente)	20	36

Regulation: Chemical vs. Clinical

Opinion differs as to the extent of diet restriction and insulin therapy needed to regulate the diabetic. Some advocate carefully controlled *chemical regulation* of blood sugar. Both diet and insulin are balanced so that all carbohydrates are metabolized, the blood sugar is kept within normal limits, and the urine is sugar free. The diet is carefully calculated for prescribed amounts of carbohydrate, protein, and fat, and all foods are weighed. Some patients find it difficult to adhere to the strict diet restrictions.

Another approach is the more liberal, "free," or *clinical regulation* of blood sugar. The diet is practically unrestricted (except for sugar and foods high in sugar) as long as there are no diabetic symptoms, no ketonuria, no more than a mild glycosuria, and correct weight is maintained. Insulin is prescribed to metabolize most of the carbohydrate in the diet.

The usual diabetic diet is liberal compared with early diets for diabetics but is not completely "free." This diet is planned easily with *Exchange Lists*, shown on pages 235–239. It allows a wide choice of foods and is easy for the patient to follow because it is based on household measures. Blood and urine sugar levels are moderately controlled.

Diet

Kilocalories. The amount of kilocalories needed by the diabetic should be the same as the RDA for the nondiabetic. Adjustments in kilocalories may be necessary to maintain or attain normal body weight and can be made as necessary.

Protein. The percentage of kilocalories derived from protein is usually 15 to 20 per cent. This allows the diabetic from 1 to 1.5 grams of protein per kilogram of body weight.

Carbohydrates. Carbohydrates are no longer restricted as much as they once were. The recommended allowance is 50 to 55 per cent of total calories from carbohydrate. Complex carbohydrates are emphasized as well as high-fiber foods. (See also "Carbohydrate Distribution" and Table 7–4.)

Fat. Approximately 30 to 35 per cent of total kilocalories for the diabetic is derived from fat. Low-fat foods, lean meats, and polyunsaturated fats are emphasized to prevent cardiovascular disease (a common complication of diabetes). Cholesterol restrictions are imposed if ordered by the physician.

Calculating the Diet. Once the diet order is received from the physician, the diet can be calculated from protein, carbohydrate, and fat content. For example, if the diet order is for 2,000 calories, it can be calculated as follows:

Protein	*Carbohydrate*	*Fat*
2,000	2,000	2,000
X .20	X .50	X .30
400 calories	1,000 calories	600 calories
÷ by 4 cal/gm	÷ by 4 cal/gm	÷ by 9 cal/gm
= 100 gm protein	= 250 gm carbohydrate	= 67 gm fat

The calculations for protein, carbohydrate, and fat must now be translated into a meal pattern that will fit the diabetic's life-style and insulin type. Meals are planned using Food Exchange Lists. The foods in each list are grouped in terms of similarity of composition, and supply approximately the same amount of protein, carbohydrate, and fat. One serving of any food may be exchanged for another serving in the same list. Table 7–3 shows how the calculations for carbohydrate, protein, and fat for the just mentioned 2,000-calorie diet are used in determining the number of exchanges. The Food Exchange Lists are found on pages 235–239.

Carbohydrate Distribution. Carbohydrate should be distributed among the meals and snacks according to the type of insulin prescribed (Table 7–4). For the person receiving oral hypoglycemic agents, meals and snacks should be guided by urine sugar tests. Distributing carbohydrate will help prevent hypoglycemic and hyperglycemic reactions.

Meal Planning. Once the diet has been calculated for protein, carbohydrate, and fat and the carbohydrate distribution determined, the rest of the diet can be planned to best fit the diabetic's personal needs. Factors that need to be considered in meal planning are:

1. Economic status
2. Nutritional needs
3. Food preferences
4. Occupation and work schedule
5. Religious, cultural, and social customs
6. Exercise habits

See Table 7–5 for a sample meal plan.

TABLE 7–3. Calculating a Diabetic Diet*

Foods	No. of Exchanges	List		CHO	PRO	Fat
Milk, nonfat	2-1/2	1		30	20	—
Vegetables	2	2		10	4	—
Fruit	3	3		30	—	—
Bread	12	4		180	24	—
Meat, lean	7	5		—	49	21
Fat	9	6		—	—	45
			Total grams	250	97	66

*Diet prescription = 250 gm carbohydrate (CHO), 100 gm protein (PRO), and 67 gm fat.

TABLE 7–4. Guidelines for Carbohydrate Distribution Based Upon Peak Action and Duration of Insulin Categories*

Insulin	Morning %	Midmorning %	Noon %	Midafternoon %	Evening %	H.S.† %
Rapid acting	25	10	30		25	10
Intermediate acting	20		30	10	30	10
Slow acting	20		25		35	20
Combinations (rapid/intermediate)	20	10	30	10	20	10

*From Chicago Dietetic Association and South Suburban Dietetic Association of Cook and Wills Counties, *Manual of Clinical Dietetics*, 2nd ed. W. B. Saunders Co., Philadelphia, 1981.

†H.S. = hour of sleep, or bedtime.

Food Exchange Lists*

List 1. Milk Exchanges (Includes Nonfat, Low-Fat, and Whole Milk)

One Exchange of Milk contains 12 grams of carbohydrate, 8 grams of protein, a trace of fat, and 80 calories.

This list shows the kinds and amounts of **milk** or **milk products** to use for one Milk Exchange. Those which appear in bold type are *nonfat*. Low-fat and Whole Milk contain saturated fat.

Nonfat Fortified Milk	
Skim or nonfat milk	1 cup
Powdered (nonfat dry, before adding liquid	1/3 cup
Canned, evaporated — skim milk	1/2 cup
Buttermilk made from skim milk	1 cup
Yogurt made from skim milk (plain, unflavored)	1 cup
Low-Fat Fortified Milk	
1% fat fortified milk (omit 1/2 Fat Exchange)	1 cup
2% fat fortified milk (omit 1 Fat Exchange)	1 cup
Yogurt made from 2% fortified milk (plain, unflavored) (omit 1 Fat Exchange)	1 cup
Whole Milk (omit 2 Fat Exchanges)	
Whole milk	1 cup
Canned, evaporated whole milk	1/2 cup
Buttermilk made from whole milk	1 cup
Yogurt made from whole milk (plain, unflavored)	1 cup

Continued on following page

Food Exchange Lists (*Continued*)

List 2. Vegetable Exchanges

One Exchange of Vegetables contains about 5 grams of carbohydrate, 2 grams of protein, and 25 calories.

This List shows the kind of **vegetables** to use for one Vegetable Exchange. One Exchange is 1/2 cup.

Asparagus
Bean Sprouts
Beets
Broccoli
Brussels Sprouts
Cabbage
Carrots
Cauliflower
Celery
Cucumbers
Eggplant
Green Pepper
Greens:
- **Beet**
- **Chards**
- **Collards**
- **Dandelion**
- **Kale**

Greens:
- **Mustard**
- **Spinach**
- **Turnip**

Mushrooms
Okra
Onions
Rhubarb
Rutabaga
Sauerkraut
String Beans, green or yellow
Summer Squash
Tomatoes
Tomato Juice
Turnips
Vegetable Juice Cocktail
Zucchini

The following **raw vegetables** may be used as desired:

Chicory
Chinese Cabbage
Endive
Escarole
Lettuce
Parsley
Radishes
Watercress

Starchy Vegetables are found in the Bread Exchange List.

List 3. Fruit Exchanges

One Exchange of Fruit contains 10 grams of carbohydrate and 40 calories. This List shows the kinds and amounts of **fruits** to use for one Fruit Exchange.

Apple	1 small
Apple Juice	1/3 cup
Applesauce (unsweetened)	1/2 cup
Apricots, fresh	2 medium
Apricots, dried	4 halves
Banana	1/2 small
Berries	
Blackberries	1/2 cup
Blueberries	1/2 cup
Raspberries	1/2 cup
Strawberries	3/4 cup
Cherries	10 large
Cider	1/3 cup
Dates	2
Figs, fresh	1
Figs, dried	1
Grapefruit	1/2
Grapefruit Juice	1/2 cup
Grapes	12
Grape Juice	1/4 cup
Mango	1/2 small
Melon	
Cantaloupe	1/4 small
Honeydew	1/8 medium
Watermelon	1 cup
Nectarine	1 small
Orange	1 small
Orange Juice	1/2 cup
Papaya	3/4 cup
Peach	1 medium
Pear	1 small
Persimmon, native	1 medium
Pineapple	1/2 cup
Pineapple Juice	1/3 cup
Plums	2 medium
Prunes	2 medium
Prune Juice	1/4 cup
Raisins	2 tablespoons
Tangerine	1 medium

Cranberries may be used as desired if no sugar is added.

Food Exchange Lists (*Continued*)

List 4. Bread Exchanges (Includes **Bread, Cereal,** and **Starchy Vegetables**)

One Exchange of Bread contains 15 grams of carbohydrate, 2 grams of protein, and 70 calories.

This list shows the kinds and amounts of **Breads, Cereals, Starchy Vegetables,** and Prepared Foods to use for one Bread Exchange. Those which appear in **bold type** are low-fat.

Cereal	
Bran Flakes	1/2 cup
Other ready-to-eat unsweetened Cereal	3/4 cup
Puffed Cereal (unfrosted)	1 cup
Cereal (cooked)	1/2 cup
Grits (cooked)	1/2 cup
Rice or Barley (cooked)	1/2 cup
Pasta (cooked), Spaghetti, Noodles, Macaroni	1/2 cup
Popcorn (popped, no fat added)	3 cups
Cornmeal (dry)	2 Tbsp
Flour	2-1/2 Tbsp
Wheat Germ	1/4 cup

Crackers	
Arrowroot	3
Graham, 2-1/2" sq.	2
Matzo, 4" × 6"	1/2
Oyster	20
Pretzels, 3-1/8" long × 1/8" dia.	25
Rye Wafers, 2" × 3-1/2"	3
Saltines	6
Soda, 2-1/2" sq.	4

Dried Beans, Peas, and Lentils	
Beans, Peas, Lentils (dried and cooked)	1/2 cup
Baked Beans, no pork (canned)	1/4 cup

Starchy Vegetables	
Corn	1/3 cup
Corn on Cob	1 small
Lima Beans	1/2 cup
Parsnips	2/3 cup
Peas, Green (canned or frozen)	1/2 cup
Potato, White	1 small
Potato (mashed)	1/2 cup
Pumpkin	3/4 cup
Winter Squash, Acorn or Butternut	1/2 cup
Yam or Sweet Potato	1/4 cup

Prepared Foods	
Biscuit 2" dia. (omit 1 Fat Exchange)	1
Corn Bread, 2" × 2" × 1" (omit 1 Fat Exchange)	1
Corn Muffin, 2" dia. (omit 1 Fat Exchange)	1
Crackers, round butter type (omit 1 Fat Exchange)	5
Muffin, plain small (omit 1 Fat Exchange)	1
Potatoes, French Fried, length 2" to 3-1/2" (omit 1 Fat Exchange)	8
Potato or Corn Chips (omit 2 Fat Exchanges)	15
Pancake, 5" × 1/2" (omit 1 Fat Exchange)	1
Waffle, 5" × 1/2" (omit 1 Fat Exchange)	1

List 5. Meat Exchanges — Lean Meat

One Exchange of Lean Meat (1 oz) contains 7 grams of protein, 3 grams of fat, and 55 calories.

This List shows the kinds and amounts of **Lean Meat** and other Protein-Rich Foods to use for one Low-Fat Meat Exchange.

Beef:	**Baby Beef (very lean), Chipped Beef, Chuck, Flank Steak, Tenderloin, Plate Ribs, Plate Skirt Steak, Round (bottom, top), all cuts Rump, Spare Ribs, Tripe**	1 oz
Lamb:	**Leg, Rib, Sirloin, Loin (roast and chops), Shank, Shoulder**	1 oz
Pork:	**Leg (Whole Rump, Center Shank), Ham, Smoked (center slices)**	1 oz
Veal:	**Leg, Loin, Rib, Shank, Shoulder, Cutlets**	1 oz
Poultry:	**Meat without skin of Chicken, Turkey, Cornish Hen, Guinea Hen, Pheasant**	1 oz
Fish:	**Any fresh or frozen**	1 oz
	Canned Salmon, Tuna, Mackerel, Crab, Lobster,	1/4 cup
	Clams, Oysters, Scallops, Shrimp,	5 or 1 oz
	Sardines, drained	3
Cheeses containing less than 5% butterfat		1 oz
Cottage Cheese, Dry and 2% butterfat		1/4 cup
Dried Beans and Peas (omit 1 Bread Exchange)		1/2 cup

Continued on following page

Food Exchange Lists (*Continued*)

List 5. Meat Exchanges — Medium-Fat Meat

For each Exchange of Medium-Fat Meat omit 1/2 Fat Exchange.
This List shows the kinds and amounts of **Medium-Fat Meat** and other Protein-Rich Foods to use for one Medium-Fat Meat Exchange.

Beef:	Ground (15% fat), Corned Beef (canned), Rib Eye, Round (ground commercial)	1 oz
Pork:	Loin (all cuts Tenderloin), Shoulder Arm (picnic), Shoulder Blade, Boston Butt, Canadian Bacon, Boiled Ham	1 oz
Liver, Heart, Kidney and Sweetbreads (these are high in cholesterol)		1 oz
Cottage Cheese, creamed		1/4 cup
Cheese:	Mozzarella, Ricotta, Farmer's cheese, Neufchatel,	1 oz
	Parmesan	3 Tbsp
Egg (high in cholesterol)		1
Peanut Butter (omit 2 additional Fat Exchanges)		2 Tbsp

List 5. Meat Exchanges — High-Fat Meats

For each Exchange of High-Fat Meat omit 1 Fat Exchange.
This List shows the kinds and amounts of **High-Fat Meat** and other Protein-Rich Foods to use for one High-Fat Meat Exchange.

Beef:	Brisket, Corned Beef (Brisket), Ground Beef (more than 20% fat), Hamburger (commercial), Chuck (ground commercial), Roasts (Rib), Steaks (Club and Rib)	1 oz
Lamb:	Breast	1 oz
Pork:	Spare Ribs, Loin (Back Ribs), Pork (ground), Country style Ham, Deviled Ham	1 oz
Veal:	Breast	1 oz
Poultry:	Capon, Duck (domestic), Goose	1 oz
Cheese:	Cheddar Types	1 oz
Cold Cuts		4-1/2" × 1/8" slice
Frankfurter		1 small

List 6. Fat Exchanges

One Exchange of Fat contains 5 grams of fat and 45 calories.
This List shows the kinds and amount of **Fat-Containing Foods** to use for one Fat Exchange. To plan a diet low in Saturated Fat select only those Exchanges which appear in **bold type**. They are **Polyunsaturated.**

Margarine, soft, tub or stick†	1 teaspoon
Avocado (4" in diameter)‡	1/8
Oil, Corn, Cottonseed, Safflower, Soy, Sunflower	1 teaspoon
Oil, Olive‡	1 teaspoon
Oil, Peanut‡	1 teaspoon
Olives‡	5 small
Almonds‡	10 whole
Pecans‡	2 large whole
Peanuts‡	
Spanish	20 whole
Virginia	10 whole
Walnuts	6 small
Nuts, other‡	6 small
Margarine, regular stick	1 teaspoon
Butter	1 teaspoon
Bacon fat	1 teaspoon
Bacon, crisp	1 strip
Cream, light	2 tablespoons
Cream, sour	2 tablespoons

Food Exchange Lists *(Continued)*

Cream, heavy	1 tablespoon
Cream Cheese	1 tablespoon
French dressing§	1 tablespoon
Italian dressing§	1 tablespoon
Lard	1 teaspoon
Mayonnaise§	1 teaspoon
Salad dressing, mayonnaise type§	2 teaspoons
Salt pork	3/4-inch cube

*The exchange lists from the *Exchange Lists for Meal Planning* were prepared by committees of the American Diabetes Association, Inc. and the American Dietetic Association in cooperation with the National Institute of Arthritis, Metabolism and Digestive Diseases and the National Heart and Lung Institute, National Institutes of Health, Public Health Service, U.S. Department of Health, Education and Welfare. Copyright American Diabetes Association, Inc., The American Dietetic Association, 1976.

†Made with corn, cottonseed, safflower, soy, or sunflower oil only.

‡Fat content is primarily monounsaturated.

§If made with corn, cottonseed, safflower, soy, or sunflower oil can be used on fat modified diet.

Patient Counseling

Individualized counseling and instruction is very important for the diabetic person. Family support is also necessary, so family members should be included in the counseling for the child as well as for the adult diabetic. The following is a list of the points to be emphasized when counseling diabetics:

1. Understanding the need for dietary restrictions in the control of diabetes and prevention of complications (cardiovascular disease, renal disease, blindness, and neuropathy).
2. Adapting the instruction to the patient's background and intelligence level.
3. Demonstrating portion sizes with the use of meal tray, food models, or measuring cups and spoons.
4. Avoiding foods with high sugar content.
5. Regularly spaced meals and snacks.
6. Preparing food using only the foods allowed in the meal pattern.
7. Reading labels for carbohydrate, protein, and fat content.
8. Adjusting recipes to fit into allowed foods or using recipes from diabetic cookbooks.
9. Adjusting carbohydrate intake under special circumstances (Table 7-6).
10. Preventing insulin shock and diabetic coma.

WHAT ARE INSULIN SHOCK AND DIABETIC COMA?

Insulin Shock

Insulin shock (insulin reaction) occurs when there is too much insulin. It can be the result of omitting foods from the diet, increased activity and exercise, or an error in insulin injection. The result is a hypoglycemia, a lowering of the blood sugar level. The onset is usually sudden. The diabetic begins to perspire and experiences hunger and nervousness, and the skin is pale, cold, and clammy. If the hypoglycemia is not promptly treated, the diabetic becomes mentally confused and disoriented. If this situation is prolonged, unconsciousness results.

TABLE 7–5. Sample Meal Plan for a Diabetic*

Meal Plan	Menu
Breakfast	
1 nonfat milk exchange	1 cup skim milk
1 fruit exchange	1/2 cup orange juice
2 bread exchanges	2 slices whole-wheat toast
1 meat exchange	1 poached egg
2 fat exchanges	2 tsp margarine
	Coffee
Lunch	
1 nonfat milk exchange	1 cup nonfat milk
1 fruit exchange	1 small apple
3 bread exchanges	2 ounces of ham on 2 slices of whole-wheat bread with 3 tsp mayonnaise
1 vegetable exchange	1/2 cup tomato juice
2 meat exchanges	6 saltine crackers
3 fat exchanges	
Midafternoon	
1 bread exchange	2 graham crackers
1 fruit exchange	1/3 cup apple juice
Dinner	
1/2 nonfat milk exchange	1/2 cup skim milk
1 vegetable exchange	1/2 cup carrots
4 bread exchanges	1/3 cup corn
3 meat exchanges	1/2 cup mashed potato
3 fat exchanges	2 slices whole-wheat bread
	3 ounces baked chicken
	3 tsp margarine
	Coffee
Bedtime	
1 meat exchange	1 ounce of Swiss cheese
2 bread exchanges	12 saltine crackers
1 fat exchange	Decaffeinated coffee
	2 Tbsp light cream

*Diet Prescription = 2,000 calories, 250 gm carbohydrate, 100 gm protein, and 67 gm fat.
Insulin = Lente (intermediate).
Carbohydrate distribution = 20 per cent breakfast, 30 per cent (each) lunch and dinner, and 10 per cent (each) midafternoon and evening snacks.

The diabetic is given juice, candy, sugar, or nondietetic soda to relieve the hypoglycemia (see Table 7–6). If the person becomes unconscious, an intravenous solution of glucose is administered.

Diabetic Coma

Diabetic coma (acidosis, ketoacidosis) occurs when there is too little insulin to meet the body's needs. It can result from an overconsumption of food, illness, or an error in insulin injection. In this condition, the blood sugar level becomes elevated. There is glycosuria and ketonuria. Since ketones are acid products, they will lower the pH of the blood if allowed to accumulate. The person experiences drowsiness, lethargy, and sometimes nausea.

TABLE 7-6. Diet Dilemmas for Insulin Users*

Condition	Remedy	Adjust Meal Pattern for Additional CHO
Insulin Reaction	10† grams CHO If lasts more than 15 min., take more CHO	No
Exercise		
Light: (i.e., 1/2-mile walk)	Do not increase food intake	No
Moderate: (i.e., golf, bowling)	10–15‡ grams CHO per hour of exercise	No
Vigorous: (i.e., skating, running)	20–30§ grams CHO per hour of exercise	No
Delayed Meal	15–30 grams CHO will prevent reaction 1–2 hrs	Yes Deduct from meal pattern
Illness	50–75 grams CHO every 6–8 hours	Replaces meal pattern

*Data obtained from B. El-Beheri-Burgess, "Diet Dilemmas for Insulin Users," *Diabetes Forecast*, Vol. 35, No. 5, Sept.–Oct. 1982, p. 10.

†10 grams CHO (examples):	‡15 grams CHO (examples):	§30 grams CHO (examples):
4 Lifesavers	6 saltines	1/2 cup sherbet
4 oz orange juice	8 oz nondietetic soda	12 oz nondietetic soda
4 oz nondietetic soft drink	4 oz apple juice	12 vanilla wafers
2 tsp honey	6 vanilla wafers	8 oz apple juice
2 tsp sugar	2 graham cracker squares	

The skin becomes hot and dry. There is a fruity odor to the breath (acetone). Breathing is deep and labored.

Coma and death will result if the patient is not treated promptly with insulin and fluids.

Study Questions and Activities

1. Why is weight control important for the diabetic?
2. Calculate a diabetic diet that is 1,500 kilocalories, 50 per cent carbohydrate, 20 per cent protein, and 30 per cent fat. Determine the Exchange List servings that will compose this diet.
3. Write a sample meal plan for the diet in question 2.
4. Bring some food labels into class. How can they be calculated into a diabetic's diet?
5. Why is exercise beneficial to the diabetic?

Weight Control: Overweight and Underweight (High- and Low-Kilocalorie Diets)

WHY IS WEIGHT CONTROL DESIRABLE FOR HEALTH?

Overweight, once considered a sign of success and prosperity, is now considered a form of malnutrition and a major problem in preventive health care. Excess weight places undue strain on the body, lowering resistance to infection and increasing the susceptibility to diabetes, cardiovascular and renal disorders, and other degenerative diseases. Changes in some body functions may also occur. It reduces life expectancy. Surgery is a greater risk for an obese person. Excess weight during pregnancy predisposes to complications during pregnancy and at childbirth. Statistics also show that very obese persons are accident-prone. Obesity handicaps a person physically and may cause emotional and psychological problems.

Underweight associated with undernutrition can be a health problem because of lowered resistance to disease, accompanied by fatigue and impaired body efficiency. It may be a symptom or a predisposing factor in disease. It is especially serious in younger individuals, as underweight persons are more subject to tuberculosis. In children, it may result in retarded growth. Additional kilocalories over and above those needed for basal metabolism and activity are required to meet growth needs during infancy, childhood, and pregnancy.

WHAT IS DESIRABLE WEIGHT AND HOW IS IT DETERMINED?

Revised height-weight tables (Appendix A–4, page 329) indicate "desirable" weights, those associated with lowest mortality rates, based on the weights of individuals approximately 25 years of age. They take into consideration differences in body frame—small, medium, or large—and height. Unlike older tables, they do not consider increases of weight with age to be ideal. Rather, the proper weight for one's height and body build at age 25 is recognized to be the ideal one to be maintained for the remainder of life. These tables are published by the Metropolitan Life Insurance Company following extensive research on their insurance policyholders, relating weight to health and longevity.

Although useful, height-weight tables cannot determine the degree of body fat. This is measured with calipers, usually using the thickness of skinfolds on the upper arm or abdomen. These measurements can then be used to calculate percentages of body fat. The fat under the skin in these regions is roughly proportional to body fat. A skinfold more than an inch thick indicates overweight; under a half inch reflects underweight.[3] Skinfold measurements should be taken by trained professionals.

It is possible for a person to be "overweight" according to height-weight tables but not possess too much body fat. A professional football player is a good example of an individual who may be overweight in terms of height-weight tables but who carries his extra weight in muscle mass, not fat tissue.

It is also possible for a person to be within the ideal range of weight in a height-weight table but still possess too much fat tissue.

The practice of measuring body fat percentages is of more value than height-weight tables, since it can also determine if a person is dieting sensibly. If "crash" diets are used, there is a loss in the lean body tissue (muscle mass) with little if any decrease in fat tissue. The measurement of fat percentages is being used with increased frequency.

HOW IS THE NORMAL DIET MODIFIED IN ENERGY (KILOCALORIES)?

The energy value of the normal diet may be modified for therapeutic purposes by decreasing the kilocalorie value below the allowance recommended for maintenance, so that some of the body fat will be utilized for energy. Conversely, the kilocalorie value may be increased above the maintenance requirement to allow fat to be stored. In either case, the protein, minerals, and vitamins must meet or exceed the recommended dietary allowances. A further modification may be made in the consistency of either diet as needed. Table 7-7 shows one way of determining kilocalories needed for weight loss and weight gain.

WHAT IS OVERWEIGHT AND WHAT CAUSES IT?

Definition. Ten per cent above desirable weight is defined as slight overweight; 20 per cent above desirable weight is considered obese; and 100 pounds or more above desirable weight is considered gross overweight.

Causes. There are many causes of overweight. Most commonly, overweight is a result of excessive food intake (because of family customs, social eating, or emotional problems), a sedentary occupation and leisure activities,

TABLE 7-7. Calculating Kilocalories for Weight Loss and Weight Gain

Determine Energy Needs:

1. Compute basal energy expenditure (BEE).* This is the number of calories expended (burned) in a resting state.
2. Multiply BEE by 1.2 to determine calories expended with daily activity.
3. Subtract 500 to determine kilocalorie requirement for *weight loss.*
4. Add 500 to determine kilocalorie requirement for *weight gain.*

EXAMPLE: A woman 5 feet 6 inches tall, 35 years old, weighing 190 lbs ($W = 190 \times .45 = 85.5$ kg; $H = 66 \times 2.54 = 168$ cm).

How many calories per day will promote weight loss?

1. BEE women $= 655 + (9.6 \times 85.5) + (1.7 \times 168) - (4.7 \times 35) = 1{,}600$ kilocalories.
2. $1600 \times 1.2 = 1920$ kilocalories expended with daily activity.
3. $1920 - 500 = 1420$ kilocalories to promote weight loss.

*BEE formula

BEE men $= 66 + (13.7 \times W) + (5 \times H) - (6.8 \times A)$

BEE women $= 655 + (9.6 \times W) + (1.7 \times H) - (4.7 \times A)$

NOTE: W = Weight in kilograms (pounds $\times .45$ = kg)

H = Height in centimeters (inches $\times 2.54$ = cm)

A = Age in years

From G. L. Blackburn, B. R. Bistrian, B. S. Maini, et al., "Nutritional and Metabolic Assessment of the Hospitalized Patient," *Journal of Parenteral and Enteral Nutrition,* Vol. 1, No. 1, 1977, p. 11.

skipping meals and overeating at other times, glandular disorders (although this cause is rare), decreased energy demand with aging process coupled with decreased activity level, or hereditary influences of bone structure and muscle mass.

HOW IS OVERWEIGHT TREATED?

Dietary Treatment. Calories are restricted after energy needs have been determined by the Basal Energy Expenditure (BEE) formula,[4] which calculates the number of kilocalories expended (burned) in a resting state. The formula used is (BEE × 1.2) − 500 = number of kilocalories required for weight loss (see Table 7–7). Caloric intake must be less than output so that the body will draw on its reserves of fat. These levels of caloric restrictions will help mobilize and utilize fat tissue, thus decreasing body weight.

In general, most women can lose weight best on a diet containing 1,000 to 1,200 calories. Men lose on a diet containing 1,500 to 1,800 calories. These caloric levels will allow for a 1- to 2-pound weight loss per week.

Vitamin and mineral supplementation should be ordered on caloric levels below 1,200 calories.

Calorie levels can be planned by use of the Food Exchange Lists (see pp. 235–239). An individually suited meal pattern is then planned. Table 7–8 gives some guidelines for amounts of food necessary to achieve various calorie levels. Table 7–9 provides a sample menu for 1,200 calories.

Using the Food Exchange Lists will result in a proper balance of carbohydrate, protein, and fat in the diet. Fad diets manipulate the components of a balanced diet into an unbalanced one to achieve weight loss. One of the most popular fad diets is the low-carbohydrate diet which appears from time to time under different names. The principle behind this diet is to reduce carbohydrate intake and allow for generous amounts of protein and fat consumption. This diet is also referred to as a ketogenic diet. Inadequate amounts of carbohydrates in the diet will result in an incomplete oxidation of fats and thus the accumulation of ketones. Ketosis, anorexia, dehydration, and sodium loss result from a low-carbohydrate diet.[5] There is no greater actual fat loss or sparing of body protein with this diet than with isocaloric diets.[6–10]

Potential hazards of this diet include hyperlipidemia, elevated serum uric acid levels, fatigue, and postural hypotension.[6,11] It should not be used by pregnant women.[5]

There are many other fad diets (fasting, liquid protein, etc.), candies and pills that may be used. They all have potential health risks and are not recommended.

TABLE 7–8. Amounts of Food Needed for Various Calorie Levels

Food	1,000 Calories	1,200 Calories	1,500 Calories	1,800 Calories
Milk	1-1/2 cups skim	1-1/2 cups skim	2 cups whole	2-1/2 cups whole
Fruit	3 servings	3 servings	3 servings	4 servings
Vegetables	2 servings	2 servings	2 servings	2 servings
Bread	3 servings	6 servings	7 servings	9 servings
Meat	5 ounces	5 ounces	5 ounces	5 ounces
Fats	3 servings	3 servings	3 servings	4 servings

TABLE 7–9. Sample Menu for 1,200 Calories

Breakfast	Lunch	Dinner
1/2 cup orange juice	1/2 ripe banana	2 ounce lean beef patty
1 poached egg	Turkey sandwich	1/2 cup mashed potato
1 slice toast with 1 tsp butter	1 tsp mayonnaise	1 slice whole-wheat bread
3/4 cup Special K	1/2 cup tomato juice	1/2 cup diced carrots
1/2 cup skim milk	1/2 cup skim milk	1 tsp butter
Coffee with sugar substitute	Lettuce with lo-cal salad dressing	1/2 cup diced pineapple
		1/2 cup skim milk
		Tea with sugar substitute

WHY DON'T "FAD" REDUCING DIETS WORK?

Permanent weight loss is successful weight loss. It is achieved only through learning control over food intake. Many persons are easily allured by dieting gimmicks because they feel helpless in their ability to control their intake of food. They refuse to make food choices, and so are able to rely on the rigidness of a fad diet regimen. When the desired weight loss is achieved, they usually will not maintain their weight without the crutch of the fad diet. This can be very costly and sometimes very dangerous to health, since most fad diets are nutritionally inadequate.

Fast weight loss usually results in depletion of muscle tissue and dehydration. It is easily reversed to weight gain once a normal diet is resumed.

It often takes many fad diet attempts before some individuals realize that there is no short cut to permanent weight loss.

WHAT IS BEHAVIOR MODIFICATION?

Some individuals will find it difficult to adhere to calorie-restricted diets. Calorie-restricted diets work best for those whose eating habits are good but who just need to reduce amounts of foods.

Behavior modification techniques may be needed for those individuals who eat in response to stress or emotional situations. They need to learn to reestablish "hunger" as their cue for initiating eating.

The individual is asked to keep a food diary to find out what specific factors are triggering eating behavior. Table 7–10 shows how a food diary may be used. Many variations of this diary may also be effective.

CAN OVERWEIGHT BE TREATED SURGICALLY?

Surgical techniques have been developed for the morbidly obese person in whom other treatments for obesity have failed. Two of the most common are the jejunoileal bypass and the gastric bypass.

In the *jejunoileal bypass* (Fig. 7–1) most of the ileum is bypassed by attaching the jejunum to only a very small part of the terminal ileum. Weight loss occurs because fewer nutrients and calories are absorbed. There are many complications and side effects from this type of surgery. Some of these include hepatic failure, urinary calculi, diarrhea, vitamin deficiencies, and electrolyte imbalances.[5]

In the *gastric bypass* (Fig. 7–2) the stomach is stapled into two parts: a small functioning section and a larger nonfunctioning section. The smaller functioning section is then connected to the jejunum. Thus, the person can only consume small portions of food at one time. Nausea and vomiting are

TABLE 7–10. Food Diary*

For________________________________ Date________________________________

Time	Minutes Spent Eating	Place	Physical Position	With Whom	Activity	Degree of Hunger	Foods Eaten	Feelings

*Guidelines for food diary:

Time. Certain times of the day may trigger eating behavior. By writing down times when foods are consumed, it will become apparent if a pattern has developed. If certain times of the day are troublesome, some alternative behavior must be developed to replace eating (i.e., exercise, reading, etc.).

Minutes Spent Eating. Mealtime should last at least 20 minutes, since this is when fullness is usually experienced. Eating slowly is a major step in learning permanent weight control. Putting your fork down between each bite is one suggestion that will help prolong mealtime.

Place. Eating should be done only in a place designed for eating, i.e., kitchen, dining room, or restaurant. The person should not eat in other rooms of the house or in the car.

Physical Position. One should be in a sitting position while eating. Standing at the kitchen counter preparing food is a trouble spot for many persons.

With Whom. Notice if there are certain individuals that one associates with who are "food oriented," i.e., all occasions are centered around eating some kind of food. Be prepared to refuse food if you are not hungry.

Activity. One should not engage in any other activities besides pleasant conversation while eating. It is easy to overconsume food while watching television or reading.

Degree of Hunger. Learning to eat only when you are hungry and stopping when you feel full is the most important behavior that will ensure permanent weight loss. If one is not hungry when sitting down to a meal, delay the meal until hunger is evident.

Foods Eaten. Writing down foods when consumed provides a better picture of total food intake than recalling them from memory at the end of the day. It is easy to forget the nibbling between meals.

Feelings. Oftentimes emotional upsets trigger eating behavior. Feelings of loneliness, boredom, or fatigue may result in overconsumption of foods. The person must learn to respond only to hunger cues to initiate eating behavior.

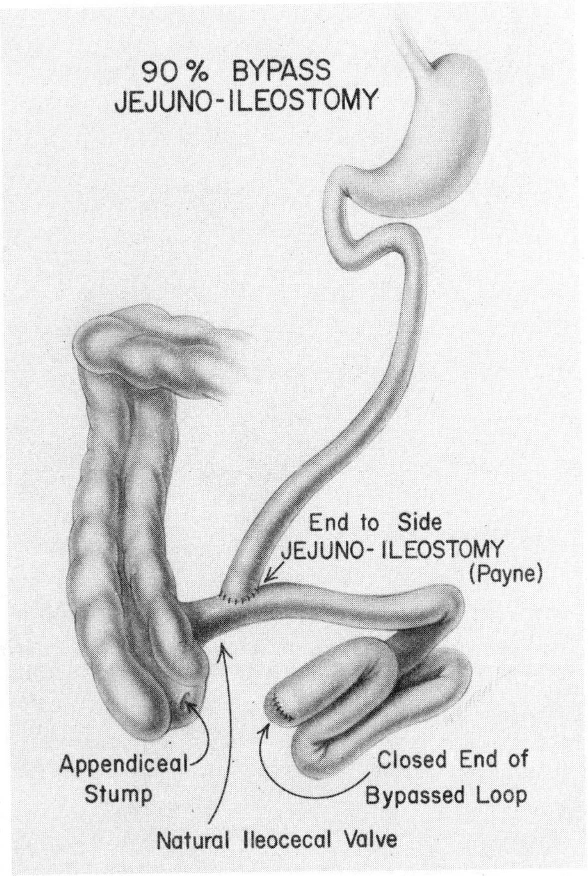

Figure 7–1. Jejunoileal bypass: end-to-side intestinal bypass. (From E. Mason, *Surgical Treatment of Obesity*. W. B. Saunders Co., Philadelphia, 1981.)

experienced for a period after surgery.[12] There are fewer postoperative complications with this surgery than with the jejunoileal bypass; however, the weight loss is less in comparison.

WHAT IS THE IMPORTANCE OF EXERCISE IN WEIGHT REDUCTION?

Exercise is a necessary component of daily living but the all too often forgotten one. Exercise will help to decrease body fat and tone muscle tissue (Figure 7–3). It helps to relieve stress and thus discourages overeating for some individuals.

The amount of exercise for persons with health problems will depend upon the physician's advice.

HOW CAN ONE FAMILY MEMBER DIET WHILE OTHERS EAT NORMALLY?

Table 7–11 shows how a normal 3,000-kilocalorie diet may be modified to give one family member a 1,200 kilocalorie diet without preparing separate meals. Some items are omitted, some served in smaller portions, and some served in modified form—skim milk instead of whole milk, black coffee instead of coffee with cream and sugar.

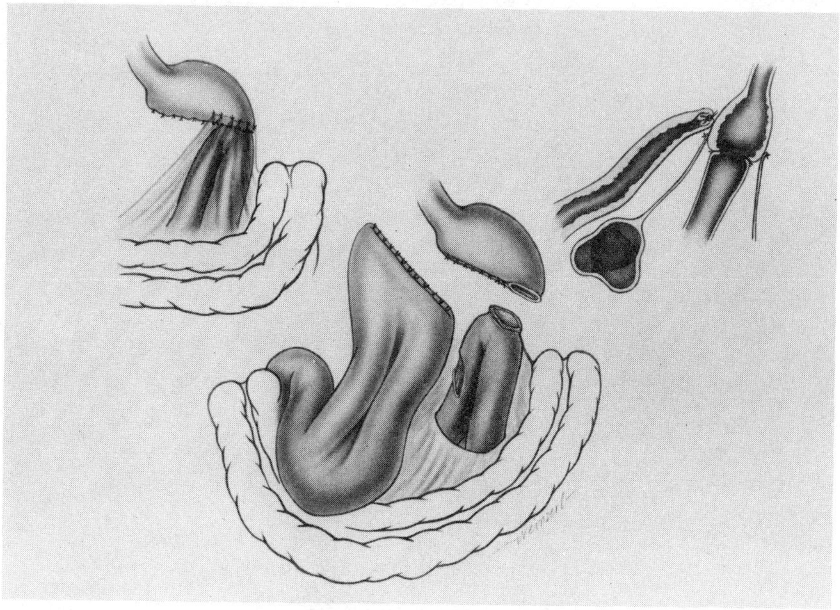

Figure 7–2. Division of the stomach in gastric bypass. (From E. Mason, *Surgical Treatment of Obesity*. W. B. Saunders Co., Philadelphia, 1981.)

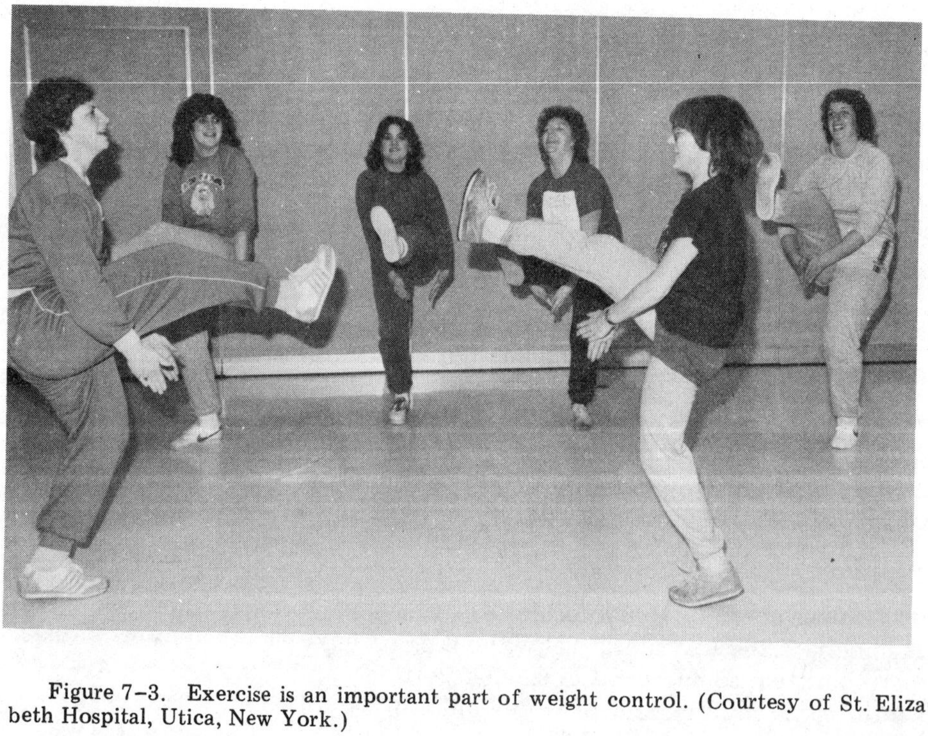

Figure 7–3. Exercise is an important part of weight control. (Courtesy of St. Elizabeth Hospital, Utica, New York.)

TABLE 7-11. Modified 3,000-Kilocalorie Diet*

1,200 Kilocalories		3,000 Kilocalories	
		Breakfast	
Orange juice	1/2 cup	Orange juice	1/2 cup
Soft-cooked egg	1 egg	Soft-cooked egg	1 egg
Whole-wheat toast	1 slice	Bacon	2 medium strips
Butter or margarine	1 teaspoon	Whole-wheat toast	2 slices
Skim milk	1 cup	Butter or margarine	2 teaspoons
Coffee (black), if desired		Whole milk	1 cup
		Coffee	1 cup
		Cream	1 tablespoon
		Sugar	1 teaspoon
		Lunch	
		Tomato soup with milk	1 cup
Sandwich:		Sandwich:	
Enriched bread	2 slices	Enriched bread	3 slices
Boiled ham	1-1/2 ounces	Boiled ham	3 ounces
Mayonnaise	2 teaspoons	Mayonnaise	2-1/2 teaspoons
Mustard		Mustard	
Lettuce	1 large leaf	Lettuce	2 large leaves
Celery	1 small stalk	Celery	1 small stick
Radishes	4 radishes	Radishes	4 radishes
Dill pickle	1/2 large	Dill pickle	1/2 large
Skim milk	1 cup	Apple	1 medium
		Whole milk	1 cup
		Dinner	
Roast lamb	3 ounces	Roast lamb	4 ounces
Rice, converted	1/2 cup	Rice, converted	2/3 cup
Spinach	3/4 cup	Spinach, buttered	2/3 cup
Lemon	1/4 medium	Lemon	1/4 medium
Salad:		Salad:	
Peaches, canned	1 half peach	Peaches, canned	2 halves
Cottage cheese	2 tablespoons	Cottage cheese	2 tablespoons
Lettuce	1 large leaf	Lettuce	1 large leaf
		Rolls, enriched	2 small
		Butter or margarine	1 teaspoon
		Plain cake, iced	1 piece, 3 by 3 by 2 inches
		Between-Meal Snack	
Apple	1 medium	Saltines	4 saltines
		Peanut butter	2 tablespoons
		Whole milk	1 cup

*Excerpted from *Food and Your Weight.* Home and Garden Bulletin No. 74. U.S. Department of Agriculture, Washington, D.C., 1973, p. 10.

WHAT IS UNDERWEIGHT AND WHAT CAUSES IT?

Definition. Ten to 15 per cent or more below the desirable weight is considered underweight.

Causes. There are many reasons an individual may weigh less than is desirable. Among them are food intake insufficient for needs in quality and quantity because of poor absorption and utilization of food, wasting disease (e.g., cancer), increased metabolic rate (e.g., fevers, infection, hyperthyroidism, or burns), mental strain and worry, and excessive activity.

HOW IS UNDERWEIGHT TREATED?

Dietary Treatment. A high-kilocalorie diet is used to restore and maintain normal weight. Kilocalories in excess of expenditure will result in storage of fatty tissue [(BEE × 1.2) + 500]. If 1,000 kilocalories per day above caloric requirements are consumed, approximately 2 pounds will be gained each week. Meals should be planned according to the Basic Four Food Groups. Additional amounts of the basic foods, particularly those with high-energy value, should be added to each meal or in an extra small evening meal or between-meal snacks. Two slices of bread generously spread with butter, peanut butter, or cheese and two glasses of milk consumed during the day can easily add about 500 calories. With further increases in servings of bread, cereals, cream, eggs, and fruit juices, an additional 1,000 kilocalories may be obtained. Adding dry skim milk powder to milk used for drinking or in cereals, puddings, milk shakes, or casseroles will help increase calories and nutrients.

Concentrated fats and sweets should be avoided when appetite is poor, since they will quickly cause satiety.

Mineral and vitamin supplements are used to replenish body stores to optimum levels quickly and to correct, if present, any signs of deficiency diseases.

Thyroid Disturbances
(High- and Low-Kilocalorie Diets)

WHAT IS HYPOTHYROIDISM AND HOW IS IT TREATED?

Definition. In this disorder there is a deficiency in thyroid gland activity. The metabolic rate may be 15 to 30 per cent below normal. It is caused by underproduction of thyroxine or iodine deficiency.

Treatment. *Calorie-restricted diet.* Because of the decrease in the metabolic rate, the individual with hypothyroidism burns fewer kilocalories, and obesity may result. Kilocalorie-restricted diets (see p. 244) and medication are used together to help correct this condition.

WHAT IS HYPERTHYROIDISM AND HOW IS IT TREATED?

Definition. This disorder is characterized by excessive functional activity of the thyroid gland. The metabolic rate may be increased from 15 to 75 per cent above normal. Its cause is unknown.

Treatment. *High-kilocalorie diet.* Because the patient's metabolic rate is greatly increased, a high-kilocalorie diet is necessary to restore lost weight and to maintain desirable weight. Drugs and surgery may be necessary to correct the condition.

Study Questions and Activities

1. Collect information about a fad reducing regimen. Evaluate the information collected for (a) nutritional deficiencies, (b) health hazards, (c) cost, and (d) long-term effectiveness.

2. Why is obesity such a problem in the United States?

3. Keep a Food Diary (see Table 7–10) for one day. What does it tell you about your eating habits?

4. Plan a 1,000-kilocalorie diet and a 3,500-kilocalorie diet.

REFERENCES

1. Chicago Dietetic Association and South Suburban Dietetic Association of Cook and Wills Counties, *Manual of Clinical Dietetics,* 2nd ed. W. B. Saunders Co., Philadelphia, 1981.
2. National Diabetes Data Group, "Classification and Diagnosis of Diabetes Mellitus and Other Categories of Glucose Intolerance, *Diabetes,* Vol. 28, 1979, p. 1039.
3. E. M. Hamilton and E. Whitney, *Nutrition: Concepts and Controversies.* West Publishing Co., St. Paul, 1979, p. 185.
4. G. L. Blackburn, B. R. Bistrian, B. S. Maini, et al., "Nutrition and Metabolic Assessment of the Hospitalized Patient," *Journal of Parenteral and Enteral Nutrition,* Vol. 1, No. 1, 1977, p. 11.
5. R. B. Friedmen, P. Kindy, and J. A. Reinke, "What to Tell Your Patients About Weight-Loss Methods," *Postgraduate Medicine,* Vol. 72, No. 4, Oct. 1982.
6. *Nutrition and Your Health: Dietary Guidelines for Americans.* Home and Garden Bulletin No. 232, U.S. Departments of Agriculture and Health and Human Services, Washington, D.C., 1980.
7. T. B. Van Itallie, "Dietary Approaches to the Treatment of Obesity," *Psychiatric Clinics of North America,* Vol. 1, 1978, pp. 609–620.
8. S. C. Werner, "Comparison Between Weight Reduction on a High-Calorie, High-Fat Diet and on an Isocaloric Regimen High in Carbohydrate," *New England Journal of Medicine,* Vol. 252, 1955, pp. 661–664.
9. J. Yudkin, "The Low-Carbohydrate Diet in the Treatment of Obesity," *Postgraduate Medicine,* Vol. 51, No. 5, 1972, pp. 151–154.
10. M. Baird, R. L. Parsons, and A. N. Howard, "Clinical and Metabolic Studies of Chemically Defined Diets in the Management of Obesity," *Metabolism,* Vol. 23, 1968, pp. 645–657.
11. American Medical Association Council on Foods and Nutrition, "A Critique of Low-Carbohydrate Ketogenic Weight Reduction Regimes. A Review of Dr. Atkins' Diet Revolution," *Nutrition Review,* Vol. 32, No. 1, 1974, p. 15.
12. E. E. Mason, K. J. Printen, T. J. Blommers, et. al., "Gastric Bypass for Obesity after Ten Years' Experience," *International Journal of Obesity,* Vol. 2, 1978, pp. 197–206.

ADDITIONAL REFERENCES

DIABETES MELLITUS

Diabetes Outlook, Vol. 16, No. 2, May–July 1981.

B. El-Beheri-Burgess, "Diet Dilemmas for Insulin Users," *Diabetes Forecast,* Vol. 35, No. 5, Sept.–Oct. 1982, p. 10.

E. A. Sims and D. F. Sims, "No More Neglect," *Diabetes Forecast,* Vol. 34, No. 4, July–Aug. 1982, p. 22.

8

Cardiovascular and Renal Disease

CHAPTER OUTLINE

ATHEROSCLEROSIS AND HYPERLIPIDEMIA
- Characteristics
- Risk Factors
- Dietary Treatment

CARDIAC DISORDERS AND HYPERTENSION
- Types, Causes, and Symptoms of Cardiac Disorders
- Dietary Treatment

RENAL DISEASE
- Functions of the Kidney
- Causes and Types of Renal Disorders
- Dietary Treatment

OBJECTIVES

- ☐ To understand the relation of diet to atherosclerosis, hyperlipidemia, cardiac and renal disorders, and hypertension.
- ☐ To learn how the basic normal diet is modified for therapeutic treatment.

TERMS TO UNDERSTAND

Arteriosclerosis
Atherosclerosis
Compensated
Congestive heart failure
Decompensated
Edema
Endocardium
Hypercholesterolemia
Hyperglycemia
Hyperlipidemia
Hypertension
Meniere's disease
Myocardium
Pericardium
Sodium
Toxemia

Atherosclerosis and Hyperlipidemia

WHAT IS ATHEROSCLEROSIS?

Atherosclerosis is a complex disease of the arteries—a form of arteriosclerosis, or hardening of the arteries. The passageways through the arteries become roughened and narrowed by fatty deposits so that blood cannot flow freely. Atherosclerosis is thought to be a cause of heart attack (coronary thrombosis or myocardial infarction, or plain "coronary"), and cerebral vascular accident (stroke).

Factors in Development[1]

The American Heart Association advises that the nature of coronary heart disease is such that prevention is the primary means by which a reduction in morbidity and mortality will be accomplished. Therefore, it appears prudent to follow a diet aimed at lowering serum lipid concentrations. For most individuals, this can be achieved by lowering intake of calories, cholesterol, and saturated fats. Many persons in the United States have consumed diets similar to those recommended by the AHA for more than 15 years without harmful effects. Worldwide population studies have yielded similar findings.

The AHA identifies 10 risk factors associated with coronary disease:

1. Hypertension
2. Cigarette smoking
3. Hyperlipidemia
4. Diabetes
5. Obesity
6. Male sex
7. Heredity
8. Advancing age
9. Personality traits
10. Sedentary life-style

Studies have shown that in populations habitually subsisting on a low-fat and low-cholesterol diet, or one that is low in saturated fats and cholesterol, there is a low incidence of coronary disease. At a serum cholesterol level of 260 mg/100 ml, a level common in American adults, the risk for developing coronary heart disease is about twice that of persons with a serum level of 210 mg/100 ml. At higher serum cholesterol levels the risk for coronary heart disease is even greater. To be maximally effective for prevention of atherosclerosis, a diet that effects reduction of serum lipids will need to be consumed throughout life. It should be palatable, effective, economically feasible, and nutritionally adequate.

What Dietary Measures Does the Heart Association Suggest to Reduce the Risk of Heart Disease?

The AHA gives the following general dietary recommendations to reduce the risk of heart disease.[1]

1. An adjustment of caloric intake to achieve and maintain ideal body weight. Correction of obesity or avoidance of obesity is strongly recommended.

2. A reduction in total fat calories achieved by a substantial reduction in dietary saturated fatty acids. It is desirable to reduce the level of fat in the diet to 35 per cent of total energy intake, with 10 per cent as saturated fatty acids and 10 per cent of total calories as polyunsaturated fatty acids. Nutritional labeling is of value to the consumer when planning such a modification of diet.

3. A substantial reduction in dietary cholesterol. It is recommended that the adult consume less than 300 mg of cholesterol daily. High-quality proteins from vegetable sources can be substituted for the reduced animal protein, a rich source of cholesterol.

4. An increase in dietary carbohydrate. When fat in the diet is reduced, carbohydrates make up the difference in calories. Vegetables, fruits, and cereals will tend to lower serum triglycerides.

5. Dietary sodium: Experimental animal studies suggest that it is wise to avoid excess sodium in the diet. The physician should be the one to determine the level of sodium restriction for the patient with hypertension, congestive heart failure, or edema.

6. Other dietary factors. Since alcohol can contribute a great number of calories to the diet, obesity and hyperlipidemia could result. Fiber, trace minerals, hardness of water, vitamins, and coffee may also have significant roles in the development of coronary heart disease, but there is insufficient evidence at this time to permit specific recommendations regarding these dietary factors.

Refer to Figure 8–1 to determine your own risk factors in developing heart disease.

How Can Diet Intake of Cholesterol-Rich Foods and Amount and Type of Fat Be Controlled?[2]

1. Eat no more than three egg yolks a week, including eggs in cooking.
2. Limit the use of shrimp and organ meats.
3. Use fish, chicken, turkey, and veal in most of the meat meals for the week; use moderate-sized portions of beef, lamb, pork, and ham less frequently.
4. Choose lean cuts of meat, trim visible fat, and discard the fat that cooks out of the meat.
5. Avoid deep fat frying; use cooking methods that help to remove fat, e.g., baking, boiling, broiling, roasting, and stewing.
6. Restrict the use of fatty "luncheon" and "variety" meats like sausages and salami.
7. Instead of butter and cooking fats that are solid or completely hydrogenated, use liquid vegetable oils and margarines that are rich in polyunsaturated fats.
8. Instead of whole milk and cheeses made from whole milk and cream, use skimmed milk and skimmed milk cheeses.

H E A R T

Everyone plays the game of health whether he wants to or not. What is your score? Add up the numbers in each category that most nearly describe you.

Heredity	1 No known history of heart disease	2 One relative with heart disease over 60 years	3 Two relatives with heart disease over 60 years	4 One relative with heart disease under 60 years	6 Two relatives with heart disease under 60 years
Exercise	1 Intensive exercise, work and recreation	2 Moderate exercise, work and recreation	3 Sedentary work & intensive recreational exercise	5 Sedentary work & moderate recreational exercise	6 Sedentary work & light recreational exercise
Age	1 10–20	2 21–30	3 31–40	4 41–50	6 51–65
Lb	0 More than 5 lb below standard weight	1 ± 5 lb standard weight	2 6–20 lb overweight	4 21–35 lb overweight	6 36–50 lb overweight
Tobacco	0 Nonuser	1 Cigar or pipe	2 10 cigarettes or fewer per day	4 20 cigarettes or more per day	6 30 cigarettes or more per day
Habits of eating Fat	1 0% No animal or solid fats	2 10% Very little animal or solid fats	3 20% Little animal or solid fats	4 30% Much animal or solid fats	5 40% Very much animal or solid fats

Your risk of heart attack:
4–9 Very remote
10–15 Below average
16–20 Average
21–25 Moderate
26–30 Dangerous
31–35 Urgent danger — reduce score!

Other conditions — such as stress, high blood pressure, and increased blood cholesterol — detract from health and should be evaluated by your physician.

Figure 8–1. Risk factors in heart disease. (Courtesy of the School of Health, Loma Linda University.)

Remember also to (1) meet your daily needs for protein, vitamins, minerals, and other nutrients, (2) control calories and maintain a desirable weight, (3) avoid eating excessive amounts of foods containing saturated fat and cholesterol by lowering your total intake of such foods, and (4) eat less total fat and substitute margarine and polyunsaturated fats whenever possible.

Table 8–1 gives dietary modifications of the Basic Four Food Groups, Table 8–2 gives diet plans and Table 8–3 provides sample menus for 1,200- and 1,800-kilocalorie fat-controlled meals.

WHAT ARE THE TYPES OF HYPERLIPIDEMIA AND THE DIET MODIFICATIONS?

Hyperlipidemia is a term that refers to an elevation of specific lipoproteins, cholesterol, and triglycerides. When one or more lipoproteins are elevated, the condition is called hyperlipoproteinemia, of which there are five types: I, IIa and b, III, IV, and V. The following characteristics apply to all of the dietary modifications for hyperlipoproteinemia.

TABLE 8–1. Dietary Modification of the Basic Four in Treatment of Cardiovascular Disease*

Every day, select foods from each of the basic food groups in lists 1–5, and follow the recommendations for number and size of servings.

	RECOMMENDED	AVOID OR USE SPARINGLY
1 MEAT POULTRY FISH DRIED BEANS and PEAS NUTS - EGGS **1 serving . . .** **3-4 ounces of cooked meat or fish (not including bone or fat) or 3-4 ounces of a vegetable listed here** **Use 2 or more servings (a total of 6-8 ounces) daily**	**Chicken • turkey • veal • fish • in most of your meat meals for the week.**	Duck • goose
	Shellfish: clams • crab • lobster • oysters • scallops. Use a 4-ounce serving as a substitute for meat.	Shrimp is moderately high in cholesterol. Use a 4-ounce serving in a meat meal no more than once a week.
	Beef • lamb • pork • ham • less frequently. Choose lean ground meat and lean cuts of meat • trim all visible fat before cooking • bake, broil, roast, or stew so that you can discard the fat which cooks out of the meat.	Heavily marbled and fatty meats • spare ribs • mutton • frankfurters • sausages • fatty hamburgers • bacon • luncheon meats. Organ meats: liver • kidney • heart • sweetbreads • are very high in cholesterol. Since liver is very rich in vitamins and iron, it should not be eliminated from the diet completely. Use a 4-ounce serving in a meat meal no more than once a week.
	Nuts and dried beans and peas: Kidney beans • lima beans • baked beans • lentils • chick peas (garbanzos) • split peas • are high in vegetable protein and may be used in place of meat occasionally.	
	Egg whites as desired.	Egg yolks: limit to 3 per week including eggs used in cooking. Cakes, batters, sauces, and other foods containing egg yolks.

2 VEGETABLES and FRUIT

(Fresh, frozen, or canned)

1 serving . . . $1/2$ cup

Use at least 4 servings daily

RECOMMENDED

One serving should be a source of Vitamin C:
Broccoli • cabbage (raw) • tomatoes. Berries • cantaloupe • grapefruit (or juice) • mango • melon • orange (or juice) • papaya • strawberries • tangerines.

One serving should be a source of Vitamin A—dark green leafy or yellow vegetables, or yellow fruits:
Broccoli • carrots • chard • chicory • escarole • greens (beet, collard, dandelion, mustard, turnip) • kale • peas • rutabagas • spinach • string beans • sweet potatoes and yams • watercress • winter squash • yellow corn.
Apricots • cantaloupe • mango • papaya.

Other vegetables and fruits are also very nutritious; they should be eaten in salads, main dishes, snacks, and desserts, *in addition* to the recommended daily allowances of high vitamin A and C vegetables and fruits.

AVOID OR USE SPARINGLY

If you must limit your calories, use vegetables such as potatoes, corn, or lima beans sparingly. To add variety to your diet, one serving ($1/2$ cup) of any one of these may be substituted for one serving of bread or cereals.

3 BREAD and CEREALS

(Whole grain, enriched, or restored)

1 serving of bread . . . 1 slice

1 serving of cereal . . .
$1/2$ cup, cooked
1 cup, cold, with skimmed milk

Use at least 4 servings daily

RECOMMENDED

Breads made with a minimum of saturated fat:
White enriched (including raisin bread) • whole wheat • English muffins • French bread • Italian bread • oatmeal bread • pumpernickel • rye bread.

Biscuits, muffins, and griddle cakes made at home, using an allowed liquid oil as shortening.

Cereal (hot and cold) • rice • melba toast • matzo • pretzels.

Pasta: macaroni • noodles (except egg noodles) • spaghetti.

AVOID OR USE SPARINGLY

Butter rolls • commercial biscuits, muffins, donuts, sweet rolls, cakes, crackers • egg bread, cheese bread • commercial mixes containing dried eggs and whole milk.

4 MILK PRODUCTS

1 serving . . . 8 ounces (1 cup)

Buy only skimmed milk that has been fortified with Vitamins A and D.

Daily servings:
Children up to 12 . . .
3 or more cups
Teenagers . . .
4 or more cups
Adults . . .
2 or more cups

RECOMMENDED

Milk products that are low in dairy fats:

Fortified skimmed (non-fat) milk and fortified skimmed milk powder • low-fat milk. The label on the container should show that the milk is fortified with Vitamins A and D. The word "fortified" alone is not enough.

Buttermilk made from skimmed milk • yogurt made from skimmed milk • canned evaporated skimmed milk • cocoa made with low-fat milk.

Cheeses made from skimmed or partially skimmed milk, such as cottage cheese, creamed or uncreamed (uncreamed, preferably) • farmer's, baker's, or hoop cheese • mozarella and sapsago cheeses.

AVOID OR USE SPARINGLY

Whole milk and whole milk products:

Chocolate milk • canned whole milk • ice cream • all creams including sour, half and half, whipped • whole milk yogurt.

Non-dairy cream substitutes (usually contain coconut oil which is very high in saturated fat).

Cheeses made from cream or whole milk.

Butter.

Table continued on following page

5 FATS and OILS

(Polyunsaturated)

An individual allowance should include about 2-4 tablespoons daily (depending on how many calories you can afford) in the form of margarine, salad dressing, and shortening.

RECOMMENDED

Margarines, liquid oil shortenings, salad dressings and mayonnaise containing any of these polyunsaturated vegetable oils:

Corn oil • cottonseed oil • safflower oil • sesame seed oil • soybean oil • sunflower seed oil.

Margarines and other products high in polyunsaturates can usually be identified by their label which lists a recommended *liquid* vegetable oil as the *first* ingredient, and one or more partially hydrogenated vegetable oils as additional ingredients.

Diet margarines are low in calories because they are low in fat. Therefore it takes twice as much diet margarine to supply the polyunsaturates contained in a recommended margarine.

AVOID OR USE SPARINGLY

Solid fats and shortenings:

Butter • lard • salt pork fat • meat fat • completely hydrogenated margarines and vegetable shortenings • products containing coconut oil.

Peanut oil and olive oil may be used occasionally for flavor, but they are low in polyunsaturates and do not take the place of the recommended oils.

6 DESSERTS BEVERAGES SNACKS CONDIMENTS

The foods on this list are acceptable because they are low in saturated fat and cholesterol. If you have eaten your daily allowance from the first five lists, however, these foods will be in excess of your nutritional needs, and many of them also may exceed your calorie limits for maintaining a desirable weight. If you must limit your calories, limit your portions of the foods on this list as well.

Moderation should be observed especially in the use of alcoholic drinks, ice milk, sherbet, sweets, and bottled drinks.

ACCEPTABLE

Low in calories or no calories

Fresh fruit and fruit canned without sugar • tea, coffee (no cream), cocoa powder • water ices • gelatin • fruit whip • puddings made with non-fat milk • low calorie drinks • • vinegar, mustard, ketchup, herbs, spices.

High in calories

Frozen or canned fruit with sugar added • jelly, jam, marmalade, honey • pure sugar candy such as gum drops, hard candy, mint patties (not chocolate) • imitation ice cream made with safflower oil • cakes, pies, cookies, and puddings made with polyunsaturated fat in place of solid shortening • angel food cake • nuts, especially walnuts • peanut butter • bottled drinks • fruit drinks • ice milk • sherbet • wine, beer, whiskey.

AVOID OR USE SPARINGLY

Coconut and coconut oil • commercial cakes, pies, cookies, and mixes • frozen cream pies • commercially fried foods such as potato chips and other deep fried snacks • whole milk puddings • chocolate pudding (high in cocoa butter and therefore high in saturated fat) • ice cream.

*From *The Way to a Man's Heart*, Centerfold Leaflet. American Heart Association, Dallas, Texas, 1972. Copyright American Heart Association. Reprinted with permission.

TABLE 8–2. Diet Plans for 1,200- and 1,800-Calorie Fat-Controlled Meals

Foods You Should Have Each Day on 1,200-Calorie Diet	Foods You Should Have Each Day on 1,800-Calorie Diet	In Following Your Diet . . .
1 pint of *Skim Milk*	1 pint of *Skim Milk*	Use skim milk, nonfat dry milk powder, or buttermilk made from skim milk.
3 or more servings of *Vegetables*	3 or more servings of *Vegetables*	Use any vegetables or vegetable juices you wish, since they contain little or no fat. At least 1 serving a day should be a yellow or a leafy green vegetable. (A few vegetables—dried peas and beans, corn, and potatoes—have many more calories than other vegetables. For this reason they are grouped with breads and cereals and should not be counted as part of your vegetable servings.)
3 servings of *Fruit*	3 servings of *Fruit*	Use medium size servings of any kind of fresh or canned unsweetened fruit or fruit juice you wish. The only exception is avocado, which contains fat. At least one serving a day should be a citrus fruit or juice—orange, grapefruit, tangerine.
4 servings of *Breads and Cereals*	7 servings of *Breads and Cereals*	Use breads, cereals, and the high-calorie vegetables from the *Breads and Cereals List.*
6 ounces (cooked) of *Meat, Fish, or Poultry*	6 ounces (cooked) of *Meat, Fish, or Poultry*	Use the kinds and amounts of meat, fish, poultry, and meat substitutes specified on the *Meat, Fish, and Poultry List.*
Use no more than 3 egg yolks each week (or less, depending on advice from doctor)	Use no more than 3 egg yolks each week (or less, depending on advice from doctor)	Count the egg yolks used in cooking as well as those you eat at the table. Egg whites need not be counted or limited.
2 level tablespoons of *Fat* (1 teaspoon of this may be special margarine or shortening)	4 level tablespoons of *Fat* (1 tablespoon of this may be special margarine or shortening)	Use only the oils and fats given on the *Fat List.* Be sure to use your full allowance each day.
1 serving of *Sugars or Sweets* allowed only if substitute for one serving Breads and Cereals	2 servings of *Sugars and Sweets*	Use sugars, sweets, and desserts from the *Sugars and Sweets List.*

Modified from *Planning Fat-Controlled Meals for 1200 and 1800 Calories.* The American Heart Association, Dallas, Texas.

TABLE 8–3. Sample Menus for Fat-Controlled Diets*

1,200 Kilocalories	1,800 Kilocalories
Breakfast	
Chilled half grapefruit 3/4 cup dry cereal 1 cup skim milk 1 soft-boiled egg (optional) 1 slice toast 1 teaspoon special margarine Coffee or tea	Chilled half grapefruit 3/4 cup dry cereal 1 cup skim milk 1 soft-boiled egg (optional) 1 slice toast 1 teaspoon special margarine 1 tablespoon marmalade 2 tablespoons sugar for cereal, fruit, or beverage Coffee or tea
Lunch	
Tomato stuffed with chicken (use 1 tomato; 1/2 cup diced chicken; 2 teaspoons mayonnaise; capers; parsley; lettuce) 1 small hard roll 1 cup skim milk 1 small banana, sliced Coffee or tea	Tomato stuffed with chicken (use 1 tomato; 1/2 cup diced chicken; 2 tablespoons mayonnaise; capers; parsley; lettuce) 1 large or 2 small hard rolls 1 teaspoon special margarine 1 cup skim milk 1 small banana, sliced Coffee or tea
Dinner	
Baked fish fillet (4 ounces) with 1 teaspoon oil Broccoli with 1-1/2 teaspoons Hollandaise sauce (special recipe) Scalloped tomatoes (use 1/2 cup canned tomatoes; 1 slice diced bread; 1 teaspoon oil; salt; pepper; basil) 1 fresh or canned pear (unsweetened) Coffee or tea	Baked fish fillet (4 ounces) with 1 teaspoon oil and 1/4 cup bread crumbs Broccoli with 1-1/2 teaspoons Hollandaise sauce (special recipe) Scalloped tomatoes (use 1/2 cup canned tomatoes; 1 slice diced bread; 1 teaspoon oil; salt; pepper; basil) 1 slice Boston brown bread 1 teaspoon special margarine 1 canned pear, sweetened, with syrup Coffee or tea

*Modified from *Planning Fat-Controlled Meals for 1200 and 1800 Calories.* The American Heart Association, Dallas, Texas, 1981, pp. 19–20.

1. All diets meet the RDA for protein, minerals, and vitamins for everyone except women during the child-bearing years, when more iron is required.
2. All persons with hyperlipoproteinemia should reduce weight by 1 to 2 pounds per week if overweight, then maintain ideal body weight with a well-balanced diet. Weight loss often results in a lowering of blood lipids.
3. Cholesterol intake is restricted in all types except Type I.
4. The intake of saturated fat is reduced, and polyunsaturated fatty acids are preferred to saturated fatty acids.

See Table 8–4 for a summary of the types of hyperlipoproteinemia and the dietary management of them. A practical approach for planning the diets for Types I to IV is found in Table 8–5.

TABLE 8–4. Characteristics of Hyperlipoproteinemias and Diets

	Characteristics of Hyperlipoproteinemia	Calories	Daily Dietary Restrictions: *Fat, Carbohydrate, Protein*	*Cholesterol*	*Alcohol*
Type I	Elevated serum triglycerides; normal to high serum cholesterol.		25–30 gm fat for adults; 15 gm fat for children. CHO—high.	No restriction	None allowed
Type IIa and IIb	Elevated serum cholesterol and beta-lipoprotein; normal triglycerides in Type IIa; cholesterol and triglycerides are elevated in Type IIb.	Calories are not restricted in Type IIa, but often in Type IIb	Limited CHO in Type IIb. Sharp restriction of saturated fats; emphasize polyunsaturated fats.	300 mg or less	Use with discretion in Type IIa and IIb
Type III	Abnormal form of beta-lipoproteins; elevated serum cholesterol and triglycerides; overweight is frequent.	Low until desired weight is attained	Not more than 40% of kilocalories in form of CHO and fat; eliminate concentrated sweets; substitute unsaturated for saturated fat.		May be substituted for up to 2 servings bread or cereal
Type IV	Increase in endogenous triglycerides; pre-beta and triglycerides elevated; normal serum cholesterol; obesity and complications of atherosclerosis present; some abnormal glucose intolerance; some hyperuricemia.	Low until desired weight is attained	40% of kilocalories in form of CHO; eliminate concentrated sweets; substitute unsaturated fats for saturated.	300–500 mg	Use at physician's discretion
Type V	Elevated chylomicrons and pre-beta-lipoproteins; intolerance to both exogenous and endogenous sources of fat; often abnormal glucose intolerance and blood uric acid.	Low until desired weight is attained	25–30% kilocalories in form of fat; polyunsaturated fat substituted for saturated fat. 50% kilocalories as protein. Concentrated sweets contraindicated.	300–500 mg	Contraindicated

TABLE 8-5. Food Allowances for Hyperlipoproteinemias*

Food	Type I	Type IIa	IIb Type III	Type IV	Type V
Skim milk, cups	4	2	2	2	4
Meat, poultry, fish, ounces	5	6–9	6	6	6
Egg yolks as substitute for 1 ounce meat	3/week	None	None	3/week	3/week
Bread, cereals	6+	7+	7	3	10
Potato or other starchy vegetable	1+	1+	1	2	1
Vegetables Dark green or yellow, daily	5	5	2	2	Ad lib.
Fruit, servings Citrus, daily			3	3	3
Fat, teaspoons	None	6–9	12	10	9
Sugar, sweets	Ad lib.	Ad lib.	None	None	None
Low-fat dessert	Ad lib.	Ad lib.	None	None	None
Alcohol	None	With discretion	Subst.†	Subst.†	None

*Reprinted with permission of Macmillan Publishing Co., Inc., from C. H. Robinson and M. R. Lawler, *Normal and Therapeutic Nutrition*, 16th ed. Copyright 1982 by Macmillan Publishing Co., Inc. Adapted from D. S. Fredrickson, et al., *Dietary Management of Hyperlipoproteinemia.* Publ. No. (NIH) 76-110. U.S. Department of Health, Education, and Welfare, Washington, D.C., 1975.

†In these diets up to two servings of alcoholic beverages may be substituted for 2 slices bread. One slice of bread is equal to 1 ounce gin, rum, vodka, or whiskey; 1-1/2 ounces sweet or dessert wine; 2-1/2 ounces dry wine; or 5 ounces beer.

Cardiac Disorders and Hypertension

WHAT ARE THE TYPES AND CAUSES OF CARDIAC DISORDERS?

Cardiac disorders are either *acute* or *chronic.* The acute form occurs suddenly without warning, whereas in the chronic form, circulation progressively decreases. The extent of heart damage determines whether the condition is *compensated* or *decompensated.* The clinical findings and needs for each type of condition are found in Table 8-6.

In diseases of the heart, one or several parts may be damaged. The affected part may be the muscle (myocardium), the outer covering (pericardium), the lining (endocardium), the blood vessels, or the valves.

There are several causes of cardiac disease. They generally fall into one of two categories, *organic* or *functional.* Among the organic causes are congenital conditions, rheumatic fever (causing damage to the heart valves), arteriosclerosis with hypertension, and atherosclerosis. Infections, inflammation, and fatigue are considered functional causes.

WHAT IS HYPERTENSION?

Hypertension is an elevation of the blood pressure above normal and is often a symptom of cardiovascular and renal disease. It is one of the most important risk factors associated with cardiovascular disease.

TABLE 8–6. Clinical Findings and Needs in Cardiac Distress

Compensated Condition	Decompensated Condition
1. Normal circulation 2. Enlarged heart 3. Increased pulse rate 4. Some restriction of vigorous activity 5. Individualized dietary management: 1,000–1,200 kcalories if overweight 1,600–2,000 kcalories to maintain weight Complex carbohydrate to furnish bulk of kcalories Five to six small meals per day Avoid indigestible, bulky, or gas-forming foods Limit tea and coffee Good choice of foods and fluids to aid elimination Possible sodium restriction if edema is a possibility Multivitamin-mineral supplement may be prescribed	1. Poor circulation (heart cannot carry oxygen and nutrients to tissues nor carry waste products such as carbon dioxide from tissues) 2. Edema in extremities and, with increasing failure, in abdominal and chest cavities (congestive heart failure) 3. Bed rest 4. Oxygen and drug therapy 5. Individualized dietary management: Progress from liquid to soft consistency using easily digested foods Avoid very hot or iced beverages during acute stage No caffeine containing beverages Five to six small feedings Mild sodium restriction—2,000 mg Possible fluid restriction 1,000 to 1,200 kcalories until weight is appropriate Fat-controlled diet if needed 1 gm protein per kg body weight Multivitamin-mineral supplement and diuretic may be prescribed

Since obesity is a predisposing factor in hypertension, a low kilocalorie diet is often prescribed to reduce weight and to maintain weight at a normal level. Sodium restriction is often recommended. Further adjustments in protein and fluids as well as sodium intake are made if there is kidney involvement. Sodium restriction improves the effectiveness of diuretic therapy. If diuretics are taken, patients are advised to increase their potassium intake to replenish that lost in the increased urine volume. Bananas and orange juice are frequently recommended for their potassium content. Most fresh vegetables, fruits, legumes, and uncured meats are also good sources of potassium and add only a small amount of sodium to the diet. Physicians should be consulted before using a potassium substitute for salt.

Salt is often linked to hypertension simply because the sodium in salt causes the body to accumulate fluid. Any excess fluid puts greater pressure on the walls of the blood vessels, creating higher blood pressure. For many people with high blood pressure, reducing salt in the diet will often bring it within normal range.

WHAT ARE THE PURPOSES OF SODIUM-RESTRICTED DIETS AND INDICATIONS FOR THEM?

There are several reasons for restricting sodium intake. The most important are:

1. To aid the body in eliminating sodium and fluids (to prevent edema) in disorders in which fluid retention is a problem.
2. To control sodium intake.
3. To relieve elevated blood pressure.

The indications for restricting sodium intake include:

1. Hypertension
2. Congestive heart failure
3. Renal disorders with edema
4. Edema from any cause
5. Eclampsia or pre-eclampsia (toxemia) in pregnancy
6. ACTH and cortisone therapy
7. Cirrhosis of the liver
8. Meniere's disease

WHAT ARE SODIUM AND SALT AND WHERE ARE THEY FOUND?[3]

Sodium (Na), an essential mineral nutrient required daily in a small but nutritionally significant amount, is found in nearly all plants and animals used as food. Salt or sodium chloride (NaCl) is nearly half sodium. An average healthy person receives more sodium through food and water than necessary, but the excess is excreted through the kidneys. In certain disorders water is retained in the body and some sodium along with it. A reduction of the sodium in the diet under these conditions helps the body to reduce its salt content to approximately the amount it needs daily. Sodium in food is naturally present or is added during processing, cooking, or both, usually as table salt or monosodium glutamate (MSG), both of which are high in sodium. Foods labeled "low sodium" may still be high in sodium for very restricted diets. Table 8–7 shows sources of sodium in the diet.

TABLE 8–7. Sources of Sodium*

Natural Sources	Sodium Compounds Added to Foods in Processing and Preparation	Medicines and Dentifrices
Small amounts: fruits Large amounts: meat, fish, poultry, milk, milk products, eggs; canned, smoked, salted seasoned meats Small to large amounts: vegetables Read labels for sodium in cereals (some have no added sodium) High amounts: Average drinking waters, "softened" waters Low amounts: Distilled water	Salt (sodium chloride) Baking soda (sodium bicarbonate) Brine (table salt and water) Monosodium glutamate Disodium phosphate Sodium hydroxide Sodium propionate Sodium alginate Sodium benzoate Sodium sulfite Baking powder Sodium saccharin (read labels on processed foods) 1 level tsp salt (NaCl) contains about 2,300 mg sodium 1 level tsp baking soda contains about 1,000 mg sodium 1 level tsp regular baking powder contains about 370 mg sodium 1 level tsp monosodium glutamate contains 750 mg sodium	"Alkalizers" Antibiotics Cough medicines Laxatives Pain relievers Sedatives Tooth pastes and powders Mouth washes (read label)

*From *Your 500-Milligram Sodium Diet.* The American Heart Association, Dallas, Texas, 1969. Reprinted with permission of the American Heart Association.

WHAT IS A SODIUM-RESTRICTED DIET?

A sodium-restricted diet is a normal adequate diet modified in sodium content, from a very low amount of 250 milligrams to 2,000 milligrams or more.

An average diet prepared in the kitchen with some commercially prepared foods, foods salted during cooking, and some salt added at the table provides about 3,000 to 7,000 milligrams of sodium daily. For therapeutic purposes, sodium may vary from 250 milligrams daily to 2,000 milligrams or more. Diets in which sodium is limited were formerly called "low-salt" diets when salt was omitted only in the preparation of food and "salt-free" when it was allowed neither in cooking nor at the table. Such diets are now named in terms of the level of salt restriction, the most usual being the 500-mg sodium diet (strict), the 1,000-mg sodium diet (moderate), and the 2,400 to 4,500-mg sodium diet (mild restriction). Table 8–8 shows the differences between sodium-restricted diets at different sodium levels.

Sodium-restricted diets require careful planning to include just the right amounts of the foods permitted. The booklets available from local heart associations or the American Heart Association show the correct amounts of foods and sample menus for 500-mg, 1,000-mg, and mild sodium-restricted diets. Table 8–9 shows a diet plan with foods to use and not to use for the 1,800-kilocalorie, 500-mg sodium diet.[3] Table 8–10 gives two sets of menus for this diet plan.[4]

TABLE 8–8. Characteristics of Sodium-Restricted Diets

Mild Restriction (2,400 to 4,500 mg Sodium)	Moderate Restriction (1,000 mg Sodium)	Strict Restriction (500 mg Sodium)
No salt at table. Only light salting of food during cooking. About half as much salt as most people are accustomed to is about right. Canned and processed foods are already lightly salted. No foods that are very salty or that are preserved in salt or brine. No monosodium glutamate or soy sauce to be added to foods. Check with doctor about any unprescribed medicines.	Small amount of salt each day, either in cooking or at the table; alternatives: either add 1/4 *level* teasooon *only* to the 500-mg sodium diet to make it a 1,000-mg sodium diet. Or, two slices of bakery bread containing 400 mg sodium (200/slice) *and* 2 teaspoons of salted butter or margarine containing 100 mg sodium (50/slice) will provide the extra 500 mg of sodium. Drinking water if it contains no more than 5 mg sodium to each 8 oz (otherwise, use distilled). No "softened water" as it contains too much sodium.	Limited quantities of foods with natural sodium. See menus in Tables 8–9 and 8–10. The use of low-sodium milk instead of regular milk will reduce amount of sodium to 250 mg.

TABLE 8–9. Diet Plan for a 500-mg Sodium, 1,800-Kilocalorie Diet*

Foods and Amounts	Use	Do Not Use
Milk 2 glasses Each glass contains about 170 calories, 120 mg sodium. 1 glass milk = 8 oz; 1/2 cup evaporated milk = 1 glass milk.	Regular (whole) milk; evaporated milk; skim milk; powdered milk. If skim milk used, add 2 servings fat to diet for each glass milk. Substitute for not more than one glass milk a day: 2 oz meat, poultry, or fish or 6 oz yogurt (3/4 container). Count milk used in cooking from day's allowance. Check dairies for use of milk in buttermilk.	Ice cream; sherbet; malted milk; milk shake; instant cocoa mixes; chocolate milk; condensed milk; all other kinds of milk and fountain drinks. These foods are high in calories and the sodium content is unknown.
Meat, Poultry Fish 5 oz cooked. Each ounce contains average of 75 calories, 25 mg Na.	Fresh, frozen, or dietetic canned meat or poultry; beef; lamb; pork; veal; fresh tongue; liver; chicken; duck; turkey; rabbit. Fresh or dietetic (not frozen) fish: any kind except those listed at right. Substitutes for 1 oz meat, poultry, fish: an egg (limit is 1 egg a day); 1/4 cup unsalted cottage cheese; 1 oz low-sodium dietetic cheese; 2 tbsp low-sodium dietetic peanut butter. Use beef liver not more than once in two weeks.	Brains or kidneys; canned, salted, or smoked meat (bacon, bologna, chipped or corned beef, frankfurters, ham, meats koshered by salting, luncheon meats, salt pork, sausage, smoked tongue). Frozen fish fillets: canned, salted, or smoked fish (anchovies, caviar, salted cod, herring, sardines); canned tuna or salmon unless low-sodium dietetic; shellfish (clams, crabs, lobsters, oysters, scallops, shrimp). Regular cheeses, peanut butter, and salted cottage cheese.
Vegetables At least 3 servings Each starchy vegetable contains about 70 calories, 5 mg sodium. Other vegetables contain from 5 to 35 calories, about 9 mg sodium. Count as serving: about 1/2 cup vegetable.	Any fresh, frozen, or dietetic canned vegetables or vegetable juices, except those listed at right. Check label on frozen peas and lima beans—may have had salt or other sodium compound added during processing. Avoid ordering vegetables when eating out, because of salt and MSG additions.	Canned vegetables or vegetable juices unless low-sodium dietetic; frozen vegetables if processed with salt; the following vegetables in any form: artichokes, beet greens, beets, carrots, celery, chard, dandelion greens, whole hominy, kale, mustard greens, sauerkraut, spinach, white turnips.
Fruit At least 3 servings Each serving contains about 40 calories, 2 mg sodium. Size of fruit serving varies, depending on the fruit and the calories.	Any kind of fruit or fruit juice—fresh, frozen, canned, or dried—if sugar has not already been added. Substitute for fruit juice: low-sodium dietetic tomato juice. If you do want sweetened fruit or juice, add an allowed sugar substitute or the amount of sugar, honey, etc., allowed on list headed "And . . . take your choice."	Fruits canned or frozen in sugar syrup because of extra calories they contain.
Low-Sodium Breads, Cereals, and Cereal Products 7 servings Each serving contains about 70 calories, 5 mg sodium. 1 serving: 1 slice bread; 1 roll or muffin; 4 crackers or pieces melba toast; 1/2 cup cooked cereal, noodles, rice; 1-1/2 cup popcorn; 2-1/2 tablespoons flour.	Low-sodium bread, rolls, crackers; unsalted cooked cereals (farina, hominy grits, oatmeal, rolled wheat, wheat meal); dry cereals (puffed rice, puffed wheat, shredded wheat); plain unsalted matzo; unsalted melba toast; macaroni; noodles; spaghetti; rice; barley; unsalted popcorn; flour. Substitute for a serving of bread or cereal: a starchy vegetable.	Regular breads, crackers; commercial mixes; cooked cereals containing a sodium compound (read label); dry cereal other than those listed or those that have more than 6 mg sodium in 100 gm cereal (read label); self-rising corn meal or flour; potato chips; pretzels; salted popcorn.

TABLE 8-9. Diet Plan for a 500-mg Sodium, 1,800-Kilocalorie Diet* *(Continued)*

Foods and Amounts	Use	Do Not Use
Unsalted Fat 4 servings Each serving contains about 45 calories, practically no sodium. 1 serving: 1 teaspoon butter, margarine, fat, oil, mayonnaise; 1 tbsp heavy cream (sweet or sour); 2 tbsp light cream; 1 tbsp French dressing; 6 small nuts; 1/3 of a 4-inch avocado.	Unsalted butter or margarine; unsalted cooking fat or oil; unsalted French dressing; unsalted mayonnaise; heavy or light cream; unsalted nuts; avocado. Limit cream to 2 tablespoons a day.	Regular butter or margarine; commerical salad dressings or mayonnaise unless low-sodium dietetic; bacon and bacon fat; salt pork; olives; salted nuts; party spreads and dips.
And... Take Your Choice Choose 2—each choice contains about 75 calories, practically no sodium.	Each of these is one choice: 2 servings fruit; 1 serving bread, cereal, or starchy vegetable; 2 servings fat; 4 tbsp sugar, honey, syrup, jelly, jam, marmalade; candy made without salt or other sodium compounds—75 calories worth.	These choices are part of the diet. They are intended to give more freedom in planning the day's meals, but they must be included every day. Choices may be split, if desired. For example, 1 serving fruit and 2 tsp sugar make one choice.
Miscellaneous	Use as desired: regular and instant coffee, tea, coffee substitutes; lemons; limes; plain unflavored gelatin; vinegar; cream of tartar; potassium bicarbonate; sodium-free baking powder; yeast. Almost every seasoning may be used except celery, garlic, onion salt, catsup, chili sauce, prepared mustard, horseradish sauce with salt, barbecue sauces, meat sauce, meat tenderizers, soy sauce, Worcestershire sauce. Do not use celery leaves and flakes, celery seed, olives, pickles, relishes, cooking wine.	Instant coffee treated with a sodium compound as sodium hydroxide. Instant cocoa mixes, including fruit-flavored powders; fountain beverages. Malted milk; soft drinks, regular or low-calorie; any kind of commercial bouillon (cubes, powders, liquids); sodium saccharin; commercial candies; commercial gelatin desserts; regular baking powder; baking soda (sodium bicarbonate); rennet tablets; molasses; pudding mixes; seasonings noted below. See sodium compounds in Table 8-7.

*From *Your 500-Milligram Sodium Diet.* American Heart Association, Dallas, Texas, 1969. Reprinted with permission of the American Heart Association.

Do not use salt, MSG, etc. in cooking or at table.

Become a label reader to spot products that contain sodium. Canned vegetables usually contain sodium, but label may not say so.

If doctor prescribes 250 milligrams of sodium instead of 500, use low-sodium milk (whole or powdered) instead of regular milk.

For low-sodium baking, commercially prepared low-sodium baking powder is available in some stores; also available in some stores may be potassium bicarbonate to use in place of baking soda (sodium bicarbonate).

Consult the American Heart Association's *Sodium-Restricted Diet* Booklets for ways of adding flavor to sodium-restricted diets.

TABLE 8-10. Two Sample Menus for a 500-mg Sodium, 1,800 Kilocalorie Diet*

Breakfast	*Lunch*	*Dinner*
2 medium prunes with 2 tbsp juice 3/4 cup puffed wheat 1 cup milk 1 slice low-sodium toast 1 small pat unsalted butter Coffee or tea, if desired Mid-morning snack: 1/2 cup milk Mid-afternoon snack: 1 small orange Evening snack: 1 small sliced banana with 1/4 cup milk	2 oz broiled liver Baked acorn squash with 1 small pat unsalted butter Cabbage slaw with caraway seeds, green pepper, and vinegar 2 medium low-sodium muffins, 1 small pat unsalted butter Apricot bread pudding made with: 1 slice low-sodium bread, 4 dried apricot halves, 1/4 cup milk, 1 small pat unsalted butter Coffee or tea, if desired	Baked casserole of beef with whipped potato topping made with: 2 oz cooked beef, 1/2 cup broth from beef, 1/2 cup potato Green beans Tomato and cucumber salad on lettuce leaf with 1 tbsp low-sodium French dressing 2 medium low-sodium rolls 1 small pat unsalted butter Fruit gelatin made with: unflavored gelatin, lemon juice, 1/2 cup mixed fruit, artificial sweetener Coffee or tea, if desired
Breakfast	*Lunch*	*Dinner*
1/2 cup grapefruit juice 1 medium egg, scrambled 1/2 cup applesauce 2 slices low-sodium toast 1 small pat unsalted butter Coffee or tea, if desired Mid-morning snack: 1/2 cup milk 5 low-sodium crackers (2") Mid-afternoon snack: 1 small pear Coffee or tea, if desired	2 oz. sliced roast chicken 1/3 cup low-sodium bread dressing 1 tbsp cranberry sauce 1/2 cup cauliflower Lettuce salad 1 medium low-sodium roll 1 small pat unsalted butter 1 cup milk Coffee or tea, if desired Evening snack: 12 grapes Coffee or tea, if desired	Home-made bean soup made with 1/2 cup cooked dried beans 2 oz broiled halibut with lemon 1/2 cup green peas 1 small broiled tomato 1/2 baked sweet potato 1 small low-sodium cornmeal muffin 2 small pats unsalted butter Rice-raisin pudding made with 1/2 cup cooked rice, 2 tbsp raisins, 1/2 cup milk Coffee or tea, if desired

*From *Sodium-Restricted Diet: 500-Milligrams.* Leaflet, The American Heart Association, Dallas, Texas, 1969. Reprinted with permission of the American Heart Association.
Salt or other salt seasonings not allowed at the table or in preparing these foods.
You may eat the between-meal snacks at mealtime if you like.
1 small pat of butter = 1 tsp butter (1 unit).

Activities

If possible, observe patients on sodium-restricted diets at various sodium levels. Follow observations with class discussion on progress of patients.

Renal Disease

WHAT ARE THE FUNCTIONS OF THE KIDNEY AND WHAT ARE THE TYPES OF RENAL DISORDERS?

Kidney Functions. Kidneys act as a selective filter, removing waste materials of metabolism from the blood and other substances (to form urine collected in the bladder and eventually discharged from the body) and retaining other useful materials to be reabsorbed and returned to the circulation.

The filtering unit is the nephron, which contains a tuft of capillaries called the glomerulus surrounded by a membrane or funnel-like capsule which leads to a long winding tubule.

The kidney helps to maintain normal composition and volume of blood, and it maintains water balance and acid-base balance (body neutrality).

WHAT ARE THE CAUSES AND TYPES OF RENAL DISORDERS?

Causes. Renal disorders are caused by anything which alters normal kidney functioning, particularly that of the filtering unit: cysts, infections, and inflammation; cardiovascular disorders; degenerative changes; or renal calculi (kidney stones). The condition may be acute, recurrent or chronic.

Types.

1. *Nephritis* or Bright's disease is a general term to cover kidney disorders of the inflammatory type. Glomerulonephritis (acute or chronic) is a more specific term, as glomeruli are primarily affected following infections.
2. *Nephrosis* (degenerative Bright's disease).
3. *Nephrosclerosis* (arteriosclerotic Bright's disease) is due to vascular disease and hardening of renal arteries occurring in older age groups, with albuminuria and edema.
4. *Renal calculi* (nephrolithiasis or kidney stones) are calcium-, oxalate-, uric acid-, or cystine-containing stones.
5. In *renal failure* the kidney is unable to excrete waste products of metabolism, with resulting uremia.

WHAT ARE THE PRINCIPLES OF DIETARY TREATMENT FOR RENAL DISORDERS?

Calories. Adequate calories are provided, particularly when the diet is restricted in protein, so that body protein will not be used to meet energy need. Calories are restricted in overweight and obesity.

Protein. An adequate amount is provided, as long as kidney functions remain unimpaired. Amounts range from very low (20 gm) to low (40 to 50 gm) to high (100 to 125 gm) depending on the disorder. Protein is increased to meet unusual nutritional needs to make up for albumin loss in urine; restricted to various levels with lessened kidney function and retention of end products of protein metabolism in blood.

Minerals. To combat edema in hypertension, *sodium* is restricted to 500 milligrams. A low-protein diet will also be a restricted-sodium diet, because protein foods are high in sodium.

Potassium is restricted because its excretion lessens with progressive kidney damage and it is retained in the blood of patients with renal failure — usually to the 1.5 gram level. A normal diet may contain as much as 3 to 8 grams because potassium is widely distributed in foods (meats, fruits, whole-grain breads and cereals, and dark-green leafy vegetables). Cooking water and canned fruit and vegetable juices must be discarded because potassium is water soluble. A usual diet order might read: protein, 40 grams; sodium, 500 milligrams; and potassium, 1.5 grams. Diet plans have been formulated for such controlled diets as this, using Food Exchange Lists similar to those used for calculating diabetic diets.

Fluids. Fluids are restricted for patients with kidney failure; a balance must be made between intake and output.

Special Modifications to Prevent Kidney Stone Formation. Sometimes restricted calcium and phosphorus diets are used to prevent calcium stones; acid-ash to prevent calcium and magnesium stones; alkaline-ash to prevent oxalate and uric acid stones; oxalates or oxalic acid in foods to prevent oxalate stones; purines to prevent uric acid stones; and sulfur-containing protein to prevent cystine stones.

Food allowances for diets at low-protein, moderate-protein, and high-protein levels are given in Table 8–11. Sample menus for a very low–protein diet and a very high–protein diet are shown in Table 8–12.

TABLE 8–11. Food Allowances for Low-Protein, Moderate-Protein, and High-Protein Diets*

	20 gram	40 gram	60 gram	110 gram
Breakfast				
Fruit	1 serving	1 serving	1 serving	2 servings
Meat	1 ounce or 1 egg	1 ounce or 1 egg	1 ounce or 1 egg	2 ounces or 2 eggs
Bread or Substitute	1/2 cup cereal	1/2 cup cereal	1/2 cup cereal 1 slice bread	1/2 cup cereal 1 slice bread
Butter or Margarine	as desired	as desired	as desired	as desired
Milk	1/2 cup	1/2 cup	1/2 cup	1 cup
Coffee, tea	as desired	as desired	as desired	as desired
Noon				
Meat	None	1 ounce	2 ounces	3 ounces
Vegetable	1 serving	1 serving	1 serving	1 serving
Fruit	1 serving	2 servings	2 servings	2 servings
Bread or Substitute	1 serving	2 servings	2 servings	3 servings
Butter or other fat	as desired	as desired	as desired	as desired
Milk	None	None	1/2 cup	1 cup
Coffee, tea	as desired	as desired	as desired	as desired
Evening				
Meat	None	1 ounce	2 ounces	4 ounces
Vegetable	1 serving	1 serving	1 serving	2 servings
Bread or Substitute	1 serving	1 serving	1 serving	2 servings
Fruit	1 serving	1 serving	1 serving	1 serving
Milk	None	None	1/2 cup	1 cup
Butter, dressing, etc.	as desired	as desired	as desired	as desired
Coffee, tea	as desired	as desired	as desired	as desired

*Include one citrus fruit daily and one green leafy or deep-yellow vegetable every other day.

REFERENCES

1. *Diet and Coronary Heart Disease, Statement.* American Heart Association, Dallas, Texas, 1978, pp. 1–4. Reprinted with permission of the American Heart Association.
2. *The Way to a Man's Heart.* Centerfold leaflet, American Heart Association, Dallas, Texas, 1972, pp. 4–5. Reprinted with permission of the American Heart Association.
3. *Your 500-Milligram Sodium Diet.* American Heart Association, Dallas, Texas, 1969, p. 8. Reprinted with permission of the American Heart Association.
4. *Sodium Restricted Diet Books.* American Heart Association, Dallas, Texas. Reprinted with permission of the American Heart Association.
5. *Sodium Restricted Diet—500 Milligrams.* Centerfold leaflet, American Heart Association, Dallas, Texas, 1969. Reprinted with permission.

ADDITIONAL REFERENCES

C. H. Robinson and M. R. Lawler, *Normal and Therapeutic Nutrition,* 16th ed. Macmillan Publishing Co., New York, 1982.

MATERIALS AVAILABLE TO THE GENERAL PUBLIC

The American Heart Association, 7320 Greenville Avenue, Dallas, Texas 75231 has prepared and published two booklets on the planning of fat-controlled, low-cholesterol diets (available to patients on doctor's prescription only): (1) *Planning Fat-Controlled Meals for 1200 and 1800 Calories,* and (2) *Planning Fat-Controlled Meals for Approximately 2000 to 2600 Calories.*

TABLE 8-12. Sample Menus for Low-Protein and High-Protein Diets

Very Low-Protein Diet (20 grams)	Very High-Protein Diet (110 grams)
Breakfast	*Breakfast*
Chilled pineapple chunks	Orange juice
Soft-cooked egg with butter	Chilled pineapple chunks
Bran flakes with 1/2 cup milk	Fried eggs, 2
Coffee with cream, sugar	Bran flakes with 1/2 cup milk
	Sugar
Luncheon	Toast, enriched, 1 slice
Mashed potato with butter	1/2 cup milk
Spinach	Coffee with cream, sugar
Tomato juice	
Dinner roll	*Luncheon*
Butter, jelly	Cold sliced turkey, roast beef, cheese, 3 ounces
Fresh pear	Potato salad
Coffee with sugar	Tomato juice
Midafternoon	Roll
Lemonade, 1 cup	Butter
	Fresh strawberries and sliced banana
Dinner	Cupcake
Buttered rice	Milk, 1 cup
Sliced carrots with parsley	Iced tea with lemon and sugar
Grapefruit and date salad	
French dressing	*Dinner*
Biscuit with butter and honey	Baked chicken, 4 ounces
Grape ice	Mashed potato with butter
Tea or coffee with sugar	Sliced carrots with parsley
	French-style green beans
Bedtime	Grapefruit and date salad
Punch, 1 cup	French dressing
	Biscuit with butter and honey
	Baked caramel custard
	Milk, 1 cup
	Tea or coffee if desired

Also available to the general public, no prescription required, are the following leaflets: (1) *The Way to a Man's Heart* — a fat-controlled, low-cholesterol meal plan to reduce the risk of heart attack, 1972; (2) *Diet and Coronary Heart Disease Statement*, 1978; (3) *Eat Well But Wisely — To Reduce Your Risk of Heart Attack;* and (4) *Recipes for Fat-Controlled, Low-Cholesterol Meals.*

Centerfold leaflets, available to patients on a physician's prescription only:
Sodium Restricted Diet—Mild Restriction (1969)
Sodium Restricted Diet—500 Milligrams (1969)
Sodium Restricted Diet—1000 Milligrams (1970)
Booklets:
Your Mild Sodium Restricted Diet (1969)
Your 500 Milligram Sodium Diet (1969)
Your 1000 Milligram Sodium Diet (1970)

9 Diseases of the Gastrointestinal Tract

CHAPTER OUTLINE

DISEASES OF THE ESOPHAGUS
- Achalasia
- Hiatal Hernia
- Dietary Modifications

DISEASES OF THE STOMACH
- Dyspepsia
- Gastritis
- Peptic Ulcer
- Dietary Modifications

DISEASES OF THE INTESTINES
- Diarrhea
- Constipation
- Steatorrhea
- Diverticulosis
- Ulcerative Colitis
- Dietary Modifications

DISEASES OF THE LIVER AND GALLBLADDER
- Hepatitis
- Cirrhosis
- Hepatic Coma
- Cholecystitis
- Cholelithiasis
- Dietary Modifications

OBJECTIVES

To understand
- ☐ The relationship of diet in treatment of diseases of the gastrointestinal tract.
- ☐ How the normal diet is modified for these diseases.

TERMS TO UNDERSTAND

Ascites
Constipation
Detoxify
Diarrhea
Diverticulitis
Diverticulosis
Dyspepsia
Esophageal varices
Fiber
Gastritis
Gluten
Hiatus
Hyperchlorhydria
Hypochlorhydria
Jaundice
Medium-chain triglycerides
Nontropical sprue
Steatorrhea
Ulcerative colitis

Diseases of the Esophagus

REVIEW

The esophagus secretes mucus that provides lubrication for swallowing and allows food to pass from the mouth to the stomach by peristaltic contractions of its muscles.

ACHALASIA

This is a condition in which the lower few centimeters of the esophagus fail to relax and allow food to pass into the stomach. The cause of this disorder is unknown. Dilation of the esophagus with inflatable bags may become necessary. For severe cases surgery may be needed.

Dietary Modifications. A high-protein, high-calorie liquid diet (Table 9–1) is necessary to meet the nutritional requirements until normal swallowing is resumed. If this is not possible, a tube feeding or peripheral parenteral nutrition should be used.

TABLE 9–1. High-Protein, High-Calorie Liquid Diet*

Description

If a patient is to be on a liquid diet for more than a week, the high-protein, high-calorie modification should be ordered. Calories will be increased by approximately 800 and protein by 30 gm when additional liquid items are added to the three meals and interval feedings. For additional calories, butter may be added to hot liquids, powdered glucose may be dissolved in fruit juices, and stick candy may be added to the tray.

For additional protein in the diet, dry milk powder (1-1/4 cups) may be added to 1 quart of milk. Vitamins and iron may be increased by the addition of supplemental formulas or milk-base nourishments.

Approximate Composition of Sample Menu

Calories	3,041
Protein, gm	109
Fat, gm	106
Carbohydrate, gm	225

Sample Menu

Breakfast	*Luncheon*	*Dinner*
1 cup strained orange juice	3/4 cup cream of potato soup	1 cup pineapple juice
1 cup farina with 1/4 cup half-and-half	1 cup grape juice	3/4 cup strained cream of chicken soup (1/2 cup soup with 1/4 cup puréed chicken)
1 cup eggnog	1/2 cup puréed peaches	1/2 cup sherbet
1 cup milk	1/2 cup chocolate custard	3/4 cup chocolate milkshake
2 tsp sugar	1/2 cup vanilla ice cream	1/2 cup flavored gelatin
Coffee or tea with 1 oz half-and-half	1 cup milk	1/2 cup puréed pears
	1 tsp sugar	1 cup milk
	Coffee or tea with 1 oz half-and-half	1 tsp sugar
		Coffee or tea with 1 oz half-and-half
Midmorning Nourishment	*Midafternoon Nourishment*	*Evening Nourishment*
1/2 cup puréed banana	1 cup vanilla-flavored yogurt	1 cup chocolate milk

*University of Iowa Hospitals and Clinic Staff, *Recent Advances in Therapeutic Diets,* 3rd ed. Iowa State University Press, Ames, Iowa, 1979.

HIATAL HERNIA

A hiatal hernia is a protrusion of a part of the stomach through the esophageal hiatus (opening) of the diaphragm. Persons having this disorder sometimes complain of heartburn because of the reflux of gastric contents into the esophagus. Medical treatment includes antacids and sometimes surgery.

Dietary Modifications. Small frequent meals of a normal balanced diet are recommended. Known food intolerances are avoided. Eating at bedtime is discouraged. For the obese person, weight loss is indicated to help relieve pressure on the diaphragm. Sometimes when symptoms are severe, a six-feeding bland diet is used (Table 9–2).

TABLE 9–2. Restricted Bland Diet (Six Feedings)*

Food Groups	Foods Recommended	Foods That May Cause Distress
Milk and milk products (2 or more cups daily)	All milk and milk drinks	None
Vegetables (2 or more servings daily)	All vegetable juices Cooked vegetables as tolerated Salads made from allowed foods	Raw vegetables, dried peas and beans, corn Gas-forming vegetables such as broccoli, Brussels sprouts, cabbage, onions, cauliflower, cucumber, green pepper, rutabagas, turnips, and sauerkraut
Fruits (2 or more servings daily)	All fruit juices Cooked or canned fruit Avocado and banana Grapefruit and orange sections without membrane	All other fresh and dried fruit Berries and figs
Bread and cereals (4 or more servings daily)	Enriched bread and cereals	Very coarse cereals such as bran Seeds in or on breads, rolls and crackers Bread and bread products made with nuts or dried fruit Any fried breads
Potato or substitute	Potatoes Enriched rice, barley, noodles, spaghetti, macaroni, and other pastas	Potato chips, fried potatoes, fried rice, wild rice
Meats or substitutes (6 oz or more daily)	All lean, tender meats, poultry, fish and shellfish Eggs, crisp bacon Mild cheeses Smooth peanut butter Soybean and other meat substitutes	Highly seasoned cured, or smoked meats, poultry, or fish such as corned beef, luncheon meats, frankfurters and other sausages, sardines, anchovies and strong-flavored cheeses Chunky peanut butter
Fats	Butter or fortified margarine Mayonnaise All fats and oils	Salad dressings
Soups	Mildly seasoned meat stock and creamed soups made with allowed foods	All other soups

TABLE 9–2. Restricted Bland Diet (Six Feedings)* *(Continued)*

Food Groups	Foods Recommended	Foods That May Cause Distress
Sweets and desserts	Sugar, syrup, honey, jelly, seedless jam, hard candies, plain chocolate candies, molasses, marshmallows Cakes, cookies, pies, puddings, custard, ice cream, sherbet and jello made from allowed foods	All sweets and desserts containing nuts, coconut, or fruit not allowed Fried pastries such as doughnuts
Beverages	Decaffeinated coffee, fruit drinks, caffeine-free carbonated beverages	Coffee, tea, alcohol, cocoa, all carbonated beverages with caffeine
Miscellaneous	Iodized salt, flavorings Mildly flavored gravies and sauces Mild herbs and spices	Strongly flavored seasonings and condiments such as catsup, pepper, barbeque sauce, chili sauce, chili pepper, horseradish, garlic, mustard, and vinegar Olives, pickles, popcorn, nuts, and coconut

Sample Menu†

Breakfast	*Lunch*	*Dinner*
1/2 cup orange juice	2 oz beef patty	2 oz broiled chicken
1 poached egg or egg substitute	1/2 cup rice	1/2 cup mashed potatoes
1 slice toast	1/2 cup spinach	1/2 cup peas
1 tsp butter or margarine	1 slice bread	1 tsp butter or margarine
1 cup decaffeinated coffee	2 tsp butter or margarine	1 cup decaffeinated coffee
1 oz cream or nondairy creamer	4 oz milk (whole or low fat)	1 oz cream or nondairy creamer
2 tsp sugar		2 tsp sugar
Midmorning Snack	*Midafternoon Snack*	*Bedtime Snack*
1/2 cup oatmeal	6 oz vegetable soup	1/2 cup cottage cheese
8 oz milk (whole or low fat)	1/2 cup sherbet	1/2 cup apricots
2 tsp sugar	2 sugar cookies	2 saltine crackers
1/2 cup peaches	1 cup decaffeinated coffee	4 oz milk (whole or low fat)
	1 oz cream or nondairy creamer	

*The restricted bland diet is designed to decrease peristalsis and avoid irritation of the gastrointestinal tract.

From Chicago Dietetic Association and South Suburban Dietetic Association of Cook and Wills Counties, *Manual of Clinical Dietetics,* 2nd ed. W. B. Saunders Co., Philadelphia, 1981, pp. 57–60.

†Approximate composition of sample menu: Calories, 2,265; Protein, 96 gm; Fat 85 gm; Carbohydrate, 280 gm.

Diseases of the Stomach

REVIEW

The *chemical functions* of the stomach are to (1) secrete gastric juice, which contains hydrochloric acid (HCl), protein-splitting enzyme, a small amount of fat-splitting enzyme, and "intrinsic factor" to aid in the absorption of vitamin B_{12}; (2) to begin the digestion of protein; and (3) to digest emulsified fats.

The *physical function* of the stomach is peristalsis, a process of contraction and relaxation of the muscular stomach wall. Peristalsis (1) mixes food with digestive juices, and (2) passes food into the intestine for further digestion and absorption.

HOW ARE GASTRIC DISORDERS CLASSIFIED?

Organic disorders result from a change in structural tissue. Examples are pathological lesions, peptic ulcer, and carcinoma.

Functional disorders (reflex disorders) involve a change in body functions without detectable changes in structural tissue. Examples are dyspepsia (indigestion), gastritis, hyperchlorhydria, and hypochlorhydria.

DYSPEPSIA

This disorder is commonly referred to as indigestion. It is discomfort experienced after eating. It may be caused by emotional upset, overeating, or a physical impairment of the gastrointestinal tract. If dyspepsia is prolonged, tests should be performed to determine if the gastrointestinal tract is properly functioning.

Dietary Modifications. Emphasis is placed on the consumption of regular balanced meals to correct faulty eating habits. Foods known to cause distress are omitted from the diet. Other modifications will depend on the results of tests.

GASTRITIS

Gastritis is an inflammation of the lining resulting in abdominal pain, nausea, and vomiting. It may be caused by food poisoning, overeating, excessive intake of alcohol, or bacterial or viral infections. A chronic condition may be related to other disease states. It often precedes the development of ulcers or cancer.

Dietary Modifications. A six-feeding bland diet may be used when symptoms occur (see Table 9–2).

PEPTIC ULCER

A peptic ulcer is an eroded lesion in the lining (mucosa) of the stomach or duodenum. Many factors are thought to contribute to its development, including irregular and hurried eating, excessive smoking, excessive aspirin ingestion, emotional stress, and heredity. Although the actual cause of peptic ulcers is not known, possible causes include hypersecretion of hydrochloric acid, hyperactivity of stomach contents passing into the duodenum, and reflux of bile acid into the stomach from the duodenum.[1] Treatment includes rest and one or more of the following drugs: antacids (to neutralize acid), anticholinergic agents (to reduce acid secretion), and antispasmodics (to reduce gastric motility).

Dietary Modifications: Traditional vs. Liberal Approach. Much controversy exists regarding which foods help to decrease secretions of stomach acid. The traditional approach has been to give hourly feedings of milk to reduce stomach acid. "Hourly feedings of milk have been shown to produce a lower pH than regular meals."[2] However, although milk initially acts as a buffer, as it becomes partially digested it is a very potent stimulant of gastric acid.

It has not yet been determined what foods are mechanically, chemically, or thermally irritating or soothing to the gastric lining.[1] Many of the foods traditionally omitted from the diet of a person with peptic ulcers were not proved to be culprits. Many clinicians now tend to adopt a more liberal

TABLE 9-3. Liberal Bland Diet

Guideline	Rationale
Eat 3 regular meals or 6 small meals	Avoids stomach distention
Avoid caffeine-containing beverages, decaffeinated coffee[4]	Stimulates gastric secretions
Avoid alcohol	Damages stomach lining
Avoid black pepper, chili powder, cloves, nutmeg, mustard seed[5]	Irritates stomach lining
Avoid aspirin	Irritates stomach lining
Avoid cigarette smoking	Delays healing of ulcer
Eat in a relaxed atmosphere	Reduces stress

Sample Menu

Breakfast	*Lunch*	*Dinner*
Poached egg	Celery and carrot sticks	Tossed salad with blue cheese dressing
Whole-wheat toast	Macaroni and cheese casserole	Baked chicken
Orange juice	Green beans	Sliced carrots
Milk	Fresh peach	Bread and butter
	Milk	Milk
Midmorning Snack	*Midafternoon Snack*	*Evening Snack*
Fresh apple slices	Graham crackers	Cheese and wheat crackers
	Milk	

approach to ulcer disease, since the bland diet has no significant effect on the healing of ulcers.[3]

While an ulcer is bleeding, no food is allowed; instead intravenous feedings of dextrose and amino acids may be given. As the condition improves the patient usually progresses from a full liquid diet to a liberal bland diet (Table 9-3).

Diseases of the Intestines

REVIEW

The *small intestine* (1) receives food from the stomach for completion of digestion, (2) completes digestion of food with the aid of enzymes from pancreatic and intestinal juices (bile aids fat digestion), (3) propels the food mass along the intestinal tract by peristaltic action, and (4) absorbs the end products of digestion in its lower portion.

The *large intestine* (1) absorbs water and salt, (2) forms feces, and (3) propels waste products by peristalsis to the colon for excretion as feces.

DIARRHEA

This intestinal disturbance is the passage of frequent stools of liquid consistency. It may be either acute, lasting 24 to 48 hours, or chronic, lasting two weeks or longer. When this condition is acute, the nutritional losses are easily replaced as food and fluid intake returns to normal. Chronic diarrhea results in more serious nutritional losses. The absorption of fluids, electrolytes, and nutrients may be impaired because of their rapid transition through the gastrointestinal tract.

Dietary Modifications. If diarrhea is severe, no food is given for up to 48 hours. This will give the intestinal tract a chance to rest. Intravenous solutions of dextrose, amino acids, and electrolytes (and vitamins) will help replace fluids and electrolytes and provide some nutrients. Clear liquid or an elemental diet may be given after this time. Once diarrhea has diminished, there is progression to a diet that is restricted in residue and high in protein, calories, nutrients, and fluids. A restricted-residue diet (Table 9–4) is gradually replaced by the return to a regular normal diet as soon as the patient is able to tolerate it.

TABLE 9–4. Diets Varying in Residue*

Foods	Residue-Restricted Diet	Moderate-Residue Diet	Minimal-Residue Diet
Milk†	Milk, buttermilk, yogurt, cream	Same	Same
Cheese	Cottage, cream,† Cheddar	Same	Cottage, cream only†
Fat	Butter, margarine	Same	Same
Eggs	Cooked, poached, scrambled in double boiler	Same	Same
Meat, fish, fowl	Tender chicken, fish, sweetbreads, ground beef, and lamb	Same	Ground, tender meat; minced chicken and fish
Soups and broths	Broth, strained meat-based soups	Same	Broth only
Vegetables	Cooked vegetables, asparagus, peas, string beans, spinach, carrots, beets, squash, potatoes—boiled, mashed, baked	Vegetable juice; vegetable purée, cooked asparagus tips, carrots, potatoes—boiled, mashed, baked	Unseasoned vegetable juices in limited amounts†
Fruits	Fruit juices, cooked and canned fruits (without skins, seeds or fiber), bananas	Fruit juice, fruit purée, ripe bananas, cooked, peeled apples, apricots, peaches, pears, plums	Fruit juices, preferably citrus, in limited amounts†
Bread, cereals	Refined, enriched bread and cereals; macaroni, spaghetti, noodles, rice, crackers	Refined, enriched bread and cereals only; macaroni, spaghetti, noodles, rice, white crackers	As in moderately low residue
Desserts	Ices, ice cream,† junket,† cereal puddings,† custard,† gelatin, plain cake, and cookies; all without fruit and nuts	Same	Same
Beverages	Tea, coffee, carbonated beverages	Same	Tea, coffee as permitted
Condiments	Salt, moderate amounts of pepper, other mild spices, sugar	Salt and sugar	Salt and sugar

*From L. Anderson, et al., *Nutrition in Health and Disease,* 17th ed. J. B. Lippincott Co., Philadelphia, 1982, p. 448.
†If tolerated.

CONSTIPATION

Constipation is the retention of the feces in the colon beyond normal emptying time.

Atonic. This type of constipation is characterized by the loss of rectal sensibility and weak peristaltic waves. It commonly occurs in elderly or obese persons, pregnant women, and postoperative patients. Factors contributing to its occurrence include a refined food diet, irregular meals, poor fluid intake, lack of exercise, and prolonged use of cathartics.

Spastic. Spastic constipation (also known as *irritable bowel syndrome*, *spastic colitis*, and *mucous colitis*) is characterized by irregular contractions of the bowel resulting in either diarrhea or constipation. Factors contributing to its occurrence include excessive use of laxatives or cathartics, irregular eating habits, antibiotic therapy, and nervous tension.

Dietary Modifications. A high-fiber diet (Table 9–5) is used in the treatment of constipation, since it allows the feces to be easily expelled. Figure 9–1 shows how this is accomplished. When diarrhea occurs during spastic constipation, a minimal-residue diet (see Table 9–4) may be used.[6]

STEATORRHEA

Steatorrhea is diarrhea characterized by excess fat in stools. It usually indicates a more serious underlying organic disease. It may be seen in pancreatitis or following gastric or intestinal resection. It may be associated with diseases of the liver or gallbladder, or with malabsorptive diseases such as nontropical sprue or regional enteritis. It sometimes occurs after gastrointestinal radiation. All of these disorders may involve problems with fat digestion or absorption.[1]

Dietary Modifications. The treatment of steatorrhea involves the use of medium-chain triglycerides (MCT), which are fats that contain 8 to 10 carbon atoms versus 12 to 18 carbon atoms for long-chain triglycerides (LCT). They are used in the treatment of steatorrhea because they are more easily digested, absorbed, and transported than LCT. They also help reduce fecal losses of water, electrolytes, and nutrients.

When planning the diet, the emphasis is on low-fat foods to decrease the amount of LCT in the diet. Over half of the allowed fat calories is in the form of MCT. This can be accomplished with the use of commercially available products. The two principal forms of MCT are

Portagen* — a powdered formula which can be mixed and served as a supplement to meals.

MCT oil* — can replace vegetable oil in recipes.

DIVERTICULOSIS

This is the formation of outpockets of small mucosal sacs (diverticula) protruding through the wall of the intestines. They are found mainly in the sigmoid colon. Low-fiber diets favor the formation of diverticulosis because intraluminal pressure is exerted against the colon wall instead of longitudinally, resulting in pouches.

---

*Available from Mead Johnson and Co., Evansville, Indiana.

TABLE 9–5. High-Fiber Diet*

Characteristics

This diet is essentially a regular diet with fiber content increased as follows:

1. Substitute at least 4 servings whole-grain bread and cereals for refined breads and cereals.
2. Emphasize raw fruits and vegetables that are high in fiber.
3. Add 1 to 2 tablespoons bran each day.

The substitution of fibrous foods should be made gradually; for example, whole-grain breads and cereals are added first, then fibrous cooked fruits and vegetables, followed by raw fruits and vegetables.

Foods Allowed

Beverages—all
Breads—breads, muffins, or rolls made from 100 per cent whole-wheat or whole-rye flour; graham, wheat, or rye crackers; Ry-Krisp
Cereals—whole-grain such as oatmeal, rolled oats; bran flakes, granola; Grape Nuts; Shredded Wheat, wheat flakes; brown rice; bran, in moderation
Cheese—all
Desserts—all, with fruit and nuts, if tolerated
Eggs—all
Fats—all
Fruits—all, including dried; preferably raw
Meats—all
Soups—all, preferably vegetable
Sweets—jam, marmalade, preserves
Vegetables—all, especially raw; potatoes in skin
Miscellaneous—condiments and seasonings in moderation

Sample Menu

Breakfast	*Luncheon*	*Dinner*	*Bedtime Snack*
Orange sections	Vegetable soup	Brown beef stew	Milk
Oatmeal with milk and brown sugar	Club sandwich:	Onions	Fresh pear
Poached egg	Sliced turkey	Carrots	Graham crackers
Bran muffins	Bacon	Oven-browned potato	
Butter or margarine	Whole-wheat bread	Coleslaw with pineapple	
Marmalade	Lettuce and tomato	Rye bread	
Coffee	Mayonnaise	Butter or margarine	
	Baked apple with raisin stuffing	Apricot fruit crisp	
	Milk	Tea with lemon and sugar	

*Reprinted with permission of Macmillan Publishing Co., Inc., from C. H. Robinson and M. R. Lawler, *Normal and Therapeutic Nutrition*, 16th ed. Copyright 1982 by Macmillan Publishing Co., Inc.

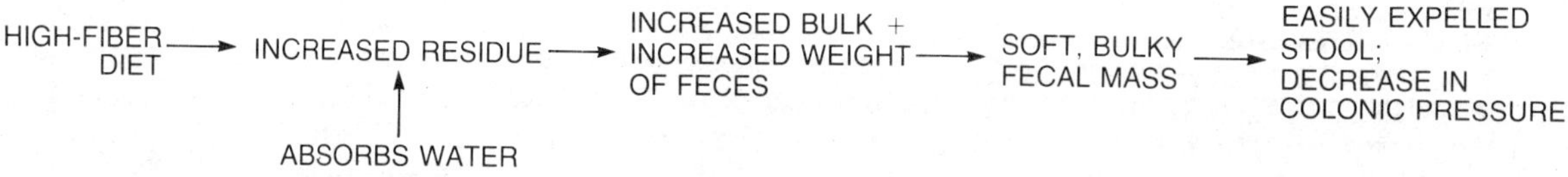

Figure 9–1. How a high-fiber diet helps correct and prevent constipation.

Dietary Modifications. The high-fiber diet (Table 9–5) is used, with omission of skins, seeds, or nuts, since they may get caught in diverticula.

DIVERTICULITIS

Diverticulitis is an inflammation of diverticula, usually resulting from food particles or materials being caught in the outpockets and attracting bacteria. Symptoms include abdominal pain, usually in the lower left quadrant, and occasionally fever.

Dietary Modifications. During the acute phase, a clear liquid diet is given and there is a progression to a restricted-residue diet (Table 9–4). Once the symptoms have disappeared, there is gradual progression to a high-fiber diet without skins, seeds, or nuts (Table 9–5).

ULCERATIVE COLITIS

Ulcerative colitis is a chronic disease characterized by inflammation and ulceration of the mucosa of large intestines. The cause of this disease is unknown. Symptoms include rectal bleeding, diarrhea, fever, anorexia, dehydration, and weight loss. Emotional upsets aggravate the condition.

Dietary Modifications. When symptoms are evident, a tube feeding of an elemental diet, peripheral parenteral nutrition (PPN), or total parenteral nutrition (TPN) may be necessary. These forms of nutritional support will provide necessary nutrients without aggravating the condition. Once solid foods are tolerated, the patient progresses to a restricted-residue diet (Table 9–4) that is high in calories, protein, vitamins, and minerals to replace nutritional losses and provide for tissue repair. Individualizing the diet to a patient's specific food tolerances is necessary to give optimal nutritional care. Vitamin and mineral supplements may be indicated to provide additional nutritional support.

GLUTEN-INDUCED ENTEROPATHY

This malabsorptive disorder is also known as nontropical sprue in adults and celiac disease in children. It is characterized by an inability to digest gluten-containing foods. Gluten is the protein portion of wheat, oats, rye, and barley. The exact cause of this disease is unknown. Symptoms include diarrhea, steatorrhea, and weight loss. If it is untreated, vitamin and mineral deficiencies will become apparent.

Dietary Modifications. A gluten-restricted diet is given, in which all products containing gluten are eliminated (Table 9–6). Once this has been accomplished, the patient's condition improves drastically. Diet counseling must include foods allowed, label reading for even small amounts of gluten in various foods, and recipes using other flours (e.g., rice, corn, and potato).

TABLE 9–6. Gluten-Restricted Diet*

Description

Wheat, rye, oats, barley, and products containing these grains are omitted from the diet in order to substantially reduce gluten intake. Corn, rice, and products made from them may be used as substitutes. Other substitutes include wheat starch; tapioca; and soybean, buckwheat, arrowroot, and potato flours.

This diet is used in the treatment of gluten-induced enteropathy. Many celiac patients may have other malabsorption problems. Therefore, the diet should contain optimal calories, protein, vitamins, and minerals. Initially, some persons may require a lactose restriction until symptoms are resolved.

NOTE: Because many processed foods contain wheat, rye, oats, barley, or flours from these grains, *labels should be read carefully.*

Approximate Composition of Sample Menu

Calories	2,313
Protein, gm	93
Fat, gm	95
Carbohydrate, gm	271

Foods Allowed and Foods to Avoid

Food Group	*Foods Allowed*	*Foods to Avoid*
Beverages	Milk, carbonated beverages, coffee, tea, decaffeinated coffee, fruit-flavored beverages	Cereal beverages; malted milk; ale; beer; beverages containing wheat, rye, oats, barley, or malt
Breads	Breads made from cornmeal; gluten-free wheat starch; corn, potato, rice, soybean, tapioca, arrowroot, and buckwheat flours	All bread and crackers containing wheat, rye, oats, or barley
Cereals	Cornmeal, rice, precooked rice cereal, dry cereals containing only rice or corn	All cooked and prepared cereals containing wheat, rye, oats, barley, or malt
Desserts	Custard; gelatin desserts; fruit ice; pudding made with cornstarch, gluten-free wheat starch, rice, or tapioca; ice cream and sherbet; cakes, cookies and other desserts made with allowed flours or starches	Cakes, cookies, pastries, or commercial pudding mixes containing restricted flours; ice cream cones; fruit sauces thickened with wheat flour; commercial ice cream or sherbet containing a wheat stabilizer
Eggs	Baked, poached, soft or hard cooked, scrambled, fried	Creamed eggs, soufflé, or fondue unless made with allowed flours
Fats	Butter, margarine, cream, vegetable oils and shortenings, lard, bacon, salad dressings thickened with allowed flours or starches	Salad dressings or gravies containing wheat, rye, oats, or barley
Fruits, fruit juices	All fresh, frozen, canned, and dried	None
Meat, fish, poultry, cheese	Baked, broiled, roasted, or steamed beef, lamb, liver, pork, veal; poultry; fish; cottage, cream, and nonprocessed cheeses	Meat, fish, poultry, or cheese products containing restricted cereals (the following foods frequently contain these cereals: meatloaf; meat patties; breaded meat, fish, or poultry; canned meat products; cold cuts unless guaranteed all meat; cheese spreads)
Potatoes or substitutes	White and sweet potatoes, rice, hominy, potato chips	Creamed or scalloped potatoes unless made with allowed flours, macaroni, noodles, spaghetti
Soups	Broth-base and cream soups made from allowed foods	Soups containing wheat, rye, oats, barley, or products made from these grains; soups thickened with wheat flour

TABLE 9–6. Gluten-Restricted Diet* *(Continued)*

Food Group	*Foods Allowed*	*Foods to Avoid*
Sugar, sweets	Sugar, syrup, honey, jelly, jam, molasses, candy, chocolate, chewing gum	Commercial candies containing wheat, rye, oats, barley, or malt
Vegetables, vegetable juices	All fresh, frozen, and canned	None
Miscellaneous	Salt (iodized), flavorings, spices, vinegar, peanut butter, coconut, popcorn, olives, pickles, catsup, mustard, chocolate, cocoa powder, gravy or cream sauce if thickened with allowed flours or starches	Pretzels

Sample Menu

Breakfast	*Luncheon*	*Dinner*
1/2 cup frozen orange juice	2 oz sliced chicken	3 oz roast beef sirloin
1/2 cup Cream of Rice cereal	1/2 cup rice	1/2 cup cubed white potato
1 egg, soft cooked	1/2 cup green beans	1/2 cup cooked carrots
1 cornmeal muffin	1/2 sliced tomato on lettuce	3/4 cup tossed lettuce salad
1 tsp butter	2 tsp mayonnaise	1 tbsp French dressing
1 tbsp grape jelly	1 slice low-protein bread	1 rice muffin
1 cup milk	1 tsp butter	2 tsp butter
2 tsp sugar	1/2 cup canned peaches	1/2 cup sherbet
Coffee or tea	1 puffed rice bar	1 cup milk
	1 cup milk	1 tsp sugar
	1 tsp sugar	Coffee or tea
	Coffee or tea	

*University of Iowa Hospitals and Clinic Staff, *Recent Advances in Therapeutic Diets,* 3rd ed. Iowa State University Press, Ames, Iowa, 1979.

Diseases of the Liver and Gallbladder

REVIEW

The liver (1) produces bile, which aids in the digestion and absorption of fat; (2) aids in the metabolism of carbohydrates, proteins, and fats; (3) stores vitamins A and D; (4) stores glycogen and releases it when needed to maintain normal blood sugar levels; (5) detoxifies harmful substances; and (6) synthesizes numerous body substances.

HEPATITIS

Hepatitis is inflammation and injury to liver cells caused by infections, drugs, or toxins. Symptoms include anorexia, fatigue, nausea, vomiting, fever, diarrhea, and weight loss.

Dietary Modifications. The symptoms during the early stage of hepatitis make it difficult for the patient to consume adequate nutrients. Peripheral parenteral nutritional support or tube feedings may be indicated until oral intake of food is tolerated. Once oral intake is resumed, a diet high in calories, protein, vitamins, and minerals with moderate fat is planned for the patient. Several small meals are usually better tolerated than three larger ones. See Table 9–7 for the diet in greater detail.

CIRRHOSIS

This is a chronic liver disease in which normal liver tissue is replaced by inactive fibrous tissue. Because liver tissue is not able to function normally, there may be jaundice, prolonged bleeding time, fatty infiltration of liver tissue, lower serum albumin levels, and other complications, depending on the severity of tissue function impairment. Symptoms sometimes include nausea, vomiting, anorexia, ascites (accumulation of fluid in the abdomen), and esophageal varices (enlargement of the veins in the esophagus because of poor portal blood circulation).

Dietary Modifications. If there are no complications, a diet adequate in all nutrients is sufficient. For the patient whose nutritional status is poor, a diet high in calories, protein, and carbohydrate is recommended. The diet outlines for hepatitis (Table 9–7) can be used. Vitamin and mineral supplements are indicated. If there is ascites, sodium should be restricted. If liver impairment is more severe, protein may have to be restricted (35 to 50 gm/day).[7]

TABLE 9–7. High-Protein, Moderate-Fat, High-Carbohydrate Diet*

Characteristics and General Rules

The caloric level may be increased by adding high-carbohydrate foods. Small amounts of cream and ice cream may be used when tolerated.

The protein intake may be increased by adding nonfat dry milk to liquid milk.

Modifications in fiber and consistency may be made by applying restrictions concerning the soft diet to the foods listed here.

Six or more small feedings may be preferred when there is lack of appetite.

When sodium restriction is ordered, all food must be prepared without salt. Low-sodium milk should replace part of all of the prescribed milk.

Include These Foods Daily

1 quart of milk
8 ounces lean meat, poultry, or fish
1 egg
4 servings vegetables, including:
  2 servings potato or substitute
  1 serving green leafy or yellow vegetable
  1–2 servings other vegetable
  One vegetable to be raw each day
3 servings fruit including:
  1 serving citrus fruit or other good source of ascorbic acid
  2 servings other fruit
1 serving enriched or whole-grain cereal
6 slices enriched or whole-grain bread
2 tablespoons butter or margarine
4 tablespoons sugar, jelly, marmalade, or jam
Additional foods to further increase the carbohydrate as the patient is able to take them.

Nutritive Value of Basic Pattern: Protein, 135 gm; fat, 106 gm; carbohydrate, 236 gm; calories, 2,590; calcium, 2.53 gm; iron, 18.3 mg; vitamin A, 18,770 I.U.; thiamine, 2.11 mg; riboflavin, 3.39 mg; niacin, 27.6 mg; ascorbic acid, 159 mg.

Typical Food Selection

Beverages—carbonated beverages, milk and milk drinks, coffee, tea, fruit juices, cocoa flavoring

TABLE 9–7. High-Protein, Moderate-Fat, High-Carbohydrate Diet* *(Continued)*

Typical Food Selection

Breads and cereals—all kinds
Cheese—cottage, cream, mild Cheddar
Desserts—angel cake, plain cake and cookies, custard, plain or fruit gelatin, fruit whip, fruit pudding, Junket, milk and cereal desserts, sherbets, ices, plain ice cream
Eggs—any way
Fat—butter, margarine, cream, cooking fat, vegetable oils
Fruits—all
Meat—lean beef, chicken, fish, lamb, liver, pork, turkey
Potato or substitute—hominy, macaroni, noodles, rice, spaghetti, sweet potato
Seasonings—salt, spices, vinegar (in moderation)
Soups—clear and cream
Sweets—honey, jam, jelly, sugar, sugar candy, syrups
Vegetables—all

Foods to Avoid

No foods are specifically contraindicated. Many patients complain of intolerance to the following groups of foods: strongly flavored vegetables; rich desserts; fried and fatty foods; chocolate; nuts; and highly seasoned foods. Although such complaints cannot always be explained on a physiologic basis, nothing is gained by giving the offending foods to the patient.

Meal Pattern	Sample Menu
Breakfast	
Fruit	1/2 grapefruit
Cereal with milk and sugar	Wheatena with milk and sugar
Egg	Scrambled egg
Whole-grain or enriched toast—2 slices	Whole-wheat toast
Butter or margarine—2 teaspoons	Margarine
Marmalade—1 tablespoon	Orange marmalade
Beverage with cream and sugar	Coffee with cream and sugar
Luncheon or Supper	
Lean meat, fish or poultry—4 ounces	Broiled whitefish
Potato or substitute	Escalloped potatoes
Cooked vegetable	Asparagus with margarine
Salad	Celery and carrot strips
Whole-grain or enriched bread—2 slices	Whole-wheat bread
Butter or margarine—2 teaspoons	Margarine
Jelly—1 tablespoon	Grape jelly
Fruit	Sliced banana
Milk	Milk
Midafternoon	
Milk with nonfat dry milk	High-protein milk with strawberry flavor
Dinner	
Lean meat, fish, or fowl—4 ounces	Roast beef
Potato	Mashed potato
Vegetable	Baked acorn squash
Whole-grain or enriched bread—2 slices	Dinner rolls
Butter or margarine—2 teaspoons	Margarine
Jelly—1 tablespoon	Apple jelly
Fruit or dessert	Raspberry sherbet
Milk—1 glass	Milk
Tea, if desired	
Evening Nourishment	
Milk beverage	High-protein milk flavored with caramel
	Bread and jelly sandwich

*Reprinted with permission of Macmillan Publishing Co., Inc., from C. H. Robinson and M. R. Lawler, *Normal and Therapeutic Nutrition*, 16th ed. Copyright 1982 by Macmillan Publishing Co., Inc.

HEPATIC COMA

When liver function becomes severely impaired, ammonia levels become abnormally high and become toxic to brain tissue. The unconsciousness that may result is known as hepatic coma. Contributing factors include gastrointestinal bleeding, excessive dietary protein, severe infection, or surgical procedures. Symptoms include confusion, irritability, delirium, and flapping tremors of the hands and feet.

Dietary Modifications. The aim of this diet is to decrease the amount of ammonia that enters the general circulation. Antibiotics are administered to decrease the ammonia production from intestinal bacteria. Protein in the diet is restricted from 0 to 20 grams (Table 9–8; see also Tables 8–11 and 8–12), depending on the severity of the condition. It is gradually increased in increments of 10 to 15 grams as liver function improves. Supplements of branched chain amino acids may be used (Hepatic-Aid). Calories must be kept high to prevent tissue breakdown. Carbohydrate and fat calories are emphasized. Sodium is restricted if ascites or edema is present. Additional vitamin and mineral supplements should be given.

REVIEW

The gallbladder (1) concentrates and stores bile, (2) releases bile triggered by hormonal stimulation from the presence of fat in the intestines, and (3) aids the digestion and absorption of fat and fat-soluble vitamins through the action of bile.

CHOLECYSTITIS

Cholecystitis is an inflammation of the gallbladder. It can be caused by a bacterial infection or stones in the gallbladder. Symptoms include pain in the upper right quadrant, nausea, vomiting, fever, and jaundice if the bile duct is blocked.

TABLE 9–8. Suggested Menu for 20-Gram Protein Diet*

Breakfast	*Dinner*	*Supper*
1/2 cup cranberry juice	1 egg, scrambled	Pineapple slice and peach half on lettuce
1/2 cup Cream of Wheat cereal	1/2 cup rice	2 slices bread, low protein
2 slices bread, low protein	1/2 cup cooked carrots	1/2 cup green beans
2 teaspoons butter	6 slices cucumber on 1 leaf lettuce	2 teaspoons butter
2 teaspoons honey	2 slices bread, low protein	1 low-protein cookie
1/4 cup whole milk	2 teaspoons butter	1 high-fat, low-protein popsicle
2 teaspoons sugar	1/2 cup sweetened canned pears	1 teaspoon sugar
3/4 cup coffee	1 teaspoon sugar	1/2 cup whole milk
	1 cup Kool-Aid	

*From P. Howe, *Basic Nutrition in Health and Disease,* 7th ed. W. B. Saunders Co., Philadelphia, 1981, p. 533.

CHOLELITHIASIS

Cholelithiasis is the formation of gallstones. Sometimes they will block the bile duct and interfere with the flow of bile. Symptoms include pain in the upper right quadrant as the gallbladder contracts, and jaundice if the bile duct is obstructed.

Dietary Modifications. During an acute attack of cholecystitis or cholelithiasis, food may be withheld for up to 24 hours. Food is gradually introduced, starting with a clear liquid diet. As food tolerance improves there is progression to a minimum-fat diet (Table 9–9) that contains approximately 30 grams of fat. As the patient's condition improves there is progression to a low-fat diet (Table 9–9) containing approximately 50 grams of fat. If surgical removal of the gallbladder or gallstones is necessary, the patient should follow a low-fat diet until surgery is performed.

After surgery, a low-fat diet should be followed for several weeks until fat digestion is normalized by bodily adjustment of bile storage to the large common duct connecting the liver and small intestine.[1] Thereafter, a normal diet is usually well tolerated.

TABLE 9–9. Low-Fat Diet: 50 Grams*

Foods Limited

Milk, skim milk: 2 cups (1 pt) daily.
Eggs: 1 poached, hard- or soft-cooked, daily.
Meats, fish or poultry: 3 oz of meat, fish, or poultry, lean and free from all visible fat and from skin of chicken, daily.
Fats: 2 pats (4 level tsp) butter, fortified margarine or oil daily.

Foods Included

Cheese: Pot cheese or uncreamed cottage cheese.
Breads: Whole-grain or enriched white preferred.
Cereals: Whole-grain preferred, except the very coarse varieties.
Cereal products: Macaroni, spaghetti, noodles, rice.
Vegetables: As tolerated (to include 1 serving green leafy or yellow vegetable daily).
Fruits: As tolerated (to include at least 1 serving citrus fruit daily). Fruit juices.
Soups: Clear soups with fat removed or soups made with skim milk.
Desserts: Angel food cake, gelatin desserts with fruits as tolerated, sherbets, and ices.
Beverages: Tea, coffee, Postum, carbonated beverages.
Sweets: Sugar, jelly, honey, hard candy, and syrup.

Foods Omitted

Meats, fish or poultry: Fat of meat, skin of chicken, bacon, scrapple, cold cuts, sausages, fatty fish (mackerel), duck, goose, fish canned in oil.
Fats: All fat except allowed butter or fortified margarine and oil.
Desserts: Except those included.
Miscellaneous: Chocolate, peanut butter, cream, nuts, pastries, fried foods, highly seasoned foods, pickled foods and pickles, rich gravies and cream sauces.

*For a minimum-fat diet, of 30 grams, omit all fats.

From M. Krause, and K. Mahan, *Food, Nutrition and Diet Therapy,* 6th ed. W. B. Saunders Co., Philadelphia, 1979, pp. 514 and 515.

Study Questions and Activities

1. How do high-fiber diets help prevent constipation and diverticulosis?
2. Why are both high- and low-protein diets used to treat liver disease?
3. Why is a low-fat diet used to treat gallbladder disease?
4. Plan a gluten-restricted menu for one day.
5. Why is a more liberal approach to peptic ulcer disease now being used?

REFERENCES

1. M. V. Krause and L. K. Mahan, *Food, Nutrition and Diet Therapy*, 6th ed. W. B. Saunders Co., Philadelphia, 1979.
2. Chicago Dietetic Association and South Suburban Dietetic Association of Cook and Wills Counties, *Manual of Clinical Dietetics*, 2nd ed. W. B. Saunders Co., Philadelphia, 1981, p. 56.
3. American Dietetic Association, "Position Paper on Bland Diet in the Treatment of Chronic Duodenal Ulcer Disease," *Journal of the American Dietetics Association.* Vol. 59, No. 3, 1971, p. 244.
4. E. J. Feldman, J. I. Isenberg, and M. J. Grossman, "Gastric Acid and Gastric Response to Decaffeinated Coffee and a Peptone Meal," *Journal of the American Medical Association,* Vol. 246, 1981, p. 248.
5. M. A. Schmeider, et al., "The Effect of Spice Ingestion Upon the Stomach," *American Journal of Gastroenterology,* Vol. 26, 1956, pp. 722–732.
6. C. H. Robinson and M. R. Lawler, *Normal and Therapeutic Nutrition,* 16th ed. Macmillan Publishing Co., Inc., New York, 1982, p. 538.
7. G. J. Gabuzda and L. Shear, "Metabolism of Dietary Protein in Hepatic Cirrhosis. Nutritional and Clinical Considerations," *American Journal of Clinical Nutrition,* Vol. 23, 1970, pp. 479–487.

ADDITIONAL REFERENCES

"Eating and Ulcers," (Editorial) *British Medical Journal,* Vol. 280, No. 1, 1980, pp. 205–206.

"'Heartburn' and 'Indigestion,'" *Nutrition and the M.D.,* Vol. 8, No. 4, 1982, p. 1.

J. I. Isenberg, "Peptic Ulcer: Epidemiology, Nutritional Aspects, Drugs, Smoking, Alcohol and Diet," *Current Concepts in Nutrition,* Vol. 9, 1980, pp. 141–151.

R. A. Levine, "An Overview of Fiber and Gastrointestinal Disease," in R. C. Kurtz, ed., *Contemporary Issues in Clinical Nutrition,* Vol. 1. Churchill Livingstone Inc., New York, 1981, p. 1.

G. G. McHardy, "Diet Therapy and Peptic Ulcer Disease," in R. C. Kurtz, ed., *Contemporary Issues in Clinical Nutrition,* Vol. 1. Churchill Livingstone Inc., New York, 1981, pp. 45–57.

C. H. Robinson and M. R. Lawler, "Diet in Diseases of Esophagus, Stomach and Duodenum," Chapter 31 in *Normal and Therapeutic Nutrition,* 16th ed. Macmillan Publishing Co., Inc., New York, 1982.

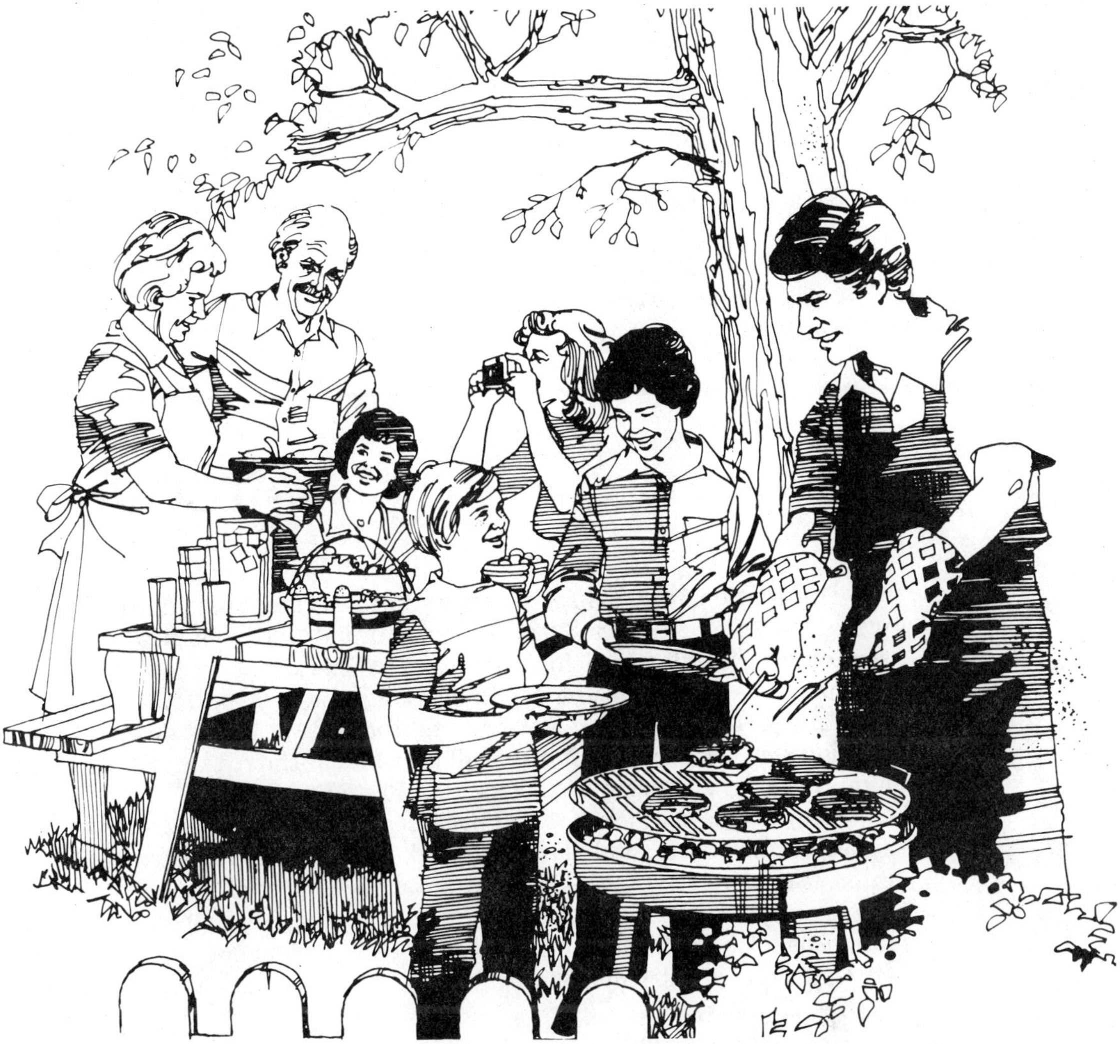

Section Three

FOOD PREPARATION AND SERVICE

OBJECTIVES

- ☐ To help the student acquire the appreciation and knowledge of the basic principles of cooking.
- ☐ To learn how to retain the nutritive value and palatability of the Basic Four Food Groups.
- ☐ To develop simple food preparation skills.
- ☐ To understand how the normal menu is modified for therapeutic diets.
- ☐ To learn the principles of food safety.

Introduction

This section includes food preparation activities that illustrate the basic principles of cooking and service for normal and therapeutic diets. The economy hints discussed in Chapter Three should be reviewed at this time to make the most out of the food budget allowance for cooking in the laboratory. Thus, principles of cooking foods high in protein and starch will be discussed so that the student will understand the reasons for certain techniques used in preparing foods from the Basic Four.

Many foods that are not ordinarily eaten raw acquire a more appetizing appearance, texture, and flavor when they are cooked. Tested recipes, accurate measurements (Table 10–1) and some basic knowledge of how foods change physically and chemically during cooking will help to produce superior products. Emphasis is on short time cooking and cooking at low temperatures to retain nutrients. See Table 10–2 for the range of temperatures used in oven cooking.

Not only are undesirable microorganisms and parasites destroyed by cooking, but foods can become more digestible by cooking, which softens the cellulose of fruits and vegetables and meat fibers, and bursts cereal and starch granules.

TABLE 10–1. Common Food Measures

3 teaspoons	= 1 tablespoon
2 tablespoons	= 1 fluid ounce
4 tablespoons	= 1/4 cup
5-1/3 tablespoons	= 1/3 cup
8 tablespoons	= 1/2 cup
10-2/3 tablespoons	= 2/3 cup
12 tablespoons	= 3/4 cup
16 tablespoons	= 1 cup
1 cup	= 8 fluid ounces
2 cups	= 1 pint
2 pints or 4 cups	= 1 quart

TABLE 10-2. Oven Temperatures

Very slow	250° and 275° F
Slow	300° and 325° F
Moderate	350° and 375° F
Hot	400° and 425° F
Very hot	450° and 475° F
Extremely hot	500° and 525° F

Many methods of food preparation help make foods and meals more interesting (Table 10-3). Microwave ovens and crock pots have become very popular in recent years; these appliances, along with the versatile food processor and the "wok," make food preparation easy and fun.

Since the main focus of this textbook is on nutrition and diet therapy and not on food preparation, only the basic cooking and serving principles of a few menu items will be discussed in this section.

TABLE 10-3. Basic Methods of Cooking

Moist Heat	Dry Heat	Frying
Boiling	Broiling	Sautéing
Simmering	Pan broiling	Pan frying
Stewing	Baking	Deep-fat frying
Braising	Roasting	
Steaming		

10 Food Preparation Basics

CHAPTER OUTLINE

GOOD WORKING HABITS

COOKING TERMS

MEASUREMENTS AND TEMPERATURES

COOKING PRINCIPLES FOR THE BASIC FOUR

GOOD WORKING HABITS

It is essential to acquire good working habits in the laboratory to assure the production of foods of high quality and to maintain efficiency and cleanliness in the work area. The following rules will help the student meet those standards:

1. Read recipe directions carefully.
2. Plan work in correct sequence.
3. Wash hands before preparing food.
4. Preheat oven for baking.
5. Assemble ingredients to be used.
6. Assemble utensils to be used, and use as few as possible.
7. Use accepted measuring equipment and methods.
8. Rinse cooking utensils as soon as used—cold water for protein foods, hot water for greasy and starchy foods.
9. Follow approved methods of dishwashing.
10. Work quietly.
11. Complete assigned housekeeping duties.

COOKING TERMS[1]

Bake To cook in a covered or uncovered container in an oven or oven-type appliance.

Barbeque To roast slowly on a spit or rack, usually basting with a highly seasoned sauce. Also, foods cooked in or served with barbeque sauce.

Baste To pour melted fat, drippings, or other liquid over food to moisten it during cooking.

Boil To cook in water, or other liquid, at boiling temperature (212° F at sea level). In a boil, bubbles rise continually and break on the surface.

Braise To cook meat or poultry slowly in steam from meat juices or added liquid trapped and held in a covered pan. Meat may be browned in a small amount of fat before braising.

Broil To cook uncovered on a rack placed directly under heat or over an open fire.

Pan-broil. To cook in uncovered pan over direct heat, pouring off fat as it accumulates.

Caramelize To heat sugar or food containing sugar until a brown color and characteristic flavor develop.

Fold To combine two mixtures (or two ingredients such as stiffly beaten egg white and sugar) by cutting down gently through the mixture, turning it over, and repeating until well mixed.

Fry To cook uncovered in fat without water.
Pan-fry or *sauté*. To cook in a small amount of fat in fry pan.
Deep-fry or *french-fry*. To cook in a deep kettle, in enough fat to cover or float food.

Grill Same as *Broil*.

Knead To press, stretch, and fold dough or other mixture to make it elastic or smooth. Bread dough becomes elastic; fondant becomes smooth and satiny.

Marinate To let foods stand in a liquid (usually a mixture of oil with vinegar or lemon juice) to add flavor or make more tender.

Parboil To boil until partly cooked.

Poach To simmer gently in liquid so food retains its shape.

Pot-roast To cook large pieces of meat by braising.

Reconstitute To restore concentrated food such as frozen orange juice or dry milk to its original state, usually by adding water.

Rehydrate To soak or cook dried foods to restore water lost in drying.

Roast To cook uncovered in heated air (usually oven) without water.

Simmer To cook in liquid just below the boiling point at temperatures of 185° to 210° F. In a simmer, bubbles form slowly and break below the surface.

Steam To cook food in steam, with or without pressure. Food is steamed in a covered container, on a rack, or in a perforated pan over boiling water.

Stew To cook in liquid just below the boiling point.

MEASURES

Correct measurement of ingredients is often an essential step in successful cookery.

Part of a cup: Use tablespoons or small measuring cup — 1/2, 1/3, 1/4 — for greater accuracy.

Brown sugar: Pack firmly into cup or spoon and level off with straight thin edge of spatula or knife.

Solid fats: When fat comes in a 1-pound rectangular form (about 2 cups), 1 cup or a fraction can be cut from the pound. Or, measure 1 cupful by packing fat firmly into cup and leveling off top with spatula or straight knife.

The water method may be used for part of a cup. To measure 1/2 cup fat, for instance, put 1/2 cup cold water in 1-cup measure. Add fat, pushing it under the water until water level rises to the 1-cup mark. Pour out water and remove fat.

Flour: Spoon flour lightly into a measuring cup until the measure is overflowing. Level off top with the straight thin edge of a spatula or knife.

Fine meals and fine crumbs: Stir instead of sifting. Measure like flour.

Baking powder, cornstarch, cream of tartar, spices: Dip spoon into container and bring it up heaping full. Level off top with straight thin edge of spatula or knife.

Dry milk: Pour dry milk from spout or opening in package, or spoon lightly into measuring cup until the measure is overflowing. Do not shake. Level off top with the straight thin edge of a spatula or knife.

COOKING PRINCIPLES FOR THE BASIC FOUR

FACTS TO REMEMBER WHEN COOKING FOODS HIGH IN PROTEIN

Meat

1. Pigments in meat change color during cooking: Rare beef is bright rose red, medium beef is pink, and well-done beef is brownish gray. Veal and pork should be well done (light gray). Lamb is pink if medium and gray if well done.
2. Some muscle proteins coagulate, except for connective tissue protein, called collagen, which changes to gelatin.
3. Fat melts, making the meat seem juicier and more tender.
4. Moisture is evaporated during cooking.
5. Drippings of meat consist of water and melted fat with some dissolved constituents of the meat.
6. Moderate heat is best for all meats, whether cooked on the top of stove, in the oven, or in the broiler.
7. The purpose of cooking meat is to improve flavor and appearance, increase digestibility, and destroy harmful bacteria.
8. It is best to broil, pan-fry, or roast tender meat cuts, and braise pot roast, or simmer less tender cuts of meat. See meat cooking guides in standard cookbooks.

Poultry

1. Age, weight, quality, and fatness determine the method of cooking.
2. Broil, fry, or roast plump young birds.
3. Braise, stew, or steam older birds or lean ones.
4. Cook at low to moderate temperatures.
5. Do not overcook.
6. Cook uncovered when frying and roasting to retain juices and prevent shrinkage.
7. Thaw frozen birds just before cooking; then stuff, if desired, and cook immediately.

Fish

1. Fat content determines method of cooking.
2. Bake or broil salmon, shad, mackerel, lake trout, and whitefish.
3. Cook in water or bake or broil and baste with melted fat; cod, flounder, haddock, pike, sea bass, perch, and carp.
4. Fry either fat or lean fish.
5. Cook just until flesh can be easily flaked.
6. Do not overcook.

Eggs

1. Coagulation of egg proteins gives firmness to breakfast eggs, thickens custards and pie fillings, and helps form the outer walls of cream puffs and popovers and air cell walls of cakes.
2. Eggs bind together ingredients.
3. Eggs help brown foods.
4. Egg whites clarify broths and coffee by enclosing particles present in the liquid.
5. A greenish color on the surface of egg yolks often occurs if eggs have been overcooked or allowed to cool slowly in the cooking water.
6. Low temperature and short cooking periods are necessary for delicate

and tender texture and attractiveness and to prevent discoloration, curdling, and shrinkage.

7. To avoid discoloration, cool eggs in cold running water immediately after hard cooking in the shell.

8. Eggs that have been stored a long time before cooking discolor more easily.

9. Use simmering water for poached and hard- and soft-cooked eggs; slow oven for baked custards and soufflés (dish may be placed in pan of water); and double boiler for soft custards.

10. Eggs beat up faster and to greater volume when brought to room temperature first.

11. In combining hot mixtures and eggs, as in custards, cream fillings, etc., pour hot mixture slowly into beaten egg, while stirring constantly.

Milk

1. Use moderately low, even temperatures when heating milk to prevent scorching.

2. Cover or stir milk while heating to prevent scum formation (scum is coagulated protein with enmeshed fat and calcium).

3. Use slow oven for milk dishes.

4. To prevent curdling when cooking with milk, thicken milk first, add other ingredients to milk gradually, and avoid overheating.

5. Albumin in milk may scorch if milk is not heated over boiling water.

6. Casein in milk may coagulate if milk is slightly acid and heated at a high temperature.

7. Homogenization decreases the stability of milk, which may then curdle more easily than nonhomogenized milk.

8. Cream whips best when it is 48 to 72 hours old and when cold.

9. Cream curdles more readily at high temperatures.

10. A deep bowl with sloping sides is best for beating air effectively into the cream.

11. Cream doubles in volume when whipped.

Cheese

1. Excessive heat causes cheese to become stringy and tough.

2. Cook cheese at low temperatures for a short period of time.

3. Aged natural or processed cheese blends best and is less likely to become stringy than cheese not aged sufficiently.

4. Use double boiler for cooking on top of the stove.

5. Place dish in pan of water for oven cooking.

6. Cheese blends more readily with sauces if grated.

7. When broiling cheese sandwiches at a high temperature, use as short a cooking time as possible.

FACTS TO REMEMBER WHEN COOKING WITH FAT

1. Fat modifies the texture of sauces.

2. Fats emulsify foods such as mayonnaise.

3. Air beaten into cakes is held in the batter by fat.

4. Frying in fat changes the color and texture of food, making it more attractive.

5. If the fat medium is not hot enough for frying, the food may become soggy and soaked with grease.

6. Use a deep kettle with a small surface for frying.

7. Fat absorption may be excessive if the dough is made more moist or sweetened with extra sugar.

8. Increased mixing time develops gluten in dough or batter and decreases both fat absorption and tenderness.

FACTS TO REMEMBER WHEN PREPARING STARCHY FOODS

1. Starch granules do not dissolve in cold water but swell and become viscous when heated in water, and become clear upon further heating.

2. Acids hydrolyze starch, and therefore fruit juices and vinegar are added to thin out starch mixtures after thickening has occurred.

3. Dry heat converts starch into dextrin, which is brownish in color—as seen in toasted bread and bread crusts.

4. Longer cooking improves the flavor of starch.

5. To insure a smooth mixture when thickening hot starchy liquids, the starch particles first must be separated by sugar (as in puddings) or by fat (as in gravy or white sauce) or by mixing the starch with water to form a paste.

Preparation Techniques for Selected Menu Items

CEREALS

Cereal cookery is largely starch cookery. Coarse cereals require longer cooking than flakes or fine cereals, but cereals may become gummy or pasty if overcooked or overstirred. The finished product should be free of lumps, neither too thick nor too thin, well flavored, and served hot.

The proportion of water to cereal in cooking varies according to the type of cereal, as shown in Table 10–4. Fruit juices or milk can be substituted for part of the water in cooking. Cereal may be cooked or served with dried or fresh fruit, butter, and brown sugar for extra food value.

The purpose of cooking cereal is to soften and rupture the cell walls (see diagram of whole-wheat grain in Figure 10–1). Quick cooking helps to conserve thiamine found in the bran (outer layers) and in the germ.

TABLE 10–4. Proportions of Water to Cereal in Cooked Cereal

Type of Cereal	Amount of Cereal	Amount of Water	Salt
Flaked	1 cup	2 cups	1/2 tsp
Whole or cracked	1 cup	4 cups	1 tsp
Granular	1 cup	5 or 6 cups	1-1/4–1-1/2 tsp
Rice	1 cup	2 cups	1/4 tsp
Macaroni	8 ounces	3 qts (drain after cooking)	1 tbsp

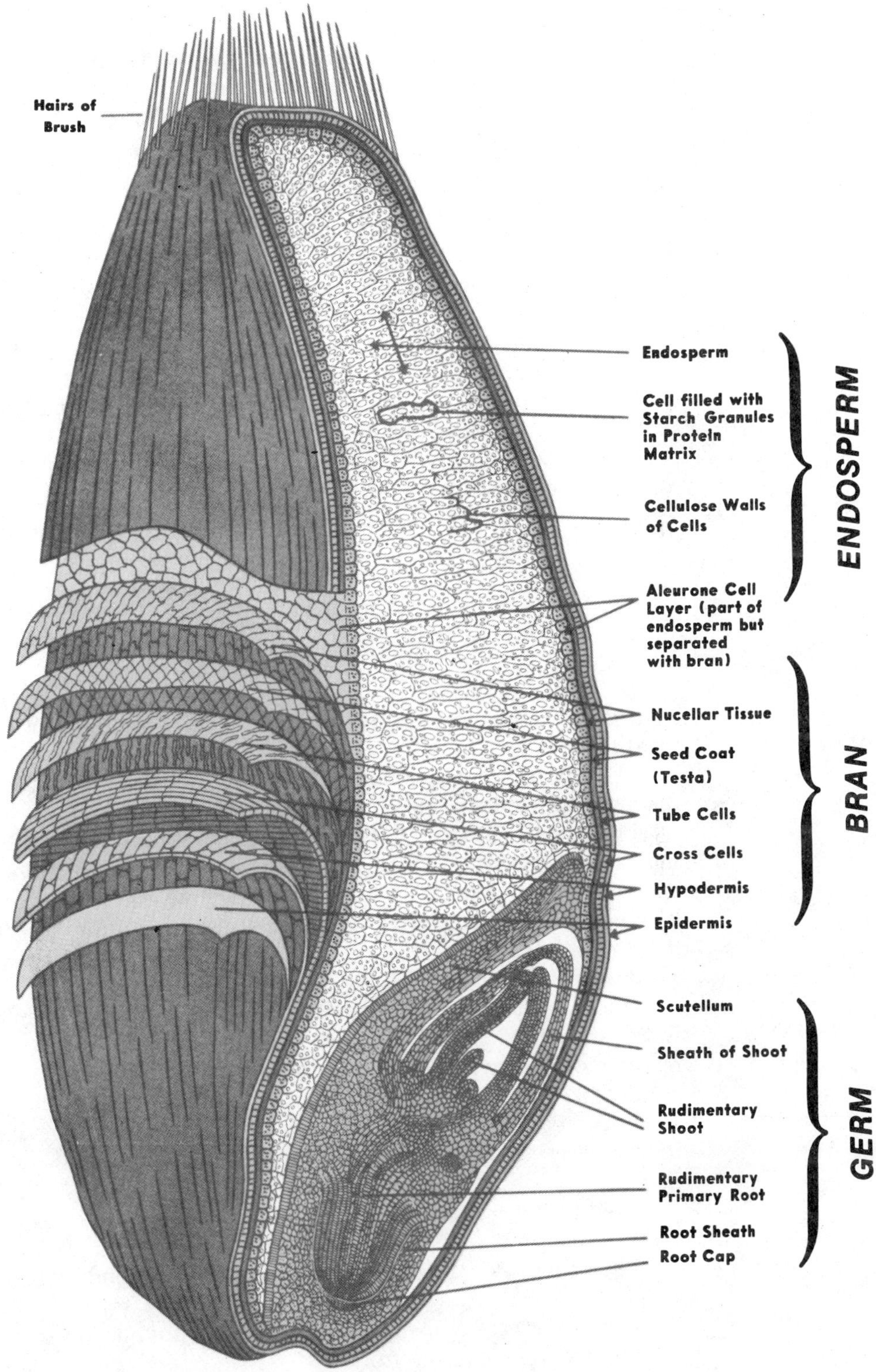

Figure 10–1. Longitudinal section of grain of wheat, enlarged approximately 35 times. (Courtesy Wheat Flour Institute.)

VEGETABLES

Pre-preparation

Use fresh vegetables that have been stored properly.

Prepare vegetables just before cooking.

Use a sharp knife to cut vegetables. A dull knife bruises the vegetable and hastens the loss of valuable nutrients.

Cooking Methods

Boiling

Use very little water. The amount depends upon the size of the pan and the amount of vegetables to be cooked. In general, use from 1/4 inch to 1 inch of water in the pan. More boiling water may be added later in cooking if necessary.

Do not add soda to vegetables. It may make them mushy, impair flavor, and destroy certain vitamins.

To shorten cooking time, bring water to boil before adding the vegetables.

Salt the water, allowing 1/2 to 3/4 teaspoon of salt for each pound of vegetable. Salting may be done at the end of cooking.

Add the vegetable.

Use a tight-fitting lid that will keep steam in the pan. Most of the vegetable must cook in steam.

Quickly bring the water to boiling point again.

Lower heat so water boils gently.

Cook vegetables only until they are tender, and serve immediately.

Baking

Potatoes, onions, carrots, tomatoes, and winter squash can be baked until tender at the temperature being used for preparing other food for the meal.

Prick potatoes either before baking to avoid bursting the skins or immediately afterwards to release steam and prevent potato from becoming soggy.

Place small pieces of fresh vegetables or partially thawed frozen vegetables into a casserole with a little fat, 1 tablespoon of water, and seasonings. Bake approximately 45 minutes covered at 325° to 350° F until tender. Or combine cooked vegetables with a white sauce, cover with buttered crumbs, and brown in 400° F oven.

Steaming

Place vegetables in the perforated container of a steamer over boiling water and cover tightly. Or place vegetables in a heavy pan with the minimum amount of water to prevent scorching ("waterless cooking").

Sprinkle salt on the vegetables in the steamer or pan.

This method is advised for white, yellow, and red vegetables, rather than for green vegetables and vegetables in the cabbage family.

Broiling

Used for both raw and leftover cooked vegetables.

Pressure Cooking

Vegetables are cut into small pieces for rapid and uniform heat penetration.

Vegetables are cooked under 5, 10, or 15 pounds of pressure.

Follow directions carefully.

After cooking, pressure is reduced to zero by putting the pan in cold water. First remove the weight from the vent and then remove the cover.

Dried beans, fibrous and mature vegetables, whole beets, and whole potatoes can be cooked satisfactorily in the pressure cooker.

Stir Frying

This technique has been adapted from Asian cooking. In stir frying, the color and nutrients of the vegetables are retained. The method is best used for tender vegetables with a high moisture content (shredded cabbage, thin diagonal pieces of asparagus, string beans or celery, pieces of spinach, etc.). The vegetable is added to 1 to 2 tablespoons of heated fat in a fry pan, the pan is covered, and the vegetables are cooked for a short time over high heat with occasional stirring. A small amount of water may be added if necessary. The vegetables should be slightly crisp.

Other popular methods of cooking vegetables include cooking in the microwave oven, deep-fat frying, braising, and pan frying.

To Prevent Color Changes

Be careful not to overcook vegetables, as excessive heat will change the pigment, which gives them their attractive color.

Cook the vegetable in an uncovered or partially covered pan for at least the first part of the cooking period. This allows the mild acids to go off in steam as cooking progresses; otherwise they stay in pan and vegetables change from a green color to olive-green. Spinach and nearly all frozen vegetables cook quickly, so they can be cooked in a covered pan.

To Prevent Development of Strong Flavors

Cook vegetables such as cabbage, cauliflower, broccoli, Brussels sprouts, or turnips in an uncovered pan to allow the substances that may develop strong flavors to go off in steam.

Cook just until the vegetable is done, as strong flavors develop with long cooking.

FRUITS

Preparation Principles

Wash carefully and remove blemishes.

Chill (except bananas and pineapple).

Serve different ways for variety.

Cut just before serving.

Juice fruits just before serving.

Whole citrus fruits have more nutritive value than strained fruit and juices.

Store fruit juices covered and chilled.

Thaw frozen fruits just before serving and do not refreeze.

If cooking fruit, cook slowly and no longer than necessary.

Cooking lessens tart flavor, causes some color changes, softens cellulose, and inverts some sugars to less sweet ones.

Simmer rather than boil fruits to lessen the loss of volatile flavors.

Cook dried fruits in the same water in which they were soaked.

Fruit Desserts (Types)

Whips — sweetened fruit pulp and beaten egg white.

Soufflés — whips baked at low temperatures.

Bread fruit puddings (fruit betty) — fruit combined with bread.

Fruit crisp — fruit topped with crumb mixture.

Fruit cobbler — fruit topped with biscuit or pastry.

Fruit pudding — fruit combined with uncooked batter before baking.

Gelatin desserts — unflavored gelatin plus fruit juices with or without the addition of fruit, nuts, marshmallows, whipped cream, etc. Flavored gelatin may be used as the base. May also serve as salad when placed on greens.

Frozen — frozen fruit juices are called ices; with beaten egg white or milk they are called sherbets.

Fruit tapioca.

SALADS

Preparation Principles

Keep salad ingredients cold, crisp, fresh, and colorful.

Put tossed salads together with a light touch.

Arrange individual salads simply.

Use clean, chilled, crisp salad greens.

Choose ingredients that provide a variety of color, flavor, shape, and texture.

Have pieces large enough to keep the food's identity.

Chill and drain canned fruits and vegetables.

Save vitamin C in vegetables by using a sharp knife for shredding, and toss with a wooden spoon and fork or two silver forks.

Prevent discoloration of fruits by dipping them in citrus or pineapple juice.

Prepare salads just ahead of serving time for best appearance, texture, flavor, and vitamin value.

Do not shred or grate ingredients ahead of time.

Add dressings just at serving time.

Do not soak prepared relishes in cold water too long.

Exhibit salads well by using unusual greens and raw vegetables, setting up an attractive relish tray, or using a cheese and cracker tray to accompany salad service.

Serving Salads

Salads may be served on individual plates, in wooden bowls, on a large platter or plate, or in an attractive serving bowl.

Chill serving dishes.

For individual or platter salads, lettuce or other greens may form a cup to hold salad, or greens may be shredded and the salad placed on top. Greens should not extend over the rim of the plate.

Dressing may be passed at the table.

Use the appropriate dressing for the salad.

Gelatin salads should be tender and firm, not rubbery or runny.

Use attractive and appropriate garnishes when needed.

Choose salad appropriate to the purpose for which it is used and in relation to other foods.

Salad Dressings

French: oil, vinegar, or lemon juice or fruit juice and seasonings in a temporary emulsion.

Mayonnaise: egg, oil, acids, and seasonings in a permanent emulsion.

Cooked: egg or flour or both used as a thickening agent with added acid.

Sour cream: alone or with variations as desired.

Main dish salads are usually served with a mayonnaise-type or cooked dressing; some with a tart French dressing.

Vegetable and vegetable fruit salads are usually served with a tart French dressing; some with a mayonnaise or cooked dressing.

Fruit salads are usually served with sweet clear French dressing; mixtures sometimes with mayonnaise and whipped cream or with thinned fruit juice.

Garnishes

Garnishes should be simple, flavorful, and not too numerous.

Vegetable salads may be garnished with any of the following: sliced cucumber (scored or plain, peeled or unpeeled), lettuce cup edge dipped in paprika, quartered or sliced tomatoes, radishes used plain or made into roses or fans, strips or rings of green or red pepper, carrot sticks or curls, quartered or sliced hard-cooked eggs.

Fruit salads may be garnished with maraschino cherries, mint leaves, strawberries, dark fruits (plums, cherries, cooked prunes), cream cheese balls, coconut, or nuts.

SANDWICHES

There are several types of sandwiches, depending on the occasion.

Hearty: to serve hot or cold, as a main dish of meal, with the use of a knife and fork or finger style, and made of meat, cheese, fish, poultry, or eggs.

Less hearty: to serve with soup course, salad, or tea.

Canapés: open sandwiches, specially garnished.

Tea: dainty sandwiches cut in various shapes and with bread crusts removed.

Sandwich fillings: sliced meat, chopped or grated vegetables, peanut butter, baked beans, tasty chopped mixtures of meat, fish, poultry, eggs, etc.

French-toasted sandwiches: many types may be French toasted (dipped in an egg-milk mixture before pan frying).

Preparation Points

Use day-old bread except for rolled sandwiches.

Slice thinly for dainty tea sandwiches and canapés; thicker for main dish sandwiches.

Remove crusts for dainty sandwiches (plan to use crusts for croutons or crumbs, or in puddings).

Spread sandwiches with softened (not melted) butter.

Cut in different shapes for eye appeal.

Have fillings fresh and crisp.

Use variety of breads: white, whole wheat, rye, nut, raisin, or fruited.

Use appropriate garnish for sandwich service when desired.

TOAST

Toast is more readily digested than untoasted bread, because starch is changed to dextrin by heat, but the dryness and hardness of toast requires mastication. The bread for toasting should be enriched or whole grain to provide maximum nutrients.

One should follow the manufacturer's directions when using an electric toaster. Bread may be broiler toasted on a rack under direct heat or oven toasted. The latter method makes the product dryer and crisper.

Toast may be served dry or buttered and served warm and covered for breakfast, or made into toast points, croutons, cinnamon toast, or milk toast. Crackers and rolls may also be toasted for variety.

CREAM SAUCES

Cream sauces or white sauces must be the right thickness for the purpose, smooth, well seasoned, and thoroughly cooked. Cream sauces promote variety in the menu because they may be used many different ways: in creamed soups, sauces, or scalloped dishes, or as the base for croquettes and soufflés. Cream sauces are an excellent way to introduce milk into the diet.

The following cooking rules must be remembered in preparing cream sauces:

1. Measure accurately.
2. Blend melted fat and flour to separate the starch grains.
3. Add liquid slowly to prevent lumping.
4. Cook slowly at low temperatures to prevent scorching and cook thoroughly.
5. Stir frequently to prevent lumps.

Types of Cream Sauces

Very thin — for cream soups.
Medium — for creamed dishes, scalloped dishes, and gravies.
Thick — for soufflés.
Very thick — for croquettes.

Activities*

1. Exhibit unusual greens and raw vegetables used in salads.
2. Display an attractive relish tray.
3. Prepare a cheese and cracker tray to accompany a salad service.
4. Demonstrate how to prepare lettuce for salads.
5. Prepare radish roses and carrot curls, etc.
6. Toss a salad with oil, vinegar, and seasonings.
7. Peel tomatoes; peel and section citrus fruits; cut fresh pineapple.
8. Prepare tomato aspic with cottage cheese.
9. Prepare a fruited gelatin.
10. Prepare a salad dressing.
11. Prepare an oven roast, pot roast, and scraped beef.
12. Make a gravy from the meat drippings.
13. Stuff and roast poultry.
14. Fry chicken.
15. Prepare an entree using a meat "analog."
16. Exhibit commonly used cuts of meat (or models or posters) and commonly used fish: whole, steaks, fillets.
17. Take a field trip to a supermarket where meat cuts and fish are sold.
18. Prepare poached eggs, omelets, egg cutlets, baked or soft custards, and junkets.

---

*If time or facilities do not permit preparation of complete menus, place proper dishes on trays for the foods not prepared. Where no actual food preparation is possible, use food models.

DEMONSTRATION TOPICS

Methods of measuring in food preparation (dry ingredients, liquids, fats).
Special cooking procedures.
Placement of utensils in oven for baking.
Storage of food in the refrigerator.

NOTE TO INSTRUCTOR

Recipes for dishes suitable to be prepared or demonstrated in food preparation classes will be found in the following references as well as in other standard cookbooks:

U.S. Department of Agriculture Yearbooks:

Food — 1959, pp. 519–554, "What and How to Cook," Recipes arranged according to the Four Food Groups in the Daily Food Guide.

Food for Us All — 1969. Recipes scattered throughout book.

Family Fare, Home and Garden Bulletin No. 1, U.S. Department of Agriculture, Washington, D.C., 1971.

I. S. Rombauer and M. R. Becker, *The Joy of Cooking*, The Bobbs-Merrill Company, Inc., Indianapolis and New York, 1975.

Betty Crocker's Cookbook. Golden Press, New York, 1969.

REFERENCE

1. *Family Fare*. Home and Garden Bulletin No. 1. U.S. Department of Agriculture, Washington, D.C., 1974, pp. 86–87.

11 Normal and Therapeutic Menu Planning

CHAPTER OUTLINE

MENU PLANNING	JUDGING MEALS
MEAL SERVICE	

MENU PLANNING

To insure an adequate daily intake of essential nutrients, menus must be planned according to the basic four food groups even if modifications for consistency and therapeutic purposes are necessary. If a diet is very restrictive and does not allow an adequate intake of nutrients, vitamin and mineral preparations should be given accordingly.

As discussed in Chapter Four, "Nutrition in the Life Cycle," everyone needs the same nutrients throughout life but in different amounts. Nutrient requirements for growth are greater than for maintenance. Athletes in training have greater energy needs than inactive persons. Recovery from illness and operations increases nutrient and energy needs. Using the basic four food groups as a daily guide for planning meals will provide all the essential nutrients needed by the body throughout the life cycle.

Milk Group. Milk, our leading source of calcium, also supplies high-quality protein, riboflavin, and vitamin A if it is whole or fortified. It is the basis for many solid and liquid foods: soups, chowders, creamed foods, and desserts. Milk and cheese together make an inexpensive main dish such as fondue or macaroni and cheese.

Cheese is an acceptable and economical meat substitute because of its high protein content. It can supplement a meal low in protein or one in which protein is of poor quality. One-half pound of cheese equals approximately one pound of meat with moderate bone and fat. Cottage cheese is an inexpensive animal protein that costs one-fourth to one-half as much as meat, has no waste, and requires no cooking. See Table 11–1 for varieties of cheese frequently used in the diet.

Breads and Cereals. This group of food supplies some protein, iron, several of the B vitamins, and calories. It can be included in the menu as a breakfast cereal, biscuits, muffins, pancakes, and hot breads. Combination dishes containing bread or cereal, as in macaroni and cheese, Spanish rice, spaghetti and meat sauce, are other ways of including this important food group in the daily menu.

Meat Group. This group is valued for protein, iron, and B vitamins. Inexpensive foods in this group include legumes and nuts. One can easily find ways to include two servings of foods from the meat group in the daily diet. Main dishes at the mid-day and evening meals are often composed of meat,

TABLE 11–1. Varieties of Cheese Commonly Used

Hard:	Cheddar, Edam, Gouda, Swiss, Parmesan
Semi-hard:	Muenster, Roquefort, Gorgonzola
Soft:	Cottage, Cream, Limburger, Camembert
Processed:	Blend of American cheese with other cheeses and pasteurized with an emulsifying agent added

fish, or poultry or alternates such as eggs, dry beans or peas, or nuts. These foods can be combined with macaroni, rice, vegetables, and potatoes.

Eggs, a popular breakfast food, are often served with ham, bacon, or sausage. At lunch or dinner, eggs can be used in casseroles, soufflés, scalloped dishes, salads, sandwich fillings, or cream sauces. Desserts containing eggs include custards, soufflés, sauces, puddings, and pie fillings.

Fruits and Vegetables. This group provides vitamins A and C and minerals, and is often used to stimulate appetite with color, aroma, texture, and taste.

Fruit is found in the menu as an appetizer, as a topping for breakfast cereals, in salads, as a garnish, and therapeutically as a juice to increase fluid intake and quench thirst. It can be served plain as a dessert, or in fruit whips, puddings, and fruit ices. It can be baked in cobblers or crisps.

Vegetables can be served cooked accompanying main dishes at mid-day or evening meals. Raw vegetables are used in salads, as relishes, or as garnishes. Combination dishes containing vegetables or fruits or both contribute to the daily quota of servings from this group.

Salads are an excellent way to introduce fruit and vegetables in the diet because they (1) provide fiber and bulk, thus stimulating peristalsis, (2) enhance meal attractiveness with flavor, color, and texture, and (3) are low in calories when served without dressings.

To plan nutritious meals, use the following guidelines:[1]

1. Plan the protein main dish from the meat group.
2. Add a bread or cereal group to complement the main dish.
3. Choose a hot or cold vegetable.
4. Select a fruit or vegetable to complement the main dish.
5. Add a dessert. Light desserts are best after a heavy meal, and vice versa.
6. Choose a beverage. Use milk to meet the requirements for the milk group.
7. Add extras (fats and sweets) after requirements from the basic four have been chosen, to complement the meal and suit family tastes.

Therapeutic Menus. It is important that the person or persons planning the meals have a thorough understanding of any diet restrictions that need to be considered. Seasonings, cooking techniques, textures, and food selections may have to be altered accordingly. See Table 11–2 for an overview of some basic diet restrictions. It is important to note that diet restriction policies

TABLE 11–2. Overview of Some Basic Diet Restrictions

Regular
No dietary or consistency restrictions. Amounts are modified to meet needs of individuals.

Soft
Consistency and texture of foods must be soft, easy to chew and swallow. It may be prescribed for persons having problems with poor dentition or dentures, or postoperatively as a progression from liquids to regular diet.

Liberal Bland
Restricts spices and caffeine-containing beverages. Other modifications depend on individual tolerances. It is prescribed for persons having peptic ulcers.

Sodium Restricted
High-sodium foods are omitted, and salt and salt seasonings are used sparingly or not at all, depending upon the level of sodium restriction. It is usually prescribed for persons with hypertension or fluid retention.

Low Fat
High-fat foods are omitted. Cooking techniques without added fat are emphasized—baking, broiling, roasting, boiling. It is usually prescribed for gallbladder or heart disease.

Calorie Restricted
Foods high in simple sugars and calories are omitted. Meals are planned using exchange lists. It is usually prescribed for overweight and diabetic persons.

will vary among health care facilities. Table 11–3 shows how the basic four food groups are modified according to various diet restrictions. Table 11–4 shows a sample day's menu of these modifications.

Cookbooks for special diets are available in many bookstores.

MEAL SERVICE

Table Setting. Attractive table settings complement carefully planned and prepared meals. Mixing and matching colors of place mats or table linen, china, and centerpieces can create a formal or informal dining atmosphere.

Whether the atmosphere is formal or informal, the following basic rules apply for table settings:

1. Use a clean tablecloth or mat of a color that looks good with the dishes.
2. Place silver, napkin, and dishes about an inch from the edge of the table.
3. Place the tines of forks and the bowls of the spoons with the hollow part up.
4. Place hemmed edges of the napkin toward the plate and edge of the table.
5. Place silverware so that pieces to be used first are farthest from the plate. Forks are placed on the left, knives and spoons on the right.
6. Place glasses above the knife. If wine glasses are used, set them to the right of the water glass.
7. Place the bread and butter plate or salad plate above the fork. If both are used, place the salad plate above the napkin. See Figure 11–1 for a sample table setting.

TABLE 11–3. Menu Modification of Basic Four Food Groups for Therapeutic Diets

Food Group	Regular	Soft	Liberal Bland	Sodium Restricted	Low Fat	Calorie Restricted
Milk	All milk and dairy products allowed	All milk and dairy products allowed	Allowed as tolerated	Milk may be limited depending on level of sodium restriction Use low sodium cheeses	Use skim milk and low-fat cheeses	Use skim milk and low-fat cheeses unless calorie level allows use of higher fat products
Meat	All meat and alternates allowed	Use soft, tender, or ground meats plain or in casseroles and soups	Avoid spicy meats and high-fat meats if not well tolerated	Avoid all processed and cured meats	Use lean meats	Use lean meats, limit to amounts prescribed in diet
Fruits and vegetables	All fruits and vegetables allowed	Use juices, soft, canned, or cooked vegetables and fruits. Chop and mash as needed.	Allowed as tolerated	Avoid dried fruits with sodium preservatives Avoid high-sodium vegetables and juices	Avoid vegetables in cream or cheese sauces	Avoid vegetables in cream or cheese sauces, fruits packed in syrup Limit to amounts prescribed in diet
Breads and cereals	All breads and cereals allowed	All breads and cereals allowed Modify in consistency as needed (milk toast, rice pudding, etc.)	Allowed as tolerated	Avoid instant hot cereals, breads with salted toppings, salted crackers Salt-free products may be used, depending on level of sodium restriction	Avoid products with added fat	Avoid products with added fat
Miscellaneous	Condiments and seasonings as desired Fats, sugar, and alcohol in moderation	Condiments and seasonings as desired Fats, sugar, and alcohol in moderation	*Omit:* Black pepper, chili powder, nutmeg, cloves, mustard seed, alcohol, and caffeine-containing beverages	Avoid salt and salt seasonings, salted snack foods, commercially canned soups	Limit use of fats and oils	Limit use of fats, oils, alcohol, and high-sugar foods

TABLE 11–4. Sample Menus for Therapeutic Diets

Meal	Regular	Soft	Liberal Bland	Sodium Restricted	Low Fat	Calorie Restricted
Breakfast	Orange juice Corn flakes Poached egg Buttered toast Milk Coffee Sugar Salt, pepper	Orange juice Cream of Wheat Poached egg Buttered toast Milk Coffee Sugar Salt, pepper	Orange juice Corn flakes Poached egg Buttered toast Milk Sugar Salt	Orange juice Shredded Wheat Poached egg SF* Buttered toast Milk Coffee Sugar Salt substitute Pepper	Orange juice Corn flakes Poached egg Toast 1 tsp butter Skim milk Coffee Sugar Salt, pepper	Orange juice Corn flakes Poached egg Toast 1 tsp butter Skim milk Coffee Sugar substitute Salt, pepper
Lunch	Vegetable soup Crackers Turkey sandwich Fresh fruit salad Vanilla pudding Milk Tea Sugar Salt, pepper	Vegetable soup Crackers Ground turkey sandwich Canned fruit salad Vanilla pudding Milk Tea Sugar Salt, pepper	Vegetable soup Crackers Turkey sandwich Fresh fruit salad Vanilla pudding Milk Salt	SF Vegetable soup SF Crackers Turkey sandwich on SF Bread Fresh fruit salad Lemon sherbet Milk Tea Sugar Salt substitute Pepper	Vegetable soup Crackers Turkey sandwich (use white meat) Fresh fruit salad Lemon sherbet Skim milk Tea Sugar Salt, pepper	Vegetable soup Crackers Turkey sandwich (use white meat) Fresh fruit salad Skim milk Tea Sugar substitute Salt, pepper
Dinner	Tossed salad with dressing Baked chicken Baked potato Buttered carrots Peach slices Dinner roll Brownie Milk Tea Sugar Salt, pepper Butter	Tomato juice Baked ground chicken Baked potato Buttered carrots Peach slices Dinner roll Brownie (no nuts) Milk Tea Sugar Salt, pepper Butter	Tossed salad with dressing Baked chicken Baked potato Buttered carrots Peach slices Dinner roll Brownie Milk Salt Butter	Tossed salad with SF dressing Baked chicken Baked potato Buttered SF carrots Peach slices Dinner roll Milk Tea Sugar Salt substitute Pepper SF butter	Tossed salad with low-calorie dressing Baked chicken (no skin) Baked potato Carrots Peach slices Dinner roll Skim milk Tea Sugar Salt, pepper 1 tsp butter	Tossed salad with low-calorie dressing Baked chicken (no skin) Baked potato Carrots Peach slices (water packed) Dinner roll Skim milk Tea Sugar substitute Salt, pepper 1 tsp butter

*SF = salt free.

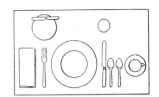

Figure 11–1. Table setting.

Beverage Service. When serving beverages the following basic rules apply:

1. Fill water glasses to 2/3 capacity.
2. Leave wine glasses empty until guests are seated.
3. Leave glasses on table while server is pouring.
4. Pick up tumbler glasses below the rim and goblet-type glasses by the stem.
5. When serving coffee or tea, empty saucers and cups are placed to the right of the table setting.

Service Order. The order of serving food will vary with the menu. An acceptable order may be appetizer, soup, salad, main course, dessert. For a buffet, all foods are served at once. Desserts may be served later at the table.

JUDGING MEALS

Learning to select, prepare, and serve meals that are nutritious and tasty is a skill that improves with experience. Table 11–5 shows a score sheet that may be used to judge meals.

TABLE 11–5. Meal Score Sheet

1. Selection (5 points each)	
a. Basic four food groups represented	________
b. Appropriate for type of meal	________
c. Colorful	________
d. Contrasting textures	________
2. Preparation (5 points each)	
a. Organized work area	________
b. Cooking techniques	________
c. Amounts prepared	________
d. Flavor and seasonings	________
3. Service (5 points each)	
a. Table setting	________
b. Appearance of food	________
c. Timing of courses	________

Possible Score = 55

Key: 1 = Very Poor
2 = Poor
3 = Satisfactory
4 = Good
5 = Excellent

Study Questions and Activities

1. Plan a dinner menu that is quick and easy to prepare. Check to make sure all food groups are represented. Can this menu be used for other diet restrictions?
2. Some diet restrictions may lead to unbalanced meals. Name two diet restrictions that fit this criterion.
3. When fat is restricted, what food groups are most affected?
4. Compare the decor of several restaurants. How does the decor affect the menu selections offered?
5. Plan, prepare, and serve a meal. Use the Meal Score Sheet (Table 11–5) to judge the meal.

REFERENCE

1. *Better Homes and Gardens' New Cookbook*, 9th ed. Meredith Corporation, Des Moines, 1981, p. 408.

ADDITIONAL REFERENCES

Betty Crocker's Cookbook. Golden Press, New York, 1969.

I. S. Rombauer and M. R. Becker, *The Joy of Cooking*, Bobbs-Merrill Co., Inc., Indianapolis, 1975.

Food Storage and Handling

12

CHAPTER OUTLINE

- PERSONAL HYGIENE
- STORING FOODS
- PREPARING AND COOKING FOODS
- FREEZING AND CANNING FOODS
- BACTERIAL FOOD POISONING

The right kinds and amounts of food in the daily diet for optimal health have been discussed in the previous chapters. The care with which these foods are handled from production through preservation, refrigeration, storage, distribution, and handling in the market and in the home will determine the final nutritive value and safety of these foods when they appear on the table. At many points along the line, the individual handling of the food helps to safeguard the food supply. Strict cleanliness of person and surroundings is the best way to prevent the contamination of foods and the spread of food-borne illness.

PERSONAL HYGIENE[1]

Anyone who has an infectious disease should be discouraged from handling, preparing, or serving food. The bacteria in infected cuts or other skin infections may be the source of food-borne illness also. Food handlers must always work with clean hands, clean hair, and clean fingernails, and wear clean clothing. Hands must be washed after using the toilet or assisting anyone using the toilet, after smoking or blowing the nose, after touching raw meat, poultry, or eggs, and before working with other food. Food should be mixed with clean utensils rather than hands; however, plastic gloves may be worn if it is easier to use the hands. Hands should be kept away from the mouth, nose, and hair. It is important to cover coughs and sneezes with disposable tissues. The same spoon should not be used more than once for tasting food while preparing, cooking, or serving.

STORING FOODS[2]

Fresh, perishable foods should be used soon after harvest or purchase. If storage is necessary, maintain the proper temperature and humidity and use fresh foods as soon as possible, before they undergo a loss of quality. Even under the best storage conditions, freshness and nutritive value can be lost if foods are stored too long.

Under poor storage conditions, foods held too long often spoil. Some kinds of spoilage are harmful to health and others are not, but it is not always possible to distinguish between the two kinds.

Indications of spoilage that make food unpalatable but not hazardous to health are the rancid odor and flavor of fats caused by oxidation, slime on the surface of meat, and the fermentation of fruit juices due to yeast growth.

Among the signals that indicate dangerous bacterial spoilage are off-odors in foods and a sour taste in bland foods.

Low temperatures are required in the storage of many perishable foods. Low temperatures retard quality losses and delay spoilage by slowing the action of enzymes naturally present and by slowing the growth of spoilage organisms that may be present.

Foods vary in the degree of temperature and in the amount of moisture needed to retain quality in storage.

Although most fresh, perishable foods keep longest and best in the refrigerator, certain varieties of apples and some root vegetables keep well in a cool basement or outdoor cellar or pit. A few fruits and vegetables can be kept successfully at room temperatures.

Green leafy vegetables keep their crispness and nutrients best in cold, moist air. On the other hand, too much moisture in the air around cherries and berries encourages the growth of mold and rot.

Temperatures in the Refrigerator

The temperature in frostless and self-defrosting refrigerators is fairly uniform throughout the cabinet, including the storage area in the door.

In refrigerators that must be defrosted manually, the coldest area outside the freezing unit is the chill tray located just below it. The area at the bottom of the cabinet is the warmest. The door and hydrator storage areas are usually several degrees higher than the rest of the refrigerator.

When air circulates in the refrigerator, the cooler air moves downward and forces the warmer air near the bottom to rise. This air motion dries out any uncovered or unwrapped food.

In most refrigerators, with the control set for normal operation, the temperature in the general storage area is usually below 40° F. The homemaker can check the temperatures in the refrigerator by placing a thermometer at different locations in the cabinet. If the temperature is above 40° F, the control should be regulated to maintain temperatures below 40° F.

Frequent opening of the refrigerator door, especially on warm, humid days, or an accumulation of thick frost on the freezing unit, raises the refrigerator's temperatures.

The freezing compartments of home refrigerators are not designed to give a temperature of 0° F—the temperature needed for prolonged storage of frozen foods. Hold frozen foods in these compartments only a few days. In refrigerator-freezers in which the temperature can be maintained at 0° F in the freezer cabinet, food may be kept for the same storage periods as in a freezer.

Use the refrigerator properly. Do not overcrowd it; allow space around food containers for air circulation. Defrost when needed.

Breads and Cereals

Breads

Store in original wrapper in bread box or refrigerator. Use within 5 to 7 days. Bread keeps its freshness longer at room temperature than in the refrigerator. In hot, humid weather, however, bread is better protected against mold in the refrigerator than in the bread box.

Breads will retain their good quality for 2 to 3 months if frozen in their original wrappers and stored in the home freezer.

Cereals, flours, spices, and sugar

Store at room temperature, away from the heat of a range or a refrigerator unit. Store in tightly closed containers to keep out dust, moisture, and insects.

During summer, buy flours and cereals in small quantities. Inspect often for weevils.

Dry mixes

Cake, pancake, cookie, muffin, and roll mixes may be held at room temperature, away from the heat of a range or a refrigerator unit.

Meat, Poultry, Fish

Store meats in the coldest part of the refrigerator.

Cold cuts

Store in the refrigerator. Unopened vacuum-sealed packages may be kept for 2 weeks. Once opened, wrap well and use within 3 to 5 days.

Cured and smoked meats

Store ham, frankfurters, bacon, and smoked sausage in the refrigerator in their original packagings. Use within 1 week for best flavor. Uncooked, cured pork may be stored longer than fresh pork, but the fat will become rancid if held too long.

Store whole ham in original wrapping up to 1 week; half a ham, for 5 days. Use ham slices within 3 days. Canned ham, unopened, will retain optimum eating quality in the refrigerator up to 1 year.

Fresh meat; roasts, steaks, chops, and ground

Cover roasts, steaks, and chops loosely and store in refrigerator. Use within 3 to 5 days.

Sausage frequently is bought frozen and it is important to keep frozen and use within 30 days. Once thawed, use within 3 to 4 days.

Ground meats, such as hamburger, are more likely to spoil than roasts, chops, or steaks because more of the meat surface has been exposed to contamination from air, handlers, and mechanical equipment. Lightly cover these meats, store them in the refrigerator, and use within 1 or 2 days.

Poultry and fish

Poultry and fish should be used within 1 or 2 days. The transparent wrap on poultry, as purchased, may be used for storage.

Variety meats

Store variety meats such as liver, kidneys, brains, and poultry giblets in the refrigerator. Use within 1 or 2 days.

Before storing poultry giblets, remove them from the separate bag in which they are packed, rewrap, and refrigerate.

Leftover cooked meats and meat dishes

Cool leftover meats and meat dishes quickly (container may be placed in cold water). Then cover and refrigerate promptly. Use within 3 to 4 days. Cooked ham should be used within a week.

Leftover stuffing

Remove leftover stuffing from chicken or turkey, cool immediately, and store separately from the rest of the bird. Use within 1 or 2 days.

Leftover gravy and broth

These are highly perishable. Cover and store in the refrigerator promptly, and use within 1 or 2 days.

Eggs

Shell eggs

Store promptly in refrigerator. Eggs retain quality well in the refrigerator; they lose their mild flavor quickly at room temperature.

To insure best quality and flavor, use eggs within a week. If eggs are held too long, the thick white may become thin and the yolk membrane may weaken and break when the shell is opened.

If eggs are cracked, use them only in foods that will be thoroughly cooked.

Cook leftover yolks with cold water and store in the refrigerator in a covered container. Extra egg whites should also be refrigerated in a covered container. Use leftover yolks and whites within 2 to 4 days.

Dried egg

Keep in refrigerator. After a package has been opened, store unused portion in an airtight container with a tight-fitting lid.

Dried egg will keep its good flavor for about a year if it is stored properly.

Milk, Cream, Cheese

Fresh milk and cream

Store in refrigeratoı at about 40° F. For best eating quality, use within 1 week. Keep covered so milk and cream will not absorb odors and flavors of other foods. Take out of refrigerator only long enough to get the amount needed. Immediately return to refrigerator.

Dry milks

Keep dry milk — either nonfat or whole — in a tightly closed container.

Nonfat dry milk will keep in good condition for several months on the cupboard shelf.

Close the container immediately after using. If dry milk is exposed to air during storage, it may become lumpy and stale.

Dry whole milk is marketed only on a small scale, chiefly for infant feeding. Because of its fat content, it does not keep as well as nonfat dry milk; after the container has been opened, dry whole milk should be tightly covered and stored in the refrigerator.

Refrigerate reconstituted dry milk like fresh fluid milk.

Evaporated milk and condensed milk

Store at room temperature until opened, then cover tightly and refrigerate like fresh fluid milk.

Cheese spreads and cheese foods

After containers of these foods have been opened, cover and store them in the refrigerator. Use within 1 to 2 weeks.

Hard cheeses such as Cheddar, Parmesan, and Swiss

Keep in the refrigerator. Wrap tightly to keep out air. Stored this way, hard cheeses will keep for several months. Cut off mold if it develops on the surface of the cheese.

Soft cheeses such as cottage, cream, and Camembert

Store tightly covered. Use cottage cheese within 3 to 5 days, others within 2 weeks.

Vegetables

The fresher the vegetable, the better it is when eaten.

With only a few exceptions vegetables keep best in the refrigerator.

The exceptions — potatoes, sweet potatoes, mature onions, hard-rind squashes, eggplant, and rutabagas — keep well in cool rather than cold storage.

Sort vegetables before storing them. Use immediately any vegetables that are bruised or soft. Discard any that show evidence of decay.

The vegetable crisper in your refrigerator performs better if it is at least two-thirds full. If crisper is less full than this, vegetables will keep better if they are put in plastic bags before being placed in the crisper. Always store vegetables in plastic bags or plastic containers if they are not stored in the crisper.

Asparagus

Do not wash before storing. Store in the refrigerator in crisper, plastic bags, or plastic containers. Use within 2 or 3 days.

Broccoli and Brussels sprouts

Store in refrigerator in crisper, plastic bags, or plastic containers. Use within 3 to 5 days.

Cabbage, cauliflower, celery, and snap beans

Store in the refrigerator in crisper, plastic bags, or plastic containers. Use cabbage within 1 or 2 weeks; use cauliflower, celery, or snap beans within 1 week.

Carrots, beets, parsnips, radishes, and turnips

Remove tops. Store in refrigerator in plastic bags or plastic containers. Use within 2 weeks.

Green peas and limas

Leave in pods and store in the refrigerator. Use within 3 to 5 days.

Lettuce and other salad greens

Wash. Drain well. Store in the refrigerator in crisper, plastic bags, or plastic containers to reduce loss of moisture. Use within 1 week.

Onions

Store *mature onions* at room temperature, or slightly cooler, in loosely woven or open-mesh containers. Stored this way, they keep several months. They sprout and decay at high temperature and in high humidity.

Keep *green onions* cold and moist in the refrigerator. Store in plastic bags. Use within 3 to 5 days.

Peppers and cucumbers

Wash and dry. Store in crisper or in plastic bags in the refrigerator. Use within 1 week.

Potatoes

Store in a dark, dry place with good ventilation away from any source of heat, with a temperature of about 45° to 50° F. Potatoes stored in this manner will keep for several months. Light causes greening, which lowers eating quality. High temperatures hasten sprouting and shriveling. If stored at room temperature, use within a week.

Rhubarb

This vegetable is often used as a fruit. It is ready to use when purchased. Refrigerate and use within 3 to 5 days.

Spinach, kale, chard, and collard, beet, turnip, and mustard greens

Wash thoroughly in cold water. Lift out of the water as grit settles to the bottom of the pan. Drain well. Store in the refrigerator in crisper or in plastic bags. Use within 3 to 5 days.

Squash, summer varieties

Store in the refrigerator in crisper, plastic bags, or plastic containers and use within 3 to 5 days.

Sweet corn

Store unhusked and uncovered in the refrigerator. Use as soon as possible for sweetest flavor.

Sweet potatoes, hard-rind squashes, eggplant, and rutabagas

Store at cool room temperature (around 60° F). Temperatures below 50° F may cause chilling injury. These will keep several months at 60° F, but only about a week at room temperature.

Tomatoes

Store ripe tomatoes uncovered in the refrigerator. Can be stored in the refrigerator for up to a week, depending on ripeness when stored. Keep unripe tomatoes at room temperature away from direct sunlight until they ripen.

Nuts

Store in airtight containers in the refrigerator or freezer. Because of their high fat content, nuts require refrigeration to delay the development of rancidity.

In general, unshelled nuts may be stored at room temperature about 6 months. Shelled nuts, in moisture- and vapor-proof wrapping, can be refrigerated up to 6 months.

Unroasted nuts keep better than roasted ones.

Peanut butter

After a jar of peanut butter has been opened, it should be kept in the refrigerator. Remove it from the refrigerator a short time before using to allow it to soften.

Fruits

Plan to use fresh fruits promptly while they are sound and flavorful. Because fruits are fragile, they need special handling to keep them from being crushed or bruised. The softened tissues of bruised and crushed fruits permit the entrance of spoilage organisms that quickly break down quality.

Sort fruits before storing. Bruised or decayed fruit will contaminate sound, firm fruit.

Apples

Store mellow apples uncovered in the refrigerator. Unripe or hard apples are best held at cool room temperature (60° to 70° F) until ready to eat. Use ripe apples within a month.

Apricots, nectarines, and peaches

These fruits may be ripe when purchased. If not, store at room temperature until flesh begins to soften. Then refrigerate and use within 3 to 5 days.

Avocados, bananas, and pears

Allow these fruits to ripen at room temperature, then refrigerate. The skin on bananas will darken but the flesh will remain flavorful and firm. Use within 3 to 5 days.

Berries and cherries

Store covered in the refrigerator to prevent moisture loss. Do not wash or stem before storing. Use within 2 to 3 days.

Cranberries

Store covered in the refrigerator. Use within 1 week.

Grapes

Grapes are ready to use when purchased. Store covered in the refrigerator. Use within 3 to 5 days.

Citrus fruits

These fruits are best stored at a cool room temperature (60° to 70° F). Use within 2 weeks. Citrus fruits may also be stored uncovered in the refrigerator.

Melons

Keep at room temperature until ripe, then refrigerate. When storing cut melon, cover and refrigerate.

Pineapples

Pineapples will not ripen further after purchase. There will not be any increase in sugars during storage. Use pineapple as soon as possible, since holding results in deterioration. Once cut, pineapple may be stored in a tightly covered container 2 to 3 days.

Canned fruits and juices

After canned fruits and canned fruit juices have been opened, cover and store them in the refrigerator. They can be safely stored in their original containers; but for better flavor retention, storage in glass or plastic is recommended.

Plums

Plums are generally ripe when sold. Refrigerate and use within 3 to 5 days.

Dried fruits

Keep in tightly closed containers. May be stored in a cool place, for about 6 months. In warm, humid weather, store in the refrigerator.

Frozen fruit juices

Cover reconstituted fruit juice concentrates and keep in the refrigerator. For best flavor, keep in glass or plastic containers.

Jellies, jams, and preserves

After these fruit products have been opened, cover and store them in the refrigerator.

Miscellaneous Foods

Honey and syrups

Store at room temperature until opened. After the containers are opened, syrups are better protected from mold in the refrigerator. However, refrigeration hastens crystal formation. If crystals form, dissolve them by placing the container of honey or syrup in hot water.

Fats and oils

Most fats and oils need protection from air, heat, and light. Fats and oils in partially filled containers keep longer if they are transferred to smaller containers in which there is little or no air space.

Butter, fat drippings, and margarine

Store, tightly wrapped or covered, in the refrigerator. These products are best used within 2 weeks.

Keep only as much butter or margarine in the butter compartment of the refrigerator as needed for immediate use. Do not let butter or margarine stand for long periods of time at room temperature; exposure to heat and light hastens rancidity.

Cooking and salad oils

Keep small quantities at room temperature and use before flavor changes. For long storage, keep oils in the refrigerator. Some of these oils may cloud and solidify in the refrigerator; this is not harmful. If warmed to room temperature, they will become clear and liquid.

Hydrogenated shortenings and lard

Most of the firm vegetable shortenings and lard have been stabilized by hydrogenation or the addition of antioxidants. These shortenings can be held at room temperature without damage to flavor. Lard that is not stabilized should be refrigerated. Keep these products covered.

Mayonnaise and other salad dressings

Keep all homemade salad dressings in the refrigerator. Purchased mayonnaise and other ready-made salad dressings should be refrigerated after jars have been opened.

PREPARING AND COOKING FOODS

GENERAL POINTERS

- Serve food soon after cooking—or refrigerate promptly. Hot foods may be refrigerated if they do not raise the temperature of the refrigerator above 45° F. Keep them in the refrigerator until served or reheated.
- Speed the cooling of large quantities of food by refrigerating them in shallow containers.
- Keep hot foods HOT (above 140° F) and cold foods COLD (below 40° F). Food may not be safe to eat if held more than 2 or 3 hours at temperatures between 60° and 125° F, the zone in which bacteria grow rapidly. Remember to count all time during preparation, storage, and serving. See the food temperature guide in Figure 12–1.
- The holding of foods for several hours in an automatic oven prior to cooking is not safe if the food is in the temperature zone of 60° to 125° F for more than 2 or 3 hours.
- Thoroughly clean all dishes, utensils, and work surfaces with soap and water after each use. It is especially important to thoroughly clean equipment and work surfaces that have been used for raw food before you use them for cooked food. This prevents the cooked food from becoming contaminated with bacteria that may have been present in the raw food. Bacteria can be destroyed by rinsing utensils and work surfaces with chlorine laundry bleach in the proportion recommended on the package. Cutting boards, meat grinders, blenders, and can openers particularly need this protection.
- Always wipe up spills with paper towels or other disposable material.

Eggs and Egg-Rich Foods

Use only fresh, clean, unbroken, and odor-free eggs in any recipes in which eggs are not thoroughly cooked, such as in egg-milk drinks, soft-cooked eggs, poached eggs, scrambled eggs, omelets, uncooked salad dressings, ice cream, meringues, soft custards, or puddings cooked on the top of the range.

Cracked or soiled eggs may contain harmful bacteria. They should be used only in foods that are to be thoroughly cooked, such as baked goods or casseroles.

Cool hot foods containing a high proportion of eggs if they are not to be served hot. Set custards and puddings in ice water and stir large batches of pudding to speed cooling. Then refrigerate promptly until time to serve.

Meat, Poultry and Fish

Thaw frozen raw meat or unstuffed raw poultry in the refrigerator, or

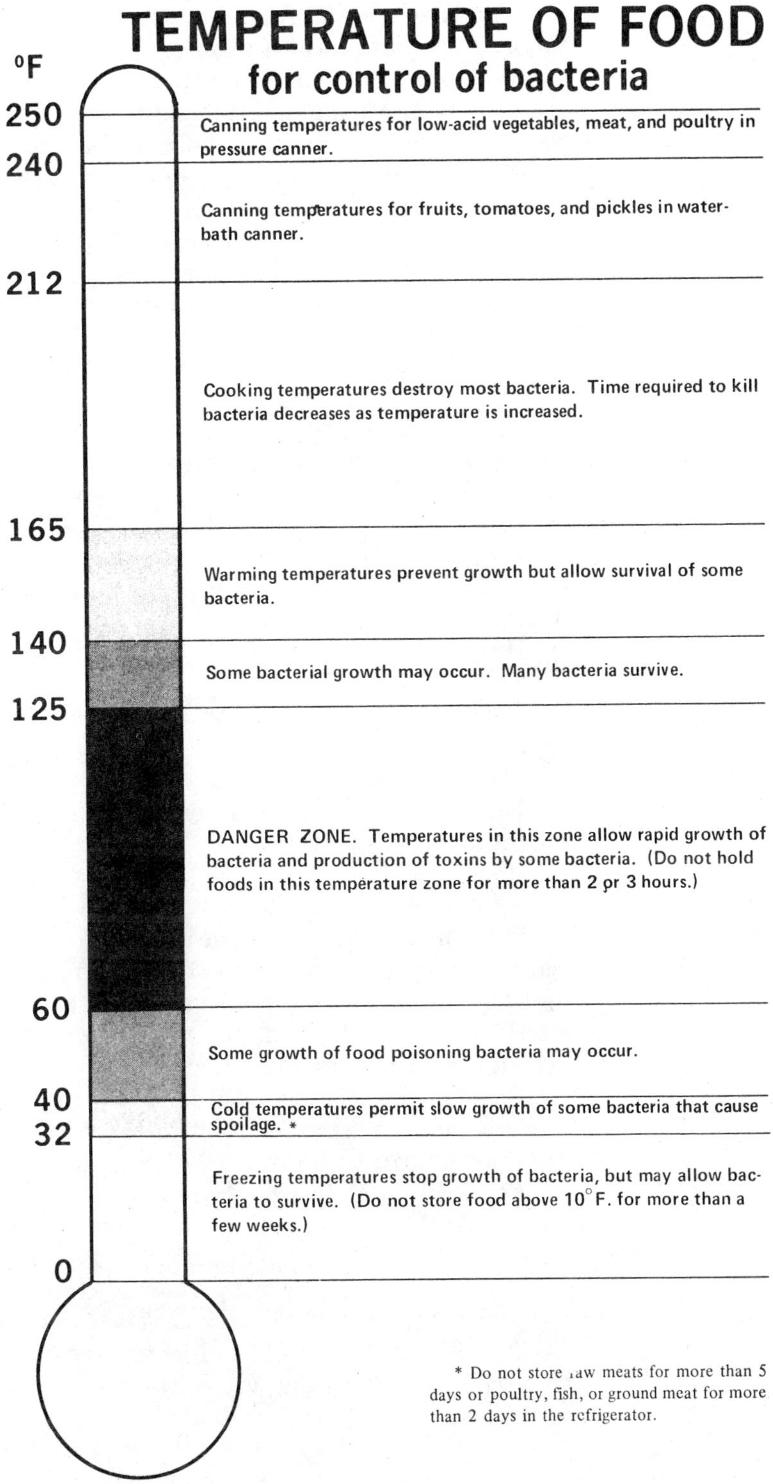

Figure 12–1. Temperature guide for storing food. (From "Keeping Food Safe to Eat — A Guide for Homemakers." Home and Garden Bulletin No. 162, U.S. Department of Agriculture, Washington, D.C.)

for a quicker method, immerse the package in its watertight wrapper in cold water. Thaw until meat is pliable.

You can cook frozen meat, poultry, or fish without thawing, but you must allow more cooking time to be sure the center of the meat is properly cooked. Allow at least one and a half times as long to cook as required for unfrozen or thawed products of the same weight and shape. Undercooked foods may not be safe to eat.

Stuff fresh or thawed meat, poultry, or fish just before roasting. Put the stuffing in lightly — without packing — to allow the stuffing to expand and heat to penetrate more quickly throughout the stuffing.

Cook meat, poultry or fish, as recommended in a reliable timetable. See Home and Garden Bulletin No. 1, "Family Fare: A Guide to Good Nutrition."

Make sure that the stuffing reaches a temperature of at least 165° F during roasting. To check the temperature of the stuffing after roasting, insert a meat thermometer in the stuffing for about 5 minutes. Cook longer if necessary. Any stuffing cooked separately in the oven should also reach 165° F.

Do not partially cook meat or poultry one day and complete the cooking the next day. Keep cooked meat, fish, or poultry hot (above 140° F) until it is served.

Heat leftovers thoroughly. Boil broth and gravies several minutes when reheating them.

Heat frozen cooked meat, poultry, or fish without thawing or thaw in the refrigerator before using.

Directions on the package of all prepared and partially prepared frozen foods must be followed exactly. Heating for the specified time assures that the food will be safe to eat.

FREEZING FOODS[1]

Strict sanitation in preparing any food for the freezer is a must. Food and utensils should be clean, because freezing does not kill the bacteria in food; it only stops their multiplication. Since bacteria continue to multiply after the food is thawed, the number of bacteria on and in foods must be held at a minimum before freezing it.

Freeze only high-quality food. Since bacteria are spread by handling, foods should be handled as little as possible. Mixtures that contain sauces and gravies favor the growth of disease causing bacteria.

Foods may safely be refrozen if they still contain ice crystals or if they are still cold — about 40° F — and have been held no longer than one or two days at refrigerator temperature after thawing. In general, if a food is safe to eat, it is safe to refreeze. *If the odor or color of any food is poor or questionable, do not taste it. Throw it out. The food may be dangerous.*

The eating quality of food is reduced by thawing and refreezing. This is true especially for fruits, vegetables, and prepared foods. The eating quality of red meats is reduced less than that of other foods.

CANNING FOODS

Commercially canned foods are considered safe because they are processed under carefully controlled conditions. However, if a canned food shows any sign of spoilage — bulging can ends, leakage, spurting liquid, off-odor, or mold — do not use it. Do not even taste it.

Home-canned vegetables, meat, and poultry may contain the toxin that causes botulism if they are not properly processed.

It is not safe to can vegetables, meat, or poultry in a boiling water bath, an oven, a steamer without pressure, or an open kettle. None of these methods will heat these products enough to kill the dangerous bacterial spores of *Clostridium botulinum* within a reasonable time.

There is no danger of botulism, however, if these foods are canned properly in a pressure canner. Be sure that the pressure canner is in perfect order and that each step of the canning process — including time and temperature directions — is followed exactly.

Tomatoes, pickled vegetables, and fruits can be processed safely in a boiling-water bath because they are more acidic than other vegetables, meat, and poultry. However, do not use overripe tomatoes for canning, since tomatoes lose acidity as they mature. Low acid tomatoes should be canned under pressure.

Heat usually makes any odor of spoilage more noticeable. Boil all home-canned vegetables and home-canned meats as follows, after opening and before tasting.

Bring home-canned vegetables to a rolling boil, then cover and boil for at least 10 minutes. Boil spinach and corn for 20 minutes. If the food looks spoiled, foams, or has an off-odor, *do not taste it;* destroy it.

Boil home-canned meat or poultry 20 minutes in a covered pan before tasting. If meat develops the characteristic odor of spoiled meat, destroy it without tasting.

BACTERIAL FOOD POISONING

Poor food-handling practices in the home often cause illness in the family, even though the foods were safe to eat when purchased or first prepared.

Lack of sanitation, insufficient cooking, and improper storage can allow bacteria in food to increase to dangerous levels. Some bacteria produce poisonous substances called toxins that cause illness when the food is eaten.

Outbreaks of illness from food contaminated by harmful bacteria are especially common during hot summer months, when perishable foods are carried on picnics and cookouts without proper refrigeration.

Certain bacteria growing in food may cause illness in one of the following ways. Disease-producting bacteria may enter the body in contaminated food and set up infections in the digestive tract and, in some cases, in the blood stream. Other bacteria may form dangerous toxins in food. Eating food in which the bacteria have grown and produced toxin causes illness.

Foods containing salmonellae can cause infection in man, called salmonellosis. The disease is difficult to control because it spreads simply and easily. Salmonella infections result from eating food in which large numbers of salmonellae are growing or from personal contact with an infested person or a carrier of the infection.

Bacteria that can produce poisonous toxins in food are *Staphylococcus aureus* and *Clostridium botulinum.* The first toxin, when eaten in food, results in so-called "staph" poisoning, probably the most common food-borne disease in the United States. The second toxin can cause botulism, the rarest and deadliest kind of food poisoning.

Another kind of bacteria involved in food-borne illness is *Clostridium perfringens.* These bacteria often cause diarrheal upsets, which are rarely fatal.

Specific information on the causes, symptoms, and prevention of bacterial food-borne illnesses is found in Table 12–1.

TABLE 12–1. Bacterial Food-borne Illness: Causes, Symptoms, and Prevention*

Name of Illness	What Causes It	Symptoms	Characteristics of Illness	Preventive Measures
Salmonellosis Examples of foods involved: Poultry, red meats, eggs, dried foods, dairy products.	Salmonellae. Bacteria widespread in nature, live and grow in intestinal tracts of human beings and animals.	Severe headache, followed by vomiting, diarrhea, abdominal cramps, and fever. Infants, elderly, and persons with low resistance are most susceptible. Severe infections cause high fever and may even cause death.	Transmitted by eating contaminated food, or by contact with infected persons or carriers of the infection. Also transmitted by insects, rodents, and pets. Onset: Usually within 12 to 36 hours. Duration: 2 to 7 days.	Salmonellae in food are destroyed by heating the food to 140° F and holding for 10 minutes or to higher temperatures for less time; for instance, 155° F for a few seconds. Refrigeration at 40° F inhibits the increase of Salmonellae, but they remain alive in foods in the refrigerator or freezer, and even in dried foods.
Perfringens poisoning Examples of foods involved: Stews, soups, or gravies made from poultry or red meat.	*Clostridium perfringens.* Spore-forming bacteria that grow in the absence of oxygen. Temperatures reached in thorough cooking of most foods are sufficient to destroy vegetative cells, but heat-resistant spores can survive.	Nausea without vomiting, diarrhea, acute inflammation of stomach and intestines.	Transmitted by eating food contaminated with abnormally large numbers of the bacteria. Onset: Usually within 8 to 20 hours. Duration: May persist for 24 hours.	To prevent growth of surviving bacteria in cooked meats, gravies, and meat casseroles that are to be eaten later, cool foods rapidly and refrigerate promptly at 40° F or below, or hold them above 140° F.
Staphylococcal poisoning (frequently called staph) Examples of foods involved: Custards, egg salad, potato salad, chicken salad, macaroni salad, ham, salami, cheese.	*Staphylococcus aureus.* Bacteria fairly resistant to heat. Bacteria growing in food produce a toxin that is extremely resistant to heat.	Vomiting, diarrhea, prostration, abdominal cramps. Generally mild and often attributed to other causes.	Transmitted by food handlers who carry the bacteria and by eating food containing the toxin. Onset: Usually within 3 to 8 hours. Duration: 1 to 2 days.	Growth of bacteria that produce toxin is inhibited by keeping hot foods above 140° F and cold foods at or below 40° F. Toxin is destroyed by boiling for several hours or heating the food in a pressure cooker at 240° F for 30 minutes.
Botulism Examples of foods involved: Canned low-acid foods, smoked fish.	*Clostridium botulinum.* Spore-forming organisms that grow and produce toxin in the absence of oxygen, such as in a sealed container.	Double vision, inability to swallow, speech difficulty, progressive respiratory paralysis. Fatality rate is high, in the United States about 65 per cent.	Transmitted by eating food containing the toxin. Onset: Usually within 12 to 36 hours or longer. Duration: 3 to 6 days.	Bacterial spores in food are destroyed by high temperatures obtained only in the pressure canner.† More than 6 hours is needed to kill the spores at boiling temperature (212° F). The toxin is destroyed by boiling for 10 to 20 minutes; time required depends on kind of food.

*From "Keeping Food Safe to Eat — A Guide for Homemakers." Home and Garden Bulletin No. 162, U.S. Department of Agriculture, Washington, D.C.

†For processing times in home canning, see Home and Garden Bulletin No. 8, "Home Canning of Fruits and Vegetables," and No. 106, "Home Canning of Meat and Poultry." U.S. Department of Agriculture, Washington, D.C.

REFERENCES

1. *Keeping Food Safe to Eat: A Guide for Homemakers*, Home and Garden Bulletin No. 162. U.S. Department of Agriculture, Washington, D.C., 1975.
2. *Storing Perishable Foods in the Home*, Home and Garden Bulletin No. 78. U.S. Department of Agriculture, Washington, D.C., 1975.

APPENDIX

1. Sources of Nutrition Information
2. Nutrition Materials
3. Growth Charts for Boys and Girls
4. 1983 Metropolitan Height and Weight Tables
5. Metric Conversions and Equivalents
6. Nutritive Values of Edible Parts of Food
7. Enteral Hyperalimentation Chart

APPENDIX 1

SOURCES OF NUTRITION INFORMATION

American Dental Association
211 East Chicago Avenue
Chicago, Ill. 60611

American Diabetes Association
18 East 48th Street
New York, N.Y. 10017
Diabetes Forecast (bimonthly)

American Dietetic Association (ADA)
430 North Michigan Avenue
Chicago, Ill. 60611
Journal of the American Diabetes Association (monthly)

American Heart Association (AHA)
7320 Greenville Avenue
Dallas, Tex. 75231

American Home Economics Association (AHEA)
2010 Massachusetts Avenue, N.W.
Washington, D.C. 20036
Journal of Home Economics (five times a year)

American Institute of Nutrition (AIN)
9650 Rockville Pike
Bethesda, Md. 20014
Journal of Nutrition (monthly)

American Medical Association (AMA)
535 North Dearborn Street
Chicago, Ill. 60610
Journal of the American Medical Association (weekly)

American Public Health Association (APHA)
1015 16th Street, N.W.
Washington, D.C. 20005
American Journal of Public Health (monthly)
The Nation's Health (monthly newspaper)

American Society of Clinical Nutrition, Inc. (ASCN)
9650 Rockville Pike
Bethesda, Md. 20014
The American Journal of Clinical Nutrition (monthly)

American Society for Parenteral and Enteral Nutrition (ASPEN)
6110 Executive Boulevard, Suite 810
Rockville, Md. 20852
Journal of Parenteral and Enteral Nutrition (bimonthly)
ASPEN Update (monthly newsletter)

Food and Drug Administration (FDA)
Consumer Information
Public Documents Distribution Center
Pueblo, Colo. 81009

Food and Nutrition Board (FNB) of National Research Council (NRC)
2101 Constitution Avenue, N.W.
Washington, D.C. 20418

National Dairy Council
6300 North River Road
Rosemont, Ill. 60018
Dairy Council Digest (bimonthly newsletter)

Nutrition Foundation, Inc.
888 17th Street, N.W.
Washington, D.C. 20006
Nutrition Reviews (monthly)

Nutrition Today Society
703 Giddings Avenue
Annapolis, Md. 21401
Nutrition Today (bimonthly)

Society for Nutrition Education (SNE)
2140 Shattuck Avenue, Suite 1110
Berkeley, Calif. 94704
Journal of Nutrition Education (quarterly)

U.S. Department of Agriculture
Institute of Home Economics
Washington, D.C. 20250
List of publications available from Office of Information

U.S. Department of Health and Human Services
Washington, D.C. 20204
List of publications available from Office of Information

APPENDIX 2

NUTRITION MATERIALS

Free or inexpensive nutrition materials are available by writing to the following addresses:

American Institute of Baking
400 East Ontario Street
Chicago, Ill. 60611

Borden Company
350 Madison Avenue
New York, N.Y. 10017

California Raisin Advisory Board
P.O. Box 5335
Fresno, Calif. 93755

Del Monte Corporation
Consumer and Education Services
Box 3757
San Francisco, Calif. 94119

Evaporated Milk Association
288 North La Salle Avenue
Chicago, Ill. 60601

Florida Citrus Commission
Box 148
Lakeland, Fla. 33802

General Foods Corporation
250 North Street
White Plains, N.Y. 10602

General Mills, Inc.
9200 Wayzata Boulevard
Minneapolis, Minn. 55426

Kellogg Company
Department of Home Economics Services
Battle Creek, Mich. 49016

Mead Johnson Nutritional Division
Evansville, Ind. 47721

Metropolitan Life Insurance Co.
Health and Welfare Division
1 Madison Avenue
New York, N.Y. 10010

National Livestock and Meat Board
Nutrition Research Department
444 North Michigan Avenue
Chicago, Ill. 60611

Peanut Association
342 Madison Avenue
New York, N.Y. 10017

Poultry and Egg National Board
250 West 57th Street
New York, N.Y. 10010

Potato Board
1385 South Colorado Boulevard
Denver, Colo. 80222

Ross Laboratories
Columbus, Ohio 43216

Sunkist Growers
P.O. Box 2706, Terminal Annex
Los Angeles, Calif. 90054

Wheat Flour Institute
309 West Jackson Boulevard
Chicago, Ill. 60606

APPENDIX 3

GROWTH CHARTS FOR BOYS AND GIRLS*

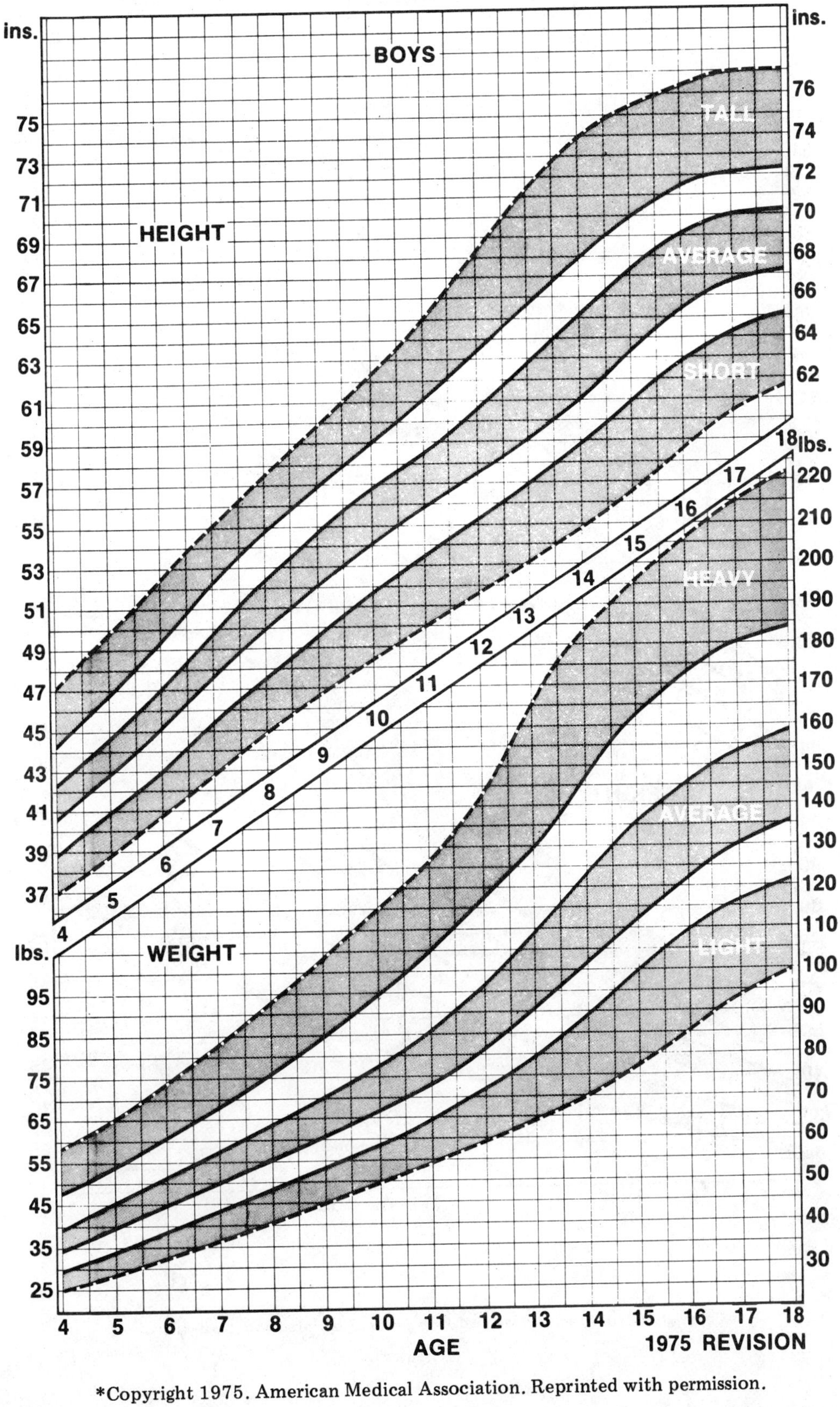

*Copyright 1975. American Medical Association. Reprinted with permission.

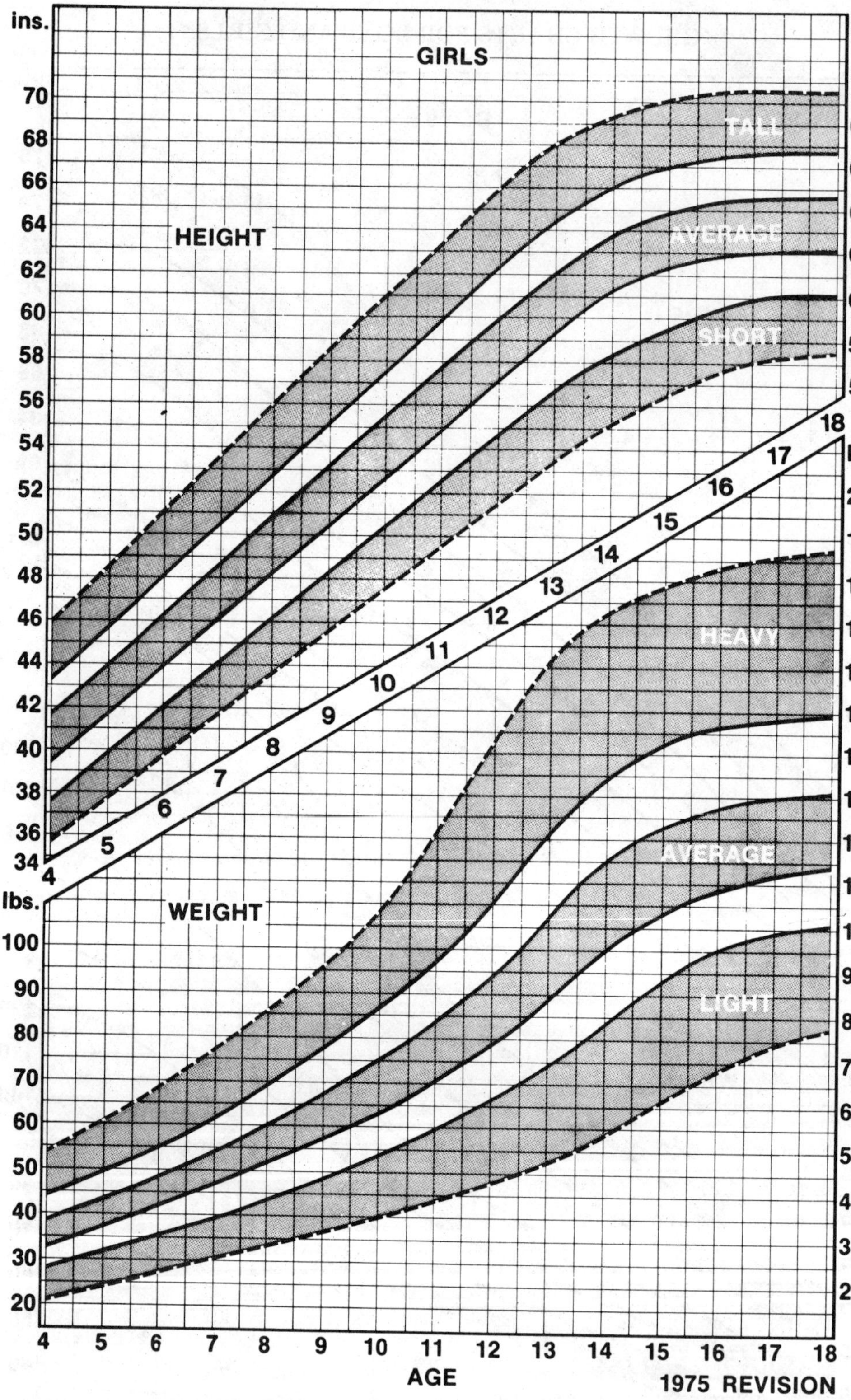
GIRLS
HEIGHT
WEIGHT
TALL
AVERAGE
SHORT
HEAVY
AVERAGE
LIGHT
ins.
70
68
66
64
62
60
58
56
54
52
50
48
46
44
42
40
38
36
34
ins.
71
69
67
65
63
61
59
57
lbs.
100
90
80
70
60
50
40
30
20
lbs.
205
195
185
175
165
155
145
135
125
115
105
95
85
75
65
55
45
35
25
4
5
6
7
8
9
10
11
12
13
14
15
16
17
18
AGE
1975 REVISION

APPENDIX 4

1983 METROPOLITAN HEIGHT AND WEIGHT TABLES

The Metropolitan Life Insurance Company has published height and weight tables as a public service. The weights are associated with greatest longevity for people aged 25 to 59, and the recently revised charts of 1983 are guidelines based on a mortality study of 4.2 million policy holders over the past 22 years. The study found that the average man is heavier than he was 20 years ago and that deaths associated with hypertension and overweight were noted to be fewer since then. It was also found that mildly elevated blood pressure can be treated effectively, so that normal life expectancy results. Longer life is still apparently associated with weighing somewhat less than what is average for one's height.

The new tables, which reflect the findings of the study, have created controversy in the medical community, since the weights are from 1 to 13 per cent higher than those published in 1959. Heart specialists are concerned that these new figures will foster a misconception that overweight or obesity may not be as detrimental to one's health after all. From the dietitian's point of view, also, it is still best to set personalized weight goals according to the needs of the individual and not based on population samples. The height and weight tables are not intended to give ideal weights.

Men (Ages 25–59)*					Women (Ages 25–59)*				
Height Feet	Height Inches	Small Frame	Medium Frame	Large Frame	Height Feet	Height Inches	Small Frame	Medium Frame	Large Frame
5	2	128–134	131–141	138–150	4	10	102–111	109–121	118–131
5	3	130–136	133–143	140–153	4	11	103–113	111–123	120–134
5	4	132–138	135–145	142–156	5	0	104–115	113–126	122–137
5	5	134–140	137–148	144–160	5	1	106–118	115–129	125–140
5	6	136–142	139–151	146–164	5	2	108–121	118–132	128–143
5	7	138–145	142–154	149–168	5	3	111–124	121–135	131–147
5	8	140–148	145–157	152–172	5	4	114–127	124–138	134–151
5	9	142–151	148–160	155–176	5	5	117–130	127–141	137–155
5	10	144–154	151–163	158–180	5	6	120–133	130–144	140–159
5	11	146–157	154–166	161–184	5	7	123–136	133–147	143–163
6	0	149–160	157–170	164–188	5	8	126–139	136–150	146–167
6	1	152–164	160–174	168–192	5	9	129–142	139–153	149–170
6	2	155–168	164–178	172–197	5	10	132–145	142–156	152–173
6	3	158–172	167–182	176–202	5	11	135–148	145–159	155–176
6	4	162–176	171–187	181–207	6	0	138–151	148–162	158–179

*Based on lowest mortality. Weight is given in pounds according to frame (in indoor clothing weighing 5 lbs [men] or 3 lbs [women], shoes with 1" heels). Source of basic data: *1979 Build Study*, Society of Actuaries and Association of Life Insurance Medical Directors of America, 1980. Copyright 1983, Metropolitan Life Insurance Company.

APPENDIX 5

METRIC CONVERSIONS AND EQUIVALENTS

Metric Conversions*

	To Change	to	Multiply by
Weight	Ounces	Grams	30†
	Pounds	Kilograms	0.45
	Grams	Ounces	0.035
	Kilograms	Pounds	2.2
Volume	Teaspoons	Milliliters	5
	Tablespoons	Milliliters	15
	Fluid ounces	Milliliters	30
	Cups	Liters	0.24
	Pints	Liters	0.47
	Quarts	Liters	0.95
	Gallons	Liters	3.8
	Milliliters	Fluid ounces	0.03
	Liters	Pints	2.1
	Liters	Quarts	1.06
	Liters	Gallons	0.26
Length	Inches	Centimeters	2.5
	Feet	Centimeters	30
	Yards	Meters	0.9
	Millimeters	Inches	0.04
	Centimeters	Feet	0.4
	Meters	Feet	3.3
	Meters	Yards	1.1

*From *Exchange Lists for Meal Planning.* American Diabetes Association, Inc., The American Dietetic Association, Chicago, 1976, p. 24. Reprinted by permission.

†The precise figure is 28.25. However, some dietitians find it more convenient to use 30.

Equivalents

1 ounce = 30 grams (approx.)
1 pound = 454 grams
1 gram = 1 milliliter
1 kilogram = 2.2 pounds
1 teaspoon = 5 milliliters
1 tablespoon = 15 milliliters
1 cup = 16 tablespoons = 240 milliliters
1 liter = 1000 milliliters
1 milligram = 1000 micrograms (mcg)

APPENDIX 6

NUTRITIVE VALUES OF THE EDIBLE PART OF FOODS*
(Dashes (-) denote lack of reliable data for a constituent believed to be present in measurable amount)

Foods, approximate measure, units, and weight (edible part unless footnotes indicate otherwise)			Nutrients in Indicated Quantity																
			A	B	C	D	E	F	G	H	I	J	K	L	M	N	O	P	Q
			Water	Food Energy	Protein	Fat	Saturated	Unsaturated Oleic	Unsaturated Linoleic	Carbohydrate	Calcium	Phosphorus	Iron	Potassium	Vitamin A value	Thiamin	Riboflavin	Niacin	Ascorbic Acid
		Grams	Percent	Calories	Grams	Grams	Grams	Grams	Grams	Grams	Milligrams	Milligrams	Milligrams	Milligrams	International units	Milligrams	Milligrams	Milligrams	Milligrams
DAIRY PRODUCTS (CHEESE, CREAM, IMITATION CREAM, MILK; RELATED PRODUCTS)																			
Cheese:																			
Cheddar: Cut pieces	1 oz.	28	37	115	7	9	6.1	2.1	.2	Trace	204	145	.2	28	300	.01	.11	Trace	0
Cottage, small curd, 4% fat	1 cup	210	79	220	26	9	6.0	2.2	.2	6	126	277	.3	177	340	.04	.34	.3	Trace
Cream	1 oz.	28	54	100	2	10	6.2	2.4	.2	1	23	30	.3	34	400	Trace	.06	Trace	0
Parmesan	1 tbsp.	5	18	25	2	2	1.0	.4	Trace	Trace	69	40	Trace	5	40	Trace	.02	Trace	0
Pasteurized Processed American	1 oz.	28	39	105	6	9	5.6	2.1	.2	Trace	174	211	.1	46	340	.01	.10	Trace	0
Swiss	1 oz.	28	37	105	8	8	5.0	1.7	.2	1	272	171	Trace	31	240	.01	.10	Trace	0
Cream:																			
Light, coffee, or table	1 tbsp.	15	74	30	Trace	3	1.8	.7	.1	1	14	12	Trace	18	110	Trace	.02	Trace	Trace
Heavy	1 tbsp.	15	58	80	Trace	6	3.5	1.4	.1	Trace	10	9	Trace	11	220	Trace	.02	Trace	Trace
Whipped topping, pressurized	1 tbsp.	3	61	10	Trace	1	.4	.2	Trace	Trace	3	3	Trace	4	30	Trace	Trace	Trace	0
Cream, sour	1 tbsp.	12	71	25	Trace	3	1.6	.6	.1	1	14	10	Trace	17	90	Trace	.02	Trace	Trace
Milk:																			
Fluid: Whole (3.3% fat)	1 cup	244	88	150	8	8	5.1	2.1	.2	11	291	228	.1	370	310[1]	.09	.40	.2	2
Low fat (2%) (No milk solids added)	1 cup	244	89	120	8	5	2.9	1.2	.1	12	297	232	.1	377	500	.10	.40	.2	2
Non fat (skim) (No milk solids added)	1 cup	245	91	85	8	Trace	.3	.1	Trace	12	302	247	.1	406	500	.09	.37	.2	2
Milk Beverages:																			
Chocolate milk (regular, commercial)	1 cup	250	82	210	8	8	5.3	2.2	.2	26	280	251	.6	417	300[2]	.09	.41	.3	2
Shake, thick, vanilla, net. wt., 11 oz.	1 container	313	74	350	12	9	5.9	2.4	.2	56	457	361	.3	572	360	.09	.61	.5	0
Milk Desserts:																			
Ice cream, hardened regular (about 11% fat)	1 cup	133	61	270	5	14	8.9	3.6	.3	32	176	134	.1	257	540	.05	.33	.1	1

*Taken from *Nutritive Value of Foods*, United States Department of Agriculture, Home and Garden Bulletin Number 72, Prepared by Agricultural Research Service, Washington, D.C., revised April 1977

[1] Vitamin A value is largely from beta carotene used for coloring

[2] Applies to product without vitamin A added

NUTRITIVE VALUES OF THE EDIBLE PART OF FOODS
(Dashes (-) denote lack of reliable data for a constituent believed to be present in measurable amount) *(Continued)*

Foods, approximate measure, units, and weight (edible part unless footnotes indicate otherwise)			Nutrients in Indicated Quantity															
			A	B	C	D	E	F	G	H	I	J	K	L	M	N	O	P	Q
			Water	Food Energy	Protein	Fat	Saturated	Unsaturated Oleic	Unsaturated Linoleic	Carbohydrate	Calcium	Phosphorus	Iron	Potassium	Vitamin A value	Thiamin	Riboflavin	Niacin	Ascorbic Acid
		Grams	Percent	Calories	Grams	Grams	Grams	Grams	Grams	Grams	Milligrams	Milligrams	Milligrams	Milligrams	International units	Milligrams	Milligrams	Milligrams	Milligrams
Milk Desserts: *(Continued)*																			
Ice milk, hardened regular	1 cup	131	69	185	5	6	3.5	1.4	.1	29	176	129	.1	265	210	.08	.35	.1	1
Sherbet (about 2% fat)	1 cup	193	66	270	2	4	2.4	1.0	.1	59	103	74	.3	198	190	.03	.09	.1	4
Custard, baked	1 cup	265	77	305	14	15	6.8	5.4	.7	29	297	310	1.1	387	930	.11	.50	.3	1
Pudding, chocolate, from mix and milk, regular, cooked	1 cup	260	70	320	9	8	4.3	2.6	.2	59	265	247	.8	354	340	.05	.39	.3	2
Yogurt:																			
With added milk solids made with low fat milk, fruit flavored	1 container (8 oz.)	227	75	230	10	3	1.8	.6	.1	42	343	269	.2	439[3]	120	.08	.40	.2	1
Egg, large, raw, whole	1 egg	50	75	80	6	6	1.7	2.0	.6	1	28	90	1.0	65	260	.04	.15	Trace	0
Butter:																			
Regular	1 tbsp.	14	16	100	Trace	12	7.2	2.9	.3	Trace	3	3	Trace	4	430[4]	Trace	Trace	Trace	0
Margarine:																			
Regular	1 tbsp.	14	16	100	Trace	12	2.1	5.3	3.1	Trace	3	3	Trace	4	470[5]	Trace	Trace	Trace	0
Oils, salad or cooking:																			
Corn	1 tbsp.	14	0	120	0	14	1.7	3.3	7.8	0	0	0	0	0	—	0	0	0	0
Salad Dressings:																			
Regular, French	1 tbsp.	16	39	65	Trace	6	1.1	1.3	3.2	3	2	2	.1	13	—	—	—	—	—
Italian	1 tbsp.	15	28	85	Trace	9	1.6	1.9	4.7	1	2	1	Trace	2	Trace	Trace	Trace	Trace	—
Mayonnaise	1 tbsp.	14	15	100	Trace	11	2.0	2.4	5.6	Trace	3	4	.1	5	40	Trace	.01	Trace	—
Tartar sauce	1 tbsp.	14	34	75	Trace	8	1.5	1.8	4.1	1	3	4	.1	11	30	Trace	Trace	Trace	Trace
FISH, SHELLFISH, MEAT, POULTRY, RELATED PRODUCTS																			
Fish sticks, breaded, cooked, frozen (4 X 1 X 1/2") or 1 fish stick	1 oz.	28	66	50	5	3	—	—	—	2	3	47	.1	—	0	.01	.02	.5	—
Haddock, breaded, fried[6]	3 oz.	85	66	140	17	5	1.4	2.2	1.2	5	34	210	1.0	296	—	.03	.06	2.7	2
Tuna, canned in oil, drained solids	3 oz.	85	61	170	24	7	1.7	1.7	.7	0	7	199	1.6	—	70	.04	.10	10.1	—
Bacon (20 slices per lb, raw), broiled or fried, crisp	2 slices	15	8	85	4	8	2.5	3.7	.7	Trace	2	34	.5	35	0	.08	.05	.8	—

Beef, cooked:																			
Cuts braised, simmered or pot roast. Lean and fat (piece 2 1/2 X 3/4")	3 oz.	85	53	245	23	16	6.8	6.5	.4	0	10	114	2.9	184	30	.04	.18	3.6	–
Ground beef, broiled Lean with 10% fat	3 oz.	85	60	185	23	10	4.0	3.9	.3	0	10	196	3.0	261	20	.08	.20	5.1	–
Roast, oven cooked, no liquid added: Lean and fat (2 pieces, 4 1/8 X 2 1/4 X 1/4")	3 oz.	85	62	165	25	7	2.8	2.7	.2	0	11	208	3.2	279	10	.06	1.9	4.5	–
Steak: Lean and fat (piece, 2 1/2 X 2 1/2 X 3/4")	3 oz.	85	44	330	20	27	11.3	11.1	.6	0	9	162	2.5	220	50	.05	.15	4.0	–
Beef, dried, chipped	2 1/2 oz. jar	71	48	145	24	4	2.1	2.0	.1	0	14	287	3.6	142	–	.05	.23	2.7	0
Beef and vegetable stew	1 cup	245	82	220	16	11	4.9	4.5	.2	15	29	184	2.9	613	2,400	.15	.17	4.7	17
Chili con carne with beans, canned	1 cup	255	72	340	19	16	7.5	6.8	.3	31	82	321	4.3	594	150	.08	.18	3.3	–
Lamb, cooked:																			
chop, rib (cut 3 per lb. with bone), broiled Lean and fat	3.1 oz.	89	43	360	18	32	14.8	12.1	1.2	0	8	139	1.0	200	–	.11	.19	4.1	–
Leg, roasted: Lean and fat (2 pcs. 4 1/8 X 2 1/4 X 1/4")	3 oz.	85	54	235	22	16	7.3	6.0	.6	0	9	177	1.4	241	–	.13	.23	4.7	–
Liver, beef, fried[7] (slice, 6 1/2 X 2 3/8 X 3/8")	3 oz.	85	56	195	22	9	2.5	3.5	.9	5	9	405	7.5	323	45,390[8]	.22	3.56	14.0	23
Pork, cured, cooked:																			
Ham, light cure, lean and fat, roasted (2 pcs. 4 1/8 X 2 1/4 X 1/4")[9]	3 oz.	85	54	245	18	19	6.8	7.9	1.7	0	8	146	2.2	199	0	.40	.15	3.1	–
Luncheon meat: Boiled ham, slice (8 per 8 oz. pkg.)	1 oz.	28	59	65	5	5	1.7	2.0	.4	0	3	47	.8	–	0	.12	.04	.7	–
Pork, fresh, cooked: Roast, oven cooked, no liquid added: Lean and fat (pc. 2 1/2 X 2 1/2 X 3/4")	3 oz.	85	46	310	21	24	8.7	10.2	2.2	0	9	218	2.7	233	0	.78	.22	4.8	–
Sausages:																			
Brown and serve (10-11 per 8 oz. pkg.) browned	1 link	17	40	70	3	6	2.3	2.8	.7	Trace	–	–	–	–	–	–	–	–	–

[3] Applies to product made with milk containing no added vitamin A
[4] Based on year-round average
[5] Based on average vitamin A content of fortified margarine
[6] Dipped in egg, milk or water, and bread crumbs, fried in vegetable shortening
[7] Regular type margarine used
[8] Value varies widely
[9] About 1/4 of the outer layer of the fat on the cut was removed. Deposits of fat within the cut were not removed

NUTRITIVE VALUES OF THE EDIBLE PART OF FOODS
(Dashes (-) denote lack of reliable data for a constituent believed to be present in measurable amount) *(Continued)*

Foods, approximate measure, units, and weight (edible part unless footnotes indicate otherwise)			A Water	B Food Energy	C Protein	D Fat	E Saturated	F Unsaturated Oleic	G Unsaturated Linoleic	H Carbohydrate	I Calcium	J Phosphorus	K Iron	L Potassium	M Vitamin A value	N Thiamin	O Riboflavin	P Niacin	Q Ascorbic Acid
		Grams	Percent	Calories	Grams	Grams	Grams	Grams	Grams	Grams	Milligrams	Milligrams	Milligrams	Milligrams	International units	Milligrams	Milligrams	Milligrams	Milligrams
Sausages: (Continued)																			
Frankfurter (8 per 1-lb. pkg.), cooked (reheated)	1 frankfurter	56	57	170	7	15	5.6	6.5	1.2	1	3	57	.8	–	–	.08	.11	1.4	–
Veal, medium fat, cooked, bone removed; cutlet (4 X 2¼ X ½"), braised or broiled	3 oz.	85	60	185	23	9	4.0	3.4	.4	0	9	196	2.7						
Poultry and poultry products:																			
Chicken, cooked:																			
Breast, fried,[10] bones removed, ½ breast (3.3 oz. with bones)	2.8 oz.	79	58	160	26	5	1.4	1.8	1.1	1	9	218	1.3	–	70	.04	.17	11.6	–
Drumstick, fried,[10] bones removed, (2 oz. with bones)	1.3 oz.	38	55	90	12	4	1.1	1.3	.9	Trace	6	89	.9	–	50	.03	.15	2.7	–
Turkey, roasted, flesh without skin: Light and dark meat pcs. (1 slice white meat, 4 X 2 X ¼" with 2 slices dark meat, 2½ X 1⅝ X ¼")	3 pcs.	85	61	160	27	5	1.5	1.0	1.1	0	7	213	1.5	312	–	.04	.15	6.5	–
FRUITS AND FRUIT PRODUCTS																			
Apple, raw, unpeeled, without cores: 2¾" diameter (about 3 per lb. with cores)	1 apple	138	84	80	Trace	1	–	–	–	20	10	14	.4	152	120	.04	.03	.1	6
Applejuice, bottled or canned	1 cup	248	88	120	Trace	Trace	–	–	–	30	15	22	1.5	250	–	.02	.05	.2	2[11]
Applesauce, canned, unsweetened	1 cup	244	89	100	Trace	Trace	–	–	–	26	10	12	1.2	190	100	.05	.02	.1	2[11]
Apricots:																			
Raw, without pits (about 12 per lb. with pits)	3 apricots	107	85	55	1	Trace	–	–	–	14	18	25	.5	301	2,890	.03	.04	.6	11

Canned in heavy syrup (halves and syrup)	1 cup	258	77	220	2	Trace	—	—	—	57	28	39	.8	604	4,490	.05	.05	1.0	10
Apricot nectar, canned	1 cup	251	85	145	1	Trace	—	—	—	37	23	30	.5	379	2,380	.03	.03	.5	36[12]
Banana without peel (about 2.6 per lb. with peel)	1 banana	119	76	100	1	Trace	—	—	—	26	10	31	.8	440	230	.06	.07	.8	12
Blueberries, raw	1 cup	145	83	90	1	1	—	—	—	22	22	19	1.5	117	150	.04	.09	.7	20
Dates: whole, without pits	10 dates	80	23	220	2	Trace	—	—	—	58	47	50	2.4	518	40	.07	.08	1.8	0
Fruit cocktail, canned, in heavy syrup	1 cup	255	80	195	1	Trace	—	—	—	50	23	31	1.0	411	360	.05	.03	1.0	5
Grapefruit, raw, med., 3¾" diameter (about 1 lb. 1 oz.) white	½ grapefruit with peel[13]	241	89	50	1	Trace	—	—	—	12	19	19	.5	166	540	.05	.02	.2	44
Grapefruit juice: canned white, unsweetened	1 cup	247	89	100	1	Trace	—	—	—	24	20	35	1.0	400	20	.07	.05	.5	84
Grapes, Thompson seedless	10 grapes	50	81	35	Trace	Trace	—	—	—	9	6	10	.2	87	50	.03	.02	.2	2
Grapes, Tokay and Emperor, seeded	10 grapes[14]	60	81	40	Trace	Trace	—	—	—	10	7	11	.2	99	60	.03	.02	.2	2
Grape juice: concentrate, Frozen, diluted with 3 parts water by vol.	1 cup	250	86	135	1	Trace	—	—	—	33	8	10	.3	85	10	.05	.08	.5	10[15]
Lemonade concentrate, frozen: Diluted with 4⅓ parts water by vol.	1 cup	248	89	105	Trace	Trace	—	—	—	28	2	3	.1	40	10	.01	.02	.2	17
Cantaloup, orange-fleshed (with rind and seed cavity, 5" diam., 2⅓ lb.)	½ melon with rind[16]	477	91	80	2	Trace	—	—	—	20	38	44	1.1	682	9,240	.11	.08	1.6	90
Honeydew (with rind and seed cavity, 6½" diam., 5¼ lb.)	1/10 melon[16] with rind	226	91	50	1	Trace	—	—	—	11	21	24	.6	374	60	.06	.04	.9	34
Orange, raw, whole, 2⅝" diam., without peel and seeds (about 2½ per lb. with peel and seeds)	1 orange	131	86	65	1	Trace	—	—	—	16	54	26	.5	263	260	.13	.05	.5	66
Orange juice: frozen concentrate, diluted with 3 parts water by vol.	1 cup	249	87	120	2	Trace	—	—	—	29	25	42	.2	503	540	.23	.03	.9	120

[10] Vegetable shortening used
[11] Applies to product without added ascorbic acid
[12] Based on product with label claim of 100% of USRDA in 6 fluid oz.
[13] Weight includes peel and membrane between sections. Without these parts, the weight of the edible portion is 118 g.
[14] Weight includes seeds. Without seeds, weight of the edible portion is 57 g.
[15] Applies to product without added ascorbic acid
[16] Weight includes rind. Without rind, the weight of the edible portion is 272 g.

NUTRITIVE VALUES OF THE EDIBLE PART OF FOODS
(Dashes (-) denote lack of reliable data for a constituent believed to be present in measurable amount) *(Continued)*

Foods, approximate measure, units, and weight (edible part unless footnotes indicate otherwise)			A	B	C	D	E	F	G	H	I	J	K	L	M	N	O	P	Q
								Nutrients in Indicated Quantity											
								Unsaturated											
			Water	Food Energy	Protein	Fat	Saturated	Oleic	Linoleic	Carbohydrate	Calcium	Phosphorus	Iron	Potassium	Vitamin A value	Thiamin	Riboflavin	Niacin	Ascorbic Acid
		Grams	Percent	Calories	Grams	Grams	Grams	Grams	Grams	Grams	Milligrams	Milligrams	Milligrams	Milligrams	International units	Milligrams	Milligrams	Milligrams	Milligrams
Peaches, canned, sliced, syrup pack (yellow-fleshed, solids and liquid)	1 cup	256	79	200	1	Trace	–	–	–	51	10	31	.8	333	1,100	.03	.05	1.5	8
Pears, raw, with skin, cored: Bartlett, 2½" diam. (about 2½ per lb. with cores and stems)	1 pear	164	83	100	1	1	–	–	–	25	13	18	.5	213	30	.03	.07	.2	7
Pears, canned, solids and liquid, syrup pack, heavy (halves or slices)	1 cup	255	80	195	1	1	–	–	–	50	13	18	.5	214	10	.03	.05	.3	3
Pineapple: canned, heavy syrup pack, solids and liquid, crushed, chunks, tidbits	1 cup	255	80	190	1	Trace	–	–	–	49	28	13	.8	245	130	.20	.05	.5	18
Pineapple juice, unsweetened, canned	1 cup	250	86	140	1	Trace	–	–	–	34	38	23	.8	373	130	.13	.05	.5	80[17]
Plums, raw, prune-type (1½" diam., about 15 per lb. with pits)	1 plum	28	79	20	Trace	Trace	–	–	–	6	3	5	.1	48	80	.01	.01	.1	1
Plums, canned, heavy syrup pack (Italian prunes), with pits and liquid	1 cup[18]	272	77	215	1	Trace	–	–	–	56	23	26	2.3	367	3,130	.05	.05	1.0	5
Prunes, dried, cooked, unsweetened, all sizes, fruit and liquid	1 cup	250	66	255	2	1	–	–	–	67	51	79	3.8	695	1,590	.07	.15	1.5	2
Prune juice, canned or bottled	1 cup	256	80	195	1	Trace	–	–	–	49	36	51	1.8	602	–	.03	.03	1.0	5
Strawberries: raw, whole, capped	1 cup	149	90	55	1	1	–	–	–	13	31	31	1.5	244	90	.04	.10	.9	88
Strawberries: frozen, sweetened, sliced, 10 oz. container	1 container	284	71	310	1	1	–	–	–	79	40	48	2.0	318	90	.06	.17	1.4	151
Tangerine, raw, 2⅜" diam., size 176, without peel (about 4 per lb. with peel and seeds)	1 tangerine	86	87	40	1	Trace	–	–	–	10	34	15	.3	108	360	.05	.02	.1	27

Watermelon, raw, 4 X 8" wedge with rind and seeds (1/16 of 32 2/3 lb. melon, 10 X 16")	1 wedge with rind & seeds[19]	926	93	110	2	1	—	—	—	27	30	43	2.1	426	2,510	.13	.13	.9	30
GRAIN PRODUCTS																			
Bagel, 3" diam. made with egg	1 bagel	55	32	165	6	2	0.5	0.9	0.8	28	9	43	1.2	41	30	.14	.10	1.2	0
Biscuit, 2" diam. (enriched flour, vegetable shortening), from home recipe	1 biscuit	28	27	105	2	5	1.5	2.0	1.2	13	34	49	.4	33	Trace	.08	.08	.7	Trace
Boston brown bread, canned, slice 3 1/4 X 1/2")[20]	1 slice	45	45	95	2	1	.1	.2	.2	21	41	72	.9	131	0[21]	.06	.04	.7	0
French bread, enriched (5 X 2 1/2 X 1")	1 slice	35	31	100	3	1	.2	.4	.4	19	15	30	.8	32	Trace	.14	.08	1.2	Trace
Raisin bread, enriched, slice (18 per loaf)	1 slice	25	35	65	2	1	.2	.3	.2	13	18	22	.6	58	Trace	.09	.06	.6	Trace
Rye bread: American, light (2/3 enriched wheat flour, 1/3 rye flour): slice (4 1/4 X 3 3/4 X 7/16")	1 slice	25	36	60	2	Trace	Trace	Trace	.1	13	19	37	.5	36	0	.07	.05	.7	0
White bread, enriched: soft crumb type, slice (18 per loaf)	1 slice	25	36	70	2	1	.2	.3	.3	13	21	24	.6	26	Trace	.10	.06	.8	Trace
Corn grits, degermed, enriched	1 cup	245	87	125	3	Trace	Trace	Trace	.1	27	2	25	.7	27	Trace[22]	.10	.07	1.0	0
Farina, quick-cooking, enriched	1 cup	245	89	105	3	Trace	Trace	Trace	.1	22	147	113[23]	([24])	25	0	.12	.07	1.0	0
Oatmeal or rolled oats	1 cup	240	87	130	5	2	.4	.8	.9	23	22	137	1.4	146	0	.19	.05	.2	0
Wheat, rolled	1 cup	240	80	180	5	1	—	—	—	41	19	182	1.7	202	0	.17	.07	2.2	0
Bran flakes (40% bran), added sugar, salt, iron, vitamins	1 cup	35	3	105	4	1	—	—	—	28	19	125	12.4	137	1,650	.41	.49	4.1	12
Corn flakes, plain, added sugar, salt, iron, vitamins	1 cup	25	4	95	2	Trace	—	—	—	21	([25])	9	0.6	30	1,180	0.29	0.35	2.9	9

[17] Based on product with label claim of 100% of USRDA in 6 fluid oz.
[18] Weight includes pits. After removal of the pits, the weight of the edible portion is 258 g.
[19] Weight includes rind and seeds. Without rind and seeds, weight of the edible portion is 426 g.
[20] Made with vegetable shortening
[21] Applies to product made with white cornmeal
[22] Applies to white varieties
[23] Applies to products that do not contain di-sodium phosphate
[24] Value may range from less than 1 mg. to about 8 mg. depending on the brand. Consult the label
[25] Value varies with the brand. Consult the label

NUTRITIVE VALUES OF THE EDIBLE PART OF FOODS
(Dashes (-) denote lack of reliable data for a constituent believed to be present in measurable amount) *(Continued)*

Foods, approximate measure, units, and weight (edible part unless footnotes indicate otherwise)			A	B	C	D	E	F	G	H	I	J	K	L	M	N	O	P	Q
			Water	Food Energy	Protein	Fat	Saturated	Unsaturated Oleic	Unsaturated Linoleic	Carbohydrate	Calcium	Phosphorus	Iron	Potassium	Vitamin A value	Thiamin	Riboflavin	Niacin	Ascorbic Acid
		Grams	Percent	Calories	Grams	Grams	Grams	Grams	Grams	Grams	Milligrams	Milligrams	Milligrams	Milligrams	International units	Milligrams	Milligrams	Milligrams	Milligrams
Wheat, shredded, plain	1 oblong biscuit or 1/2 cup spoon-size biscuits	25	7	90	2	1	–	–	–	20	11	97	.9	87	10	.06	.03	1.1	0
Wheat germ, without salt and sugar, toasted	1 tbsp.	6	4	25	2	1	–	–	–	3	3	70	.5	57	10	.11	.05	.3	1
Coffeecake, 1/6 of a cake 7 3/4 X 5 5/8 X 1 1/4"	1 piece	72	30	230	5	7	2.0	2.7	1.5	38	44	125	1.2	78	120	.14	.15	1.3	Trace
Gingerbread, piece, 1/9 of 8" square cake	1 piece	63	37	175	2	4	1.1	1.8	1.1	32	57	63	.9	173	Trace	.09	.11	.8	Trace
Plain cake with uncooked white icing 1/9 of a 9" square cake	1 piece	121	21	445	4	14	4.7	5.5	2.7	77	61	91	.8	74[26]	240	.14	.16	1.1	Trace
Brownie, home-prepared, 1 3/4 X 1 3/4 X 7/8"	1 brownie	20	10	95	1	6	1.5	3.0	1.2	10	8	30	.4	38	40	.04	.03	.2	Trace
Chocolate chip cookie from home recipe, 2 1/3" diam.	4 cookies	40	3	205	2	12	3.5	4.5	2.9	24	14	40	.8	47	40	.06	.06	.5	Trace
Vanilla wafers, 1 3/4" diam., 1/2" thick	10 cookies	40	3	185	2	6	–	–	–	30	16	25	.6	29	50	.10	.09	.8	0
Graham crackers, plain, 2 1/2" square	2 crackers	14	6	55	1	1	.3	.5	.3	10	6	21	.5	55	0	.02	.08	.5	0
Saltines, made with enriched flour	4 crackers	11	4	50	1	1	.3	.5	.4	8	2	10	.5	13	0	.05	.05	.4	0
Danish pastry (enriched flour), plain without fruit or nuts, round piece about 4 1/4" diam. X 1"	1 pastry	65	22	275	5	15	4.7	6.1	3.2	30	33	71	1.2	73	200	.18	.19	1.7	Trace
Doughnut, cake type, plain, 2 1/2" diam., 1" high	1 doughnut	25	24	100	1	5	1.2	2.0	1.1	13	10	48	.4	23	20	.05	.05	.4	Trace
Doughnut, yeast-leavened, glazed, 3 3/4" diam., 1 1/4" high	1 doughnut	50	26	205	3	11	3.3	5.8	3.3	22	16	33	.6	34	25	.10	.10	.8	0
Macaroni, enriched, cooked (cut lenghts, elbows, shells): hot, tender stage.	1 cup	140	73	155	5	1	–	–	–	32	11	70	1.3	85	0	.20	.11	1.5	0

Nutrients in Indicated Quantity

Muffin, bran, made with enriched flour from home recipe	1 muffin	40	35	105	3	4	1.2	1.4	.8	17	57	162	1.5	172	90	.07	.10	1.7	Trace
Muffin, corn (enriched, degermed cornmeal and flour), 2 3/8" diam., 1 1/2" high	1 muffin	40	33	125	3	4	1.2	1.6	.9	19	42	68	.7	54	120[27]	.10	.10	.7	Trace
Noodles (egg noodles), enriched, cooked	1 cup	160	71	200	7	2	—	—	—	37	16	94	1.4	70	110	.22	.13	1.9	0
Pancakes, (4" diam.), plain, home-made using enriched flour	1 cake	27	50	60	2	2	.5	.8	.5	9	27	38	.4	33	30	.06	.07	.5	Trace
Pie, apple, sector (1/7 of pie	1 sector	135	48	345	3	15	3.9	6.4	3.6	51	11	30	.9	108	40	.15	.11	1.3	2
Pie, banana cream, sector, 1/7 of pie	1 sector	130	54	285	6	12	3.8	4.7	2.3	40	86	107	1.0	264	330	.11	.22	1.0	1
Pie, blueberry, sector, 1/7 of pie	1 sector	135	51	325	3	15	3.5	6.2	3.6	47	15	31	1.4	88	40	.15	.11	1.4	4
Pie, cherry, sector, 1/7 of pie	1 sector	135	47	350	4	15	4.0	6.4	3.6	52	19	34	.9	142	590	.16	.12	1.4	Trace
Pie, custard, sector, 1/7 of pie	1 sector	130	58	285	8	14	4.8	5.5	2.5	30	125	147	1.2	178	300	.11	.27	.8	0
Pie, lemon meringue, sector, 1/7 of pie	1 sector	120	47	305	4	12	3.7	4.8	2.3	45	17	59	1.0	60	200	.09	.12	.7	4
Pie, mince, sector, 1/7 of pie	1 sector	135	43	365	3	16	4.0	6.6	3.6	56	38	51	1.9	240	Trace	.14	.12	1.4	1
Pizza (cheese) baked, 4 3/4" sector; 1/8 or 12" diam. pie	1 sector	60	45	145	6	4	1.7	1.5	0.6	22	86	89	1.1	67	230	0.16	0.18	1.6	4
Popcorn, popped: with oil (coconut) and salt added, large kernel	1 cup	9	3	40	1	2	1.5	.2	.2	5	1	19	.2	—	—	—	.01	.2	0
Pretzels, stick, 2 1/4" long, made with enriched flour	10 pretzels	3	5	10	Trace	Trace	—	—	—	2	1	4	Trace	4	0	.01	.01	.1	0
Rolls, enriched, brown and serve (12 per 12 oz. pkg.), browned	1 roll	26	27	85	2	2	.4	.7	.5	14	20	23	.5	25	Trace	.10	.06	.9	Trace
Hoagie or submarine, 11 1/2 X 3 X 2 1/2"	1 roll	135	31	390	12	4	.9	1.4	1.4	75	58	115	3.0	122	Trace	.54	.32	4.5	Trace
Spaghetti (enriched) with meat balls and tomato sauce from home recipe	1 cup	248	70	330	19	12	3.3	6.3	.9	39	124	236	3.7	665	1,590	.25	.30	4.0	22
Waffles made with enriched flour, 7" diam., from mix, milk and egg added	1 waffle	75	42	205	7	8	2.8	2.9	1.2	27	179	257	1.0	146	170	.14	.22	.9	Trace

[26] Applies to product made with a sodium aluminum-sulfate type baking powder
[27] Applies to product made with yellow cornmeal

NUTRITIVE VALUES OF THE EDIBLE PART OF FOODS
(Dashes (-) denote lack of reliable data for a constituent believed to be present in measurable amount) *(Continued)*

Foods, approximate measure, units, and weight (edible part unless footnotes indicate otherwise)			Nutrients in Indicated Quantity																
			A	B	C	D	E	F	G	H	I	J	K	L	M	N	O	P	Q
			Water	Food Energy	Protein	Fat	Satu-rated	Unsaturated: Oleic	Unsaturated: Linoleic	Carbo-hydrate	Calcium	Phospho-rus	Iron	Potas-sium	Vitamin A value	Thiamin	Ribo-flavin	Niacin	Ascorbic Acid
		Grams	Percent	Calories	Grams	Grams	Grams	Grams	Grams	Grams	Milli-grams	Milli-grams	Milli-grams	Milli-grams	Interna-tional units	Milli-grams	Milli-grams	Milli-grams	Milli-grams
LEGUMES (DRY), NUTS, SEEDS; RELATED PRODUCTS																			
Beans, dry:																			
Pea beans, cooked, drained (Navy)	1 cup	190	69	225	15	1	–	–	–	40	95	281	5.1	790	0	.27	.13	1.3	0
Red kidney, cooked, drained	1 cup	255	76	230	15	1	–	–	–	42	74	278	4.6	673	10	.13	.10	1.5	–
Peanut Butter	1 tbsp.	16	2	95	4	8	1.5	3.7	2.3	3	9	61	.3	100	–	.02	.02	2.4	0
Peas, split, dry, cooked	1 cup	200	70	230	16	1	–	–	–	42	22	178	3.4	592	80	.30	.18	1.8	0
SUGARS AND SWEETS																			
Candy, hard	1 oz.	28	1	110	0	Trace	–	–	–	28	6	2	.5	1	0	0	0	0	0
Fudge, chocolate, plain	1 oz.	28	8	115	1	3	1.3	1.4	.6	21	22	24	.3	42	Trace	.01	.03	.1	Trace
Jellies	1 tbsp.	18	29	50	Trace	Trace	–	–	–	13	4	1	.3	14	Trace	Trace	.01	Trace	1
Syrup, table blend, chiefly corn, light and dark	1 tbsp.	21	24	60	0	0	0	0	0	15	9	3	.8	1	0	0	0	0	0
Sugar, white granulated	1 tbsp.	12	1	45	0	0	0	0	0	12	0	0	Trace	Trace	0	0	0	0	0
VEGETABLE AND VEGETABLE PRODUCTS																			
Asparagus, green, cuts and tips, 1½ to 2" lengths, from frozen, cooked and drained	1 cup	180	93	40	6	Trace	–	–	–	6	40	115	2.2	396	1,530	.25	.23	1.8	41
Beans, green snap, cooked and drained cuts from frozen	1 cup	135	92	35	2	Trace	–	–	–	8	54	43	.9	205	780	.09	.12	.5	7
Beets, cooked, drained, peeled, diced or sliced	1 cup	170	91	55	2	Trace	–	–	–	12	24	39	.9	354	30	.05	.07	.5	10
Black-eyed peas, immature seeds, cooked and drained from frozen	1 cup	170	66	220	15	1	–	–	–	40	43	286	4.8	573	290	.68	.19	2.4	15
Broccoli, cooked, drained from frozen stalks, medium size	1 stalk	180	91	45	6	1	–	–	–	8	158	112	1.4	481	4,500	.16	.36	1.4	162

Brussels sprouts, cooked, drained, frozen	1 cup	155	89	50	5	Trace	—	—	—	10	33	95	1.2	457	880	.12	.16	.9	126
Cabbage, cooked, drained	1 cup	145	94	30	2	Trace	—	—	—	6	64	29	.4	236	190	.06	.06	.4	48
Carrots, cooked, drained, canned	1 cup	155	91	50	1	Trace	—	—	—	11	51	48	.9	344	16,280	.08	.08	.8	9
Cauliflower, cooked, drained from frozen	1 cup	180	94	30	3	Trace	—	—	—	6	31	68	.9	373	50	.07	.09	.7	74
Celery, Pascal type, raw pieces, diced	1 cup	120	94	20	1	Trace	—	—	—	5	47	34	.4	409	320	.04	.04	.4	11
Corn, sweet, cooked, drained from raw, ear 5 X 1³/₄"	1 ear[28]	140	74	70	2	1	—	—	—	16	2	69	.5	151	310	.09	.08	1.1	7
Corn, cream style, canned	1 cup	256	76	210	5	2	—	—	—	51	8	143	1.5	248	840[29]	.08	.13	2.6	13
Cucumber slices, ¹/₈" thick, without peel	9 small pcs.	28	96	5	Trace	Trace	—	—	—	1	5	5	0.1	45	Trace	0.01	0.01	0.1	3
Lettuce, raw, loose leaf, chopped or shredded	1 cup	55	94	10	1	Trace	—	—	—	2	37	14	.8	145	1,050	.03	.04	.2	10
Lettuce, head, pieces, chopped	1 cup	55	96	5	Trace	Trace	—	—	—	2	11	12	.3	96	180	.03	.03	.2	3
Onions, mature, raw, chopped	1 cup	170	89	65	3	Trace	—	—	—	15	46	61	.9	267	Trace[30]	.05	.07	.3	17
Peas, green, canned whole, drained solids	1 cup	170	77	150	8	1	—	—	—	29	44	129	3.2	163	1,170	.15	.10	1.4	14
Peppers, sweet (about 5 per lb., whole, stem and seeds removed, raw	1 pod	74	93	15	1	Trace	—	—	—	4	7	16	.5	157	310	.06	.06	.4	94
Potato, cooked, peeled before boiling (about 3 per lb.)	1 potato	135	83	90	3	Trace	—	—	—	20	8	57	.7	385	Trace	.12	.05	1.6	22
Potato, French fried, strip, 2 to 3¹/₂" long, prepared from raw	10 strips	50	45	135	2	7	1.7	1.2	3.3	18	8	56	.7	427	Trace	.07	.04	1.6	11
Potato, mashed, prepared from raw with milk added	1 cup	210	83	135	4	2	.7	.4	Trace	27	50	103	.8	548	40	.17	.11	2.1	21
Potato chips, 1³/₄ X 2¹/₂" oval cross section.	10 chips	20	2	115	1	8	2.1	1.4	4.0	10	8	28	.4	226	Trace	.04	.01	1.0	3
Spinach, cooked, drained from raw	1 cup	180	92	40	5	1	—	—	—	6	167	68	4.0	583	14,580	.13	.25	.9	50
Squash, cooked, summer (all varieties) diced, drained	1 cup	210	96	30	2	Trace	—	—	—	7	53	53	.8	296	820	.11	.17	1.7	21

[28] Weight includes cob. Without cob, weight is 77 g.
[29] Based on yellow varieties. For white varieties, value is trace
[30] Value based on white-fleshed varieties. For yellow-fleshed varieties, value in International units (I.U.) is 70

NUTRITIVE VALUES OF THE EDIBLE PART OF FOODS
(Dashes (-) denote lack of reliable data for a constituent believed to be present in measurable amount) *(Continued)*

Foods, approximate measure, units, and weight (edible part unless footnotes indicate otherwise)			Nutrients in Indicated Quantity																
			A	B	C	D	E	F	G	H	I	J	K	L	M	N	O	P	Q
			Water	Food Energy	Protein	Fat	Saturated	Unsaturated: Oleic	Unsaturated: Linoleic	Carbohydrate	Calcium	Phosphorus	Iron	Potassium	Vitamin A value	Thiamin	Riboflavin	Niacin	Ascorbic Acid
		Grams	Percent	Calories	Grams	Grams	Grams	Grams	Grams	Grams	Milligrams	Milligrams	Milligrams	Milligrams	International units	Milligrams	Milligrams	Milligrams	Milligrams
Squash, cooked winter (all varieties) baked, mashed	1 cup	205	81	130	4	1	—	—	—	32	57	98	1.6	945	8,610	.10	.27	1.4	27
Sweet potatoes, cooked (raw, 5 X 2"; about 2½ per lb.), boiled in skin, peeled	1 potato	151	71	170	3	1	—	—	—	40	48	71	1.1	367	11,940	.14	.09	.9	26
Tomatoes, raw, 2⅗" diam. (3 per 12 oz. pkg.)	1 tomato[31]	135	94	25	1	Trace	—	—	—	6	16	33	.6	300	1,110	.07	.05	.9	28[32]
Tomatoes, canned, solids and liquid	1 cup	241	94	50	2	Trace	—	—	—	10	14[33]	46	1.2	523	2,170	.12	.07	1.7	41
Turnip greens, cooked and drained from raw (leaves and stems)	1 cup	145	94	30	3	Trace	—	—	—	5	252	49	1.5	—	8,270	.15	.33	.7	68
Vegetables, mixed, frozen, cooked	1 cup	182	83	115	6	1	—	—	—	24	46	115	2.4	348	9,010	.22	.13	2.0	15
MISCELLANEOUS ITEMS																			
Beverage, cola type	12 fl. oz.	369	90	145	0	0	0	0	0	37	—	—	—	—	0	0	0	0	0
Olives, pickled, canned, green	4 medium	16	78	15	Trace	2	.2	1.2	.1	Trace	8	2	.2	7	40	—	—	—	—
Pickles, dill, medium, whole, 3¾" long, 1¼" thick	1 pickle	65	93	5	Trace	Trace	—	—	—	1	17	14	.7	130	70	Trace	.01	Trace	4
Popsicle, 3 fl. oz. size	1 Popsicle	95	80	70	0	0	0	0	0	18	0	—	Trace	—	0	0	0	0	0
Soup, canned, condensed, prepared with equal volume of milk:																			
Cream of chicken	1 cup	245	85	180	7	10	4.2	3.6	1.3	15	172	152	0.5	260	610	0.05	0.27	.7	2
Soup, canned, condensed with equal volume of water:																			
Tomato	1 cup	245	91	90	2	3	.5	.5	1.0	16	15	34	.7	230	1,000	.05	.05	1.2	12
Vegetarian	1 cup	245	92	80	2	2	—	—	—	13	20	39	1.0	172	2,940	.05	.05	1.0	—

APPENDIX 7

ENTERAL HYPERALIMENTATION CHART*

	Elemental and/or Peptide Formulations				
	Standard Vivonex	*High Nitrogen Vivonex*	*Criticare HN*	*Vipep*	*Vital High Nitrogen*
Calories/ml	1	1	1	1	1
Carbohydrate Source	Glucose oligosaccharides	Glucose oligosaccharides	Maltodextrin, corn starch	Corn syrup, sucrose, corn starch	Hydrolyzed corn starch, sucrose
Protein Source	L-amino acids	L-amino acids	Hydrolyzed casein peptides and amino acids	Peptides of 2–4 amino acid units, 4–14 amino acid units, free amino acids	Whey, soy and meat protein hydrolysates, free essential amino acids
Fat Source	Safflower oil	Safflower oil	Safflower oil	MCT oil, corn oil	Safflower oil, MCT oil
Protein gram/liter	22	44	38	25	42
Fat gram/liter	1	1	3	25	11
Carbohydrate gram/liter	231	210	222	176	188
Nonprotein Calories: g N	286:1	127:1	148:1	232:1	125:1
mOsm/kg Water	550[a]	810[a]	650	520	460
Na/K mEq/Liter	20/30	23/30	27/34	33/22	17/30
Vitamins, ml to meet 100% U.S. RDA	1800	3000	2000	2000	1500
Producer	Eaton	Eaton	Mead Johnson	Cutter	Ross
Flavors[b]	Varied	Varied	Unflavored	Varied	Varied
Form	Powder	Powder	Ready to use	Powder	Powder
Uses/Features	Supplement or tube feeding, lactose free, low Na, minimal pancreatic stimulus, absorbed in upper gut.	Supplement or tube feeding, lactose free, high protein, low Na, minimal pancreatic stimulus, absorbed in upper gut.	Tube feeding, lactose free, absorbed in upper gut.	Supplement or tube feeding, lactose free, absorbed in upper gut.	Supplement or tube feeding, lactose free, low Na, high protein, absorbed in upper gut.

Table continued on following page

ENTERAL HYPERALIMENTATION CHART (*Continued*)

	Elemental and/or Peptide Formulations		Special Formulations			
	Travasorb Std	*Travasorb HN*	*Travasorb Hepatic*	*Hepatic-Aid*	*Travasorb Renal*	*Amin-Aid*
Calories/ml	1	1	1.1	1.6	1.35	1.9
Carbohydrate Source	Glucose oligosaccharides	Glucose oligosaccharides	Glucose, oligosaccharides, sucrose	Maltodextrin, sucrose	Glucose, oligosaccharides, sucrose	Maltodextrin, sucrose
Protein Source	Enzymatically hydrolyzed lactalbumin peptides	Enzymatically hydrolyzed lactalbumin peptides	Crystalline L-amino acids	Crystalline amino acids	Crystalline L-amino acids	Crystalline essential amino acids
Fat Source	MCT oil, sunflower oil	MCT oil, sunflower oil	MCT oil, sunflower oil	Soybean oil, lecithin, mono and diglycerides	MCT oil, sunflower oil	Soy oil, lecithin mono and diglycerides
Protein gram/liter	30	45	28.6	43	23	19
Fat gram/liter	13.5	13.5	14	36	18	46
Carbohydrate gram/liter	190	175	209	289	271	366
Nonprotein Calories: g N	202:1	126:1	218:1	215:1	362:1	380:1
mOsm/kg Water	560[a]	560	690	1158	590	1095
Na/K mEq/Liter	40/30	40/30	19/29	14/< 5	–/–	14/< 5
Vitamins, ml to meet 100% U.S. RDA	2000	2000	2100[c]	—	2100[c]	—
Producer	Travenol	Travenol	Travenol	McGaw	Travenol	McGaw
Flavors[b]	Unflavored, orange	Unflavored	Apricot, strawberry	Varied	Apricot, strawberry	Varied
Form	Powder	Powder	Powder	Powder	Powder	Powder
Uses/Features	Supplement or tube feeding, lactose free, absorbed in upper gut.	Supplement or tube feeding, lactose free, absorbed in upper gut.	Supplement or tube feeding, high branch chain amino acid formula, lactose free, indicated in liver disease.	Supplement or tube feeding, high branch chain amino acid formula, low electrolytes, lactose free, indicated in liver disease.	Supplement or tube feeding, electrolyte free, essential amino acids, lactose free, indicated for renal disease.	Supplement or tube feeding, low electrolytes, essential amino acids only, lactose free, indicated in renal disease.

Table continued on following page

ENTERAL HYPERALIMENTATION CHART (*Continued*)

Carbohydrate, Fat, and Protein Modular Components

	Microlipid	*MCT Oil*	*Sumacal*	*Polycose*		*Controlyte*	*Moducal*	
Calories/ml	4.5	7.7	4 cal/g	4 cal/g	2 cal/ml	5 cal/g 2 cal/ml	4 cal/g	2 cal/ml
Carbohydrate Source	—	—	Maltodextrin	Hydrolysis of corn starch		Corn starch	Maltodextrin	
Protein Source	—	—	—	—	—	—	—	—
Fat Source	Safflower Oil	Fractionated coconut oil	—	—	—	Vegetable oil	—	—
Protein gram/liter	—	—	—	—	—	Trace	—	—
Fat gram/liter	500	933	—	—	—	96	—	—
Carbohydrate gram/liter	—	—	—	—	500	286	—	500
Nonprotein Calories: g N	—	—	—	—	—	—	—	—
mOsm/kg Water	80	Negligible	—	—	850	598	—	725
Na/K mEq/Liter	-/-	-/-	4/< 1 per 100g	—	25/5	.8/.4	—	15/6
Vitamins, ml to meet 100% U.S. RDA	—	—	—	—	—	—	—	—
Producer	Organon	Mead Johnson	Organon	Ross		Doyle	Mead Johnson	
Flavors[b]	Unflavored	Unflavored	Unflavored	Unflavored		Unflavored	Unflavored	
Form	Ready to use	Ready to use	Powder	Powder	Liquid	Powder	Powder	Liquid
Uses/Features	Fat emulsion supplement, low osmolality.	Fat supplement, medium chain triglycerides used in malabsorption states.	Carbohydrate supplement.	Carbohydrate supplement.		Carbohydrate and fat supplement.	Carbohydrate supplement.	

Table continued on following page

ENTERAL HYPERALIMENTATION CHART (*Continued*)

Carbohydrate, Fat, and Protein Modular Components

	Casec	*Pro-Mix*	*Propac*
Calories/ml	4 cal/g	4 cal/g	4 cal/g
Carbohydrate Source	—	—	—
Protein Source	Calcium caseinate	Whey protein	Whey protein
Fat Source	—	—	—
Protein gram/liter	—	9g/11.8g packet	15g/19.5g packet
Fat gram/liter	—	—	—
Carbohydrate gram/liter	—	—	—
Nonprotein Calories: g N	—	—	—
mOsm/kg Water	—	—	—
Na/K mEq/Liter	7/3 per 100g	7/41 per 100g	10/13 per 100g
Vitamins, ml to meet 100% U.S. RDA	—	—	—
Producer	Mead Johnson	Navaco	Organon
Flavors[b]	Unflavored	Unflavored	Unflavored
Form	Powder	Powder	Powder
Uses/Features	Protein supplement, lactose free.	Protein supplement.	Protein supplement.

*Copyright 1980, Clinical Unit, University Hospital, Boston, Massachusetts.
[a] Unflavored.
[b] Flavors may change values.
[c] Water-soluble vitamins only.

GLOSSARY

adrenal medulla — The inner core of the adrenal gland, which produces the hormones adrenalin and noradrenalin.
agar-agar — A substance extracted from algae. It is higher in fiber and therefore used to treat diarrhea.
aging — Reduced capacity to replace worn out cells.
albumin — A plasma protein responsible for regulating the osmotic force of blood.
alkali — A chemical substance with a pH greater than 7.
allergen — A substance that induces hypersensitivity.
amylase — An enzyme that hastens the hydrolysis of starch into sugar.
anabolism — The constructive phase of metabolism resulting in growth and repair.
analog — A fabricated food resembling another food in texture and flavor.
anemia — A reduction in the number of red blood cells or hemoglobin.
antagonist — A substance that renders another substance inactive.
anthropometry — The science that deals with body measurements such as size, weight, and proportions.
antibodies — Substances synthesized in the body that destroy bacteria.
antigens — Substances that react with antibodies or help in the formation of antibodies.
arteriosclerosis — Hardening and thickening of the walls of the arteries.
ascites — An accumulation of excess fluids in the abdomen.
behavior modification — Techniques used to change learned behavior.
beriberi — A deficiency disease caused by lack of thiamine.
bland — Mild in seasoning and flavor.
callus — The network of woven bone formed about the ends of broken bone.
catabolism — A destructive process that releases energy.
catheter — A tubular instrument inserted into a body channel for the administering or withdrawing of fluids.
chelosis — A condition characterized by dry scaly lips and cracks at the corners of the mouth seen in riboflavin deficiency.
chemo- — A prefix meaning chemical, chemistry.
coma — Unconsciousness.
compensation — The maintenance of an adequate blood flow without distressing symptoms.
culture — The characteristic habits of a given community in terms of its social, religious, and national background.
decompensation — The condition in which the heart cannot pump adequate blood through the circulatory system.
decubitus ulcer — Bed or pressure sore.
depapillation — A smooth appearance of the papilla (elevations on the surface of the tongue containing taste buds) resulting from B-vitamin deficiency.
detoxify — To remove toxic substances.
development — Increased ability to take on various functions.
diuretic — A substance promoting urine secretion.
dumping syndrome diet — A diet high in protein, low in sugar, and dry; used for relieving nausea, weakness, sweating, palpitation, and sometimes diarrhea in patients having a partial removal of the stomach.
edema — The presence of fluid in the intracellular spaces of the body, caused by a variety of factors.
efficient body weight — The weight at which fat reserves will allow for best performance of a sport.

electrolyte — A substance that disassociates into ions when fused or in solution so that electricity can be conducted.
enrichment — The replacement of nutrients once lost in processing.
enteral — By way of the small intestine.
enzyme — A protein that can hasten or produce a change in a substance.
epithelial — Pertaining to the cellular covering of the internal and external surfaces of the body.
esophageal varices — Enlargement of veins in the esophagus.
extracellular — Outside a cell or cells.
fetus — The unborn child.
fortification — The addition of nutrients above the natural level found in a food such as milk and margarine.
gastric — Pertaining to the stomach.
geriatrics — The branch of medicine concerned with the treatment and prevention of diseases affecting the elderly.
gerontology — A study of the problems of aging.
gingivitis — An inflammation of the gums.
gluten — The protein portion of wheat, oats, rye, and barley.
glycogen loading — A process by which the glycogen stores in the liver are increased beyond normal levels to allow for the demands for endurance in athletic competition.
growth — Increases in body height and weight as a result of cell multiplication and differentiation.
gustatory — Pertaining to taste.
heat exhaustion — A disorder resulting from excessive loss of body fluids and electrolytes.
hematocrit — The volume percentage of red blood cells in whole blood.
hemicellulose — A carbohydrate that is more soluble and more easily decomposed than cellulose.
hemoglobin — The oxygen-carrying pigment of the blood; the principal protein in the red blood cell.
hemorrhage — The loss of blood from a ruptured vessel.
hiatus — An opening.
histidinemia — A hereditary metabolic defect marked by excessive histidine in the blood and urine.
homocystinuria — A lack of enzyme resulting in homocystine in the urine.
homogenize — The process in which fat particles become so finely dispersed that they do not rise in a liquid.
hormone — Chemicals produced by cells of the body to stimulate or retard certain life processes such as growth and reproduction.
host — A human, animal, or plant that provides sustenance for another organism or tumor.
hyper- — A prefix meaning greater than normal.
hyperchlorhydria — An excess of hydrochloric acid in gastric juice.
hypercholesterolemia — An elevation of cholesterol in the blood.
hyperglycemia — An elevation of glucose in the blood.
hyperlipidemia — An elevation of specific lipoproteins, cholesterol, and triglycerides.
hyperlipoproteinemia — An excess of lipoproteins in the blood.
hypertension — High blood pressure.
hypo- — A prefix meaning less than normal.
hypochlorhydria — A deficiency of hydrochloric acid in gastric juice.
hypochromic — A lack of color in red blood cells due to a decrease of hemoglobin.
immune — Resistant to a disease.
insulin — A protein hormone formed in the pancreas and secreted into the blood for the purpose of regulating carbohydrate, lipid, and amino acid metabolism.
intracellular — Within a cell or cells.
intravenous — Within a vein.
-itis — A suffix meaning inflammation.
jejunal — Pertaining to the small intestine.
ketoacidosis — An accumulation of excess ketones (acid) that changes the pH of the blood. It is seen in uncontrolled diabetes mellitus.
ketogenic diet — A diet containing large amounts of fat and minimal amounts of protein and carbohydrate; sometimes used in treating certain types of epilepsy in children.
kwashiorkor — Protein deficiency disease.
legumes — The fruit or seed of pod-bearing plants such as peas, beans, lentils, and peanuts.
lipase — An enzyme that hastens the splitting of fats into glycerol and fatty acids.
lymphocyte — A type of white blood cell associated with the immune response and the production of antibody.
macrocyte — An abnormally large red blood cell.
marasmus — Protein-calorie malnutrition.
Meals-on-Wheels — A community-sponsored program that provides meals to the elderly who are homebound.
Meniere's disease — A disorder of the labyrinth of the inner ear that is treated with a low-sodium diet.
metabolite — A substance produced during metabolism.
microcyte — An abnormally small red blood cell.

modified skim milk — Milk in which extra protein has been added.
mucositis — Inflammation of the mucosa.
myocardium — The middle and thickest layer of the heart wall.
naso- — Prefix indicating the nose.
nutrition quack — One who practices unscientific methods in the treatment of disease or who misleads the public and promotes food fads.
nutriture — The status of the body in relation to nutrition.
oropharyngeal — Pertaining to the part of the pharynx between the soft palate and the upper edge of the epiglottis.
osmolality — The number of particles dissolved in a solution.
osteoporosis — A condition characterized by a reduction in the quantity of bone.
-ostomy — An operation in which an artificial opening is formed.
papillae — Small nipple-shaped elevations.
pasteurization — The heating of milk or other liquid to a temperature of 60° C (140° F) for 30 minutes, killing pathogenic bacteria and considerably delaying the development of other bacteria.
pectin — An indigestible carbohydrate found in many fruits.
peri- — A prefix meaning around or near.
pericardium — Fibrous and serous layers enclosing the heart and the roots of the great vessels.
periodontal — Around or near a tooth.
peripheral — By way of peripheral veins.
peripheral parenteral nutrition (PPN) — Administration of nutrients through peripheral veins.
pernicious anemia — A form of anemia caused by a lack of the intrinsic factor normally produced by the stomach mucosa.
phenylketonuria — A congenital disease due to a deficit in the metabolism of the amino acid phenylalanine.
pica — An abnormal craving for nonfood substances.
poly- — A prefix meaning many or much.
postural — Pertaining to posture.
prenatal — Preceding birth.
radiation — Electromagnetic waves (as in ultraviolet waves, x-rays, gamma rays, etc.).
refined cereal — Cereal that has had its nutritional value reduced by removal of the bran layer and germ from the grain.
renal threshold — The capacity for reabsorption by the kidneys.
restoration — The process in which the nutrients that have been lost in refining foods are replaced.
sodium — The chief cation of extracellular body fluids.
steatorrhea — Diarrhea characterized by excess fat in the stools.
steroids — An important group of body compounds that includes sex and adrenal hormones, vitamin D, and cholesterol.
sulfonylureas — Oral compounds that stimulate insulin secretion.
total parenteral nutrition (TPN) — Administration of nutrients through the superior vena cava.
toxemia — General intoxication sometimes due to absorption of bacterial products formed at an infection site. Also, a condition in late pregnancy characterized by elevated blood pressure, edema, and proteinuria.
toxin — A poisonous substance secreted by a cell.
transferase — An enzyme that hastens a transfer from one molecule to another.
transferrin — A serum globulin or protein that binds and transports iron.
trypsin — An enzyme produced in the intestine that hastens the hydrolysis of protein.
tumor — Uncontrolled multiplication of cells.
uremia — Retention in the blood of substances normally excreted by the kidneys.
xerophthalmia — Dryness and thickening of the membrane lining of the eyelid, eyeball, and cornea. It is due to a vitamin A deficiency.

INDEX

Page numbers in *italics* denote illustrations; page numbers followed by the letter t denote tables.